SOCIOLOGY
for
PHYSIOTHERAPISTS

SOCIOLOGY
for
PHYSIOTHERAPISTS

SECOND EDITION

Dibyendunarayan Bid
MPT (Ortho) PGDSPT PhD FOMT PGDHS (Acu)

Associate Professor
Sarvajanik College of Physiotherapy
Surat, Gujarat, India

Foreword
Yagna Unmesh Shukla

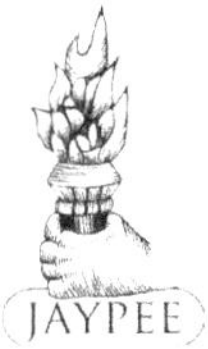

JAYPEE BROTHERS MEDICAL PUBLISHERS
The Health Sciences Publisher
New Delhi | London

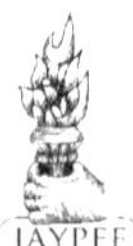 **Jaypee Brothers Medical Publishers (P) Ltd**

Headquarters

Jaypee Brothers Medical Publishers (P) Ltd
EMCA House, 23/23-B
Ansari Road, Daryaganj
New Delhi 110 002, India
Landline: +91-11-23272143
+91-11-23272703, +91-11-23282021
+91-11-23245672
Email: jaypee@jaypeebrothers.com

Corporate Office

Jaypee Brothers Medical Publishers (P) Ltd
4838/24, Ansari Road, Daryaganj
New Delhi 110 002, India
Phone: +91-11-43574357
Fax: +91-11-43574314
Email: jaypee@jaypeebrothers.com

Overseas Office

J.P. Medical Ltd
83 Victoria Street, London
SW1H 0HW (UK)
Phone: +44 20 3170 8910
Email: info@jpmedpub.com

EU GPSR Authorised Representative

Logos Europe, 9 rue Nicolas Poussin
17000, La Rochelle, France
Phone: +33 (0) 6 67 93 73 78
E-mail: Contact@logoseurope.eu

Website: www.jaypeebrothers.com
Website: www.jaypeedigital.com

© 2023, Jaypee Brothers Medical Publishers

Inquiries for bulk sales may be solicited at: jaypee@jaypeebrothers.com

Sociology for Physiotherapists

First Edition: 2016

Second Edition: **2023**

ISBN: 978-93-5696-271-2

Dedicated to

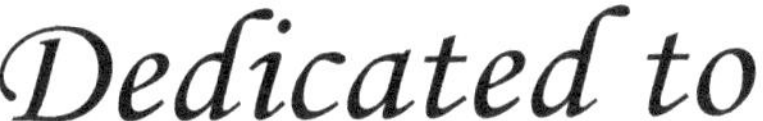

My Teachers

My Family and Friends

and

Our Wonderful Students

For Your Support and Inspiration

Foreword

Sociology is the study of human social relationships and institutions. Sociology is a social science that focuses on society, human behavior, social relationship patterns, social interaction and different aspects of culture. Studying sociology provides a better understanding of social differences and behavior and is relevant to social hierarchies and social power in everyday life. Sociology depends on the basic aspects of life and is mixed with our daily acts, social behavior, and knowledge. It is incorporated into every activity that we perform.

Physiotherapy is a branch of science that deals with healing pain with the help of different exercises and other methods. If incorporated with physiotherapy, sociology may help patients recover more efficiently and produce better results. Sociology helps physiotherapists maintain cordial relationships between personnel at different levels. Today physiotherapy is not simply an effort to cure illness. Preventive services and health promotion are also equally important aspects of physiotherapy. To be an effective agent of health promotion, knowledge of the community, facilities and resources available are essential. If the Physiotherapist is socially appropriate, they will automatically feel the patient's discomfort and help them better. It will make the Physiotherapist socially efficient, and hence dealing with patients, getting to know their pain and healing them becomes easier.

Dr Dibyendunarayan Bid has come up with his book on "*Sociology for Physiotherapists*", 2nd edition. He has written 21 chapters on different aspects of sociology in detail on Social Factors in Health and Disease, Socialization, Social Groups, Marriage, Family, Community, Cultural and Health, Social Change, Social Problems of the Disabled, Social Security, Social Worker, Social Control, Sociology of Stress, Sociology of Education, Social Welfare Programs of India, Sociology of Aging, Social Stratification, Social Organization and Social Systems, Social Structure and Sociology of Pain keeping in mind the profession. His passion for this subject is evident as this is his third book on sociology. He has done a commendable job for physiotherapists and also for society.

I recommend this book, which is an addition to sociology literature and will benefit Physiotherapists. My best wishes to Dr Dibyendunarayan Bid.

Yagna Unmesh Shukla
President, Gujarat State Council Physiotherapy
Principal, Government Physiotherapy College
Ahmedabad, Gujarat, India

Preface to the Second Edition

The demand for a comprehensive introductory sociology textbook for physiotherapy students led to the creation of this work. The *Sociology for Physiotherapists* focuses on the various aspects of society, including social relationships, institutions, social change, social organization, social problems, and social work, as they pertain to the field of sociology.

Emphasis has been placed on topics related to society and health in India, making this book suitable for meeting the syllabus requirements of physiotherapy students in universities of India. The book is not just for physiotherapy students but also for nursing, occupational therapy, speech therapy, and other paramedical students, as well as for doctors, administrators, social workers, and health personnel.

This edition features many new and engaging chapters, and a Question Bank has been added for extra practice. Feedback from readers is encouraged to improve the content in future editions.

Dibyendunarayan Did

Preface to the First Edition

The need of an introductory book in sociology to be used by physiotherapy and nursing students was sincerely felt. The present work is done to meet this demand. Since sociology is a subject dealing with society, we kept in view these factors such as social relationships, social institutions, social change, social organization, social problems and social reconstruction, while writing this book.

Special efforts have been made to present the various topics in relation to the society and health in India. This book specifically meets the requirements of syllabus of various universities in this subject for physiotherapy and nursing students. The book is primarily to serve the physiotherapy, nursing, occupational therapy, speech therapy and paramedical students. It can also be used as a handy book of sociology by doctors, administrators, social workers, paramedical and health personnel.

Five new and interesting chapters are also added: Sociology of Stress, Sociology of Aging, Drug Abuse and Drug Addiction, Social Control and Sociology of Education. Question Bank is an added feature.

Suggestions are welcome from the readers of this book to improve the content.

Dibyendunarayan Bid
Thangamani Ramalingam A

Acknowledgments

In putting this book together, numerous people gave me helpful advice. I want to thank everyone for their insightful recommendations. I am very grateful to my in-laws, Mr Swapankumar Mukherjee and Mrs Shukla Mukherjee for their unwavering support and encouragement. I owe my wife, Dr Soumita Bid, a debt of gratitude for her understanding and support.

I hereby thankfully acknowledge all the help and assistance by Shri Jitendar P Vij (Group Chairman), Mr Ankit Vij (Managing Director), Mr MS Mani (Group President), Dr Madhu Choudhary (Director-Educational Publishing), Ms Pooja Bhandari [Director-Production (Books and Journals)], Ms Sunita Katla (Executive Assistant to Group Chairman and Publishing Manager), Ms Samina Khan (Executive Assistant to Director-Educational Publishing), Mr Rajesh Sharma (Production Coordinator), Dr Sangeeta Yadav (Development Editor), Ms Seema Dogra (Cover Visualizer), Ms Neelam Kakriya (Proofreader), Mr Om Prakash Mishra (Typesetter) and Mr Sanjeev Kumar (Graphic Designer) and all the staff of the Delhi and Ahmedabad Branch of M/s Jaypee Brothers Medical Publishers (P) Ltd, New Delhi, India, who bestowed upon this work with their highly painstaking efforts in the examination of this text, its editing and printing.

Dibyendunarayan Bid

Contents

10. Social Problems 173

BPT Syllabus of Gujarat University

■ SOCIOLOGY

Objectives

At the end of the course the candidate will be able to:
1. Define the term sociology and its importance in the health delivery system.
2. Understand the basic sociological concepts, principles and social process, social institution in relation to the individual family and community and the various social factors affecting the family in the rural and urban communities in India.

Introduction

1. Meaning—definition and scope of sociology.
2. Its relation with anthropology, psychology, social psychology and ethics.
3. Methods of sociology—case study, social survey, questionnaire, interview and opinion poll methods.
4. Importance of its study with special reference to healthcare professionals.

Social Factors in Health and Disease

1. The meaning and nature of socialization.
2. The role of social factors in health and illness.

Socialization

1. Meaning and nature of socialization.
2. Primary, secondary and anticipatory socialization.
3. Agencies of socialization.

Social Groups

Concepts of social groups, influence of formal and informal groups on health and sickness, the role of primary groups and secondary groups in the hospital and rehabilitation settings.

Family

1. The family
2. Meaning and definition
3. Function
4. Types
5. Changing family patterns
6. Influence of family on individual health, family and nutrition, the effects of sickness on family and psychosomatic disease and their importance to physiotherapy.

Community

1. Rural community – meaning and features – health hazards of rural ties.
2. Urban community – meaning and features – health hazards of urbanities.

Cultural and Health

1. Concept of culture
2. Culture and behavior
3. Cultural meaning of sickness
4. Cultural and health disorders

Social Change

1. Meaning of social changes
2. Factors of social changes
3. Human adaptation and social change
4. Social change and stress
5. Social change and deviance
6. Social change and health program
7. The role of social planning in the improvement of rehabilitation

Social Problems of Disabled

Consequence of the following social problems in relation to sickness and disability, remedies to prevent this problem.
1. Population explosion
2. Poverty and unemployment
3. Beggary
4. Juvenile delinquency
5. Prostitution
6. Alcoholism
7. Problems of women in employment

Social Security

Social security and social legislation in relation to disabled.

Social Worker

Meaning of social work, role of a medical social worker.

1

Introduction to Sociology

☞ Describe the meaning and definition of sociology.
☞ What is the nature of sociology?
☞ Describe the scope of sociology.
☞ Explain the methods and techniques of sociology.
☞ What is the importance of sociology for healthcare professionals?

▨ MEANING

Sociology is one of the social sciences, and economics, psychology, anthropology, geography, and political science (among others). ***Auguste Comte***, a French philosopher, coined the term **sociology** in 1839 **(Fig. 1.1)**. He is considered the 'father of sociology'. The word *'sociology'* is derived from *'societus,'* meaning society, and the Greek word *'logos,'* meaning study or science. The etymological meaning of

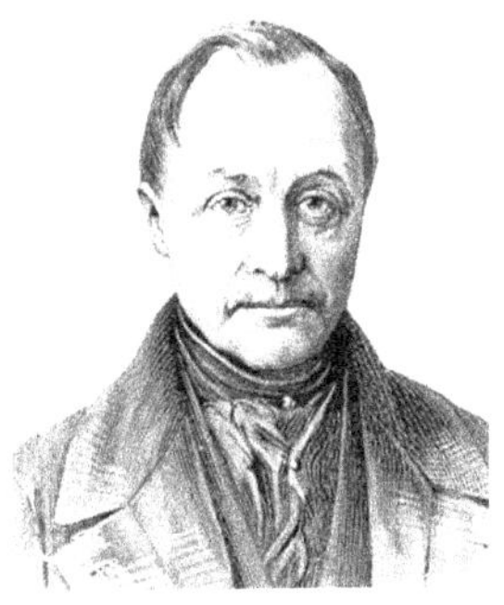

Fig. 1.1: Auguste Comte.

sociology is thus the *'science of society'.* Sociology is the youngest of all social sciences.

Sociology studies man's behavior in groups, including human interaction, social relationships, and the processes that enable human group activity.

Sociology is the scientific study of society in a nutshell. Sociologists utilize scientific tools and methodologies to figure out how and why people behave the way they do in groups. Even though social groups or societies—are made up of individuals, sociology focuses on the group instead of the individual.

■ DEFINITION OF SOCIOLOGY

Here are some definitions that some influential sociologists give:
- Sociology is the science of society, or social phenomena.

  —LF Ward
- Sociology is the study of human interaction and interrelation, their conditions, and consequences. *—M Ginsberg*
- Sociology studies the relationships between man and his human environment. *—HP Fairchild*
- *The chief interest of sociology is the people, the ideas, the customs, the other distinctively human phenomenon which surrounds the man and influence him, and which are, therefore, part of his environment.* Sociology also devotes some attention to certain aspects of the geographical environment and some natural phenomena contrasted with human phenomena. However, this interest is secondary to its preoccupation with human beings and the products of human life in an association. Our general field of study is man as he is related to other men and the creation of other men surrounding him. *— ME Jones*
- Sociology seeks to understand the principles of cohesion and order within the social structure, how it roots and grows within an environment, the moving equilibrium of changing structure and changing environment, the main trends of incessant change, and the forces that determine its direction at any given time, the harmonies and conflicts, the adjustments and mal adjustments within the structure as they are revealed in the light of human desires, and thus the practical applicability of sociology.

  —McIver

The various definitions of sociology can be summarized as follows:
- Sociology is the science of society.
- Sociology is the science of social relationships.
- Sociology is the study of social life.
- Sociology is the study of human behavior in groups.
- Sociology is the study of social actions.
- Sociology is the study of forms of social relationships.
- Sociology is the study of social groups or social systems.

■ NATURE OF SOCIOLOGY

Sociology's nature portrays the context that society creates through a predetermined and comprehensive analysis of the social practices of communities through face-to-face interactions produced by the active movement of civilization. Sociology focuses on a single aspect of society and regulates multiple dimensions of social life, including economy, science, state, family, religion, social inequality, culture, etc.

As a branch of social science, sociology has its method of investigation. It has its roots grounded in a pragmatic approach to observing social reality. Sociology as a subject gives knowledge about society and its functions and describes the nature of social interaction and the specific nature of each community.

The crucial characteristics of sociology are:

- **Sociology is an independent science:** Sociology has established itself as a distinct and separate scientific discipline. It differs from philosophy, political philosophy, and history in terms of its approach to research and inquiry. Sociology has its own specific field of study, boundaries, and methods that differentiate it as a unique science.

- **Sociology is a social science, not a physical science:** Sociology is part of the social science family, not the physical science family. It focuses on man, his social behaviors, social activities, and social life as a social science. It is closely related to other social sciences such as history, political science, economics, philosophy, anthropology, and so on as a part of the social science family.

- **Sociology is a categorical and not a normative discipline:** According to the author, sociology confines its observations to what exists rather than what ought to exist or what should be. Sociology, as a science, is deafeningly mute on the subject of value does not make any sort of value determination. It takes an amoral approach rather than a moral or immoral one. It is ethically neutral, but this does not imply that sociological information is useless or without application; instead, it means that sociology is incapable of dealing with issues of good and evil, right and wrong, and moral and immoral behavior.

- **Sociology is pure science and not an applied science:** Pure science's primary goal is to obtain knowledge, and it does not matter whether that knowledge is valuable or useful; applied science's goal is to apply that knowledge to real-life situations and put it to use. Each pure science could have its field of application. Physics, e.g., is pure science, while engineering is its application. As a pure science, sociology applies in areas such as administration, diplomacy, social work, etc. Each pure science could have multiple applications. Sociology is a pure science since its primary goal is to learn about human society rather than use it.

- **Sociology is a generalizing and not a particularizing or individualizing science:** Sociology tries to discover the general laws or principles about human interaction or situation, nature, form, content, and structure of the human group of societies. It does not study every event that takes place in society. It is not possible as well. The basics of the study of selected events are generalized. A sociologist, e.g., makes broad generalizations about the nature of secondary groups. He might conclude that secondary groupings are more substantial, less stable, and not necessarily minimal. Sociologists do this by observing and researching a few secondary groups rather than all of them.

- **Sociology is a general science and not a special social science:** Sociology is a broad and nonspecialized field of study. It's about how people connect and live their lives. Other Social Sciences, such as Political Science, History, and Economics, investigate man and human interaction, but not exclusively. Sociologists focus on specific aspects of human interaction and activity, whereas economists are experts in the study of economic activities. Political science focuses on issues such as elections and other political actions. On the other hand, sociology looks at human behaviors broadly.

- **Finally, sociology is both a rational and empirical science:** Scientific information can be divided into two categories. One approach, known as empiricism, is empiricists' approach to facts derived through observation and experimentation. On the other hand, rationalism emphasizes reason and theories derived from logical inference. The empiricist gathers facts, whereas the rationalist organizes and coordinates them. The construction of knowledge necessitates the use of ideas and facts. Both are important in sociological research.

The nature of sociology depends upon the people in society and the forms of families, such as nuclear families, joint families, and extended ones. The activities of these family types are explained by sociology. Each society has its caste system; usually, marriage occurs with the same caste people. However, some societies encourage marriages between people from different castes or religions with a broad-mind and a positive attitude.

■ SCOPE

In its broadest sense, sociology is the study of human interactions and interrelations, as well as their conditions and outcomes. As a result, sociology studies the entire life of man in society, including all activities by which he maintains himself in the struggle for survival, the rules and regulations that govern his interactions with others, the systems of knowledge and belief, art and morals, and any other capacities and habits acquired and developed while participating in society's activities. Nonetheless, this topic is far too broad for any scientist to cover adequately. As a result, efforts have been made to define and limit sociology.

Sociology has a broad scope. It is a general and unique science, as it is the subject of all social sciences. Their point of view distinguishes them from one another. As a result, economics studies society from an economic perspective, political sciences from a political perspective, and history from a historical perspective. Sociology is the study of social relationships and society as a whole.

McIver accurately observes that the selective interest is what sets each discipline apart. Sociology is distinguished by its emphasis on studying relationships, which gives it a unique identity despite its close association with other fields.

Sociology investigates all aspects of society, including social traditions, social processes, social morphology, social control, social pathology, and the impact of extra-social factors on social relationships, among other topics. Delimiting the scope of sociology is neither possible nor necessary because doing so would be "a brave attempt to confine an enormous mass of slippery material into a relatively simple system of pigeonholes" (Sprott).

Physiotherapists, nurses, and indeed all health professionals must have a sociologically informed approach to health care because 'Sociology demystifies the nature of health and illness, highlights the social causes of disease and death, exposes power-factors and ethical dilemmas in the production of health care, and either directly or indirectly helps to create a discerning practitioner capable of more focused and competitive care' (Morrall, 2001).

■ SOCIOLOGY AND ANTHROPOLOGY

Sociology and anthropology are so close together that they often appear as two names for the same field of inquiry. Anthropology comprises two Greek words: Anthropos, which means "man," and logos, which means "study." Thus, anthropology is the study of man, which studies human growth according to its original meaning. Anthropology has thus a vast field of study. Anthropology has been divided into three divisions:

i. **Physical anthropology** deals with the bodily characteristics of early man and our primitive contemporaries;

ii. **Cultural anthropology** investigates the cultural remains of ancient man and the living cultures of some of the primitive contemporaries;

iii. **Social anthropology** deals with the institutions and human relationships of primitive people of the past and present.

Anthropology thus devotes its attention entirely to studying man and his culture as they developed in the past. On the other hand, sociology examines the same phenomena as they exist. "The sociological attitude has tended towards the practical and present," writes Kluckhohn, "while the anthropological attitude has tended towards pure understanding and the past."

Sociology is heavily reliant on the information provided by anthropology. Cultural anthropology and sociology's historical component are the same. Anthropology has made a significant contribution to sociology research. Sociology must rely on anthropology to understand current social phenomena from our knowledge of the past. On the fundamental basis that cultural sociology has developed, sociology has borrowed cultural areas, traits, interdependent traits, cultural lag, and other conceptions from social anthropology. Linton and Kardiner have had a significant impact on sociology, and it is clear from their research that each society has its own culture, and the personalities of its members are shaped by it.

Similarly, Malinowski's research has been beneficial to sociology. He has given the study of culture a practical perspective. According to Franz Boas and Otto Kinberg's research, there is no link between anatomical characteristics and mental superiority. Anthropology has proven that the concept of racial superiority is false.

According to **Hoebel**, *"Sociology and Social Anthropology are the same in their broadest sense."* **AL Kroeber** has called sociology and anthropology twin sisters. **Evans Pritchard** considers social anthropology to be a branch of sociology.

Similarly, sociologists' specific findings have aided anthropologists. Morgan and his followers, e.g., have deduced the existence of primitive communism from our modern society's understanding of private property. "When one considers the entire United States, one notices that the social links between sociology and anthropology are closer than those between anthropology and political science" (Robert Redfield).

Despite their interdependence, the fields of study for these two sciences are pretty different. "However, the two academic disciplines have grown up independently and deal with quite different problems, employing markedly different research methods" (Keesing). To begin with, anthropology is the study of society as a whole. It investigates the country's political and legal issues, family structure, religion, art, industries, and occupations. Only the specific aspects of sociology are studied. Sociologists are interested in how people interact with one another. Second, anthropology studies small and static cultures, whereas sociology studies large and dynamic civilizations. That is why anthropology has progressed more quickly and effectively than sociology. Third, anthropology and sociology are distinct disciplines in that the former studies man and his cultures as they developed in the past, while the latter studies the same phenomena as they exist today.

"The sociological attitude has tended toward the practical and present" (Kluckhohn). "While the anthropological attitude has tended toward pure understanding and the past." Last but not least, sociology is concerned with social philosophy and social planning, whereas anthropology is not. It makes no recommendations for the future.

■ SOCIOLOGY AND SOCIAL PSYCHOLOGY

Social psychology studies man's mental processes as a social being. It focuses on the effects of group life on individual cognitive development, the impact of the individual mind on the group, and the development of groups' mental lives within themselves and in their interactions. Sociology is the scientific study of society's various social groups.

Social psychology must rely on sociology to fully comprehend human nature and behavior. Sociology provides information about the structure, organization, and culture of the societies in which people live. "We might say that while our main focus is on the individual's interaction with others, such interaction can only be understood within the social life and cultural matrix in which it occurs" (Kimball Young). For their part, sociologists must develop social psychology. They recognize the significance of psychological variables in explaining, among other things, changes in social structure.

LaPierre and ***Farnsworth*** wrote, *"Social psychology links psychology and sociology."* As a result of the close relationship between the two, ***Karl Pearson*** has not accepted the two as separate sciences. In other words, ***MacIver***, *"Sociology in special gives aid to psychology, just as Psychology gives special aid to sociology."* It is currently widely understood that a scientific study of social phenomena must have a psychological foundation and that psychological facts about human nature should not be taken at face value but instead investigated by direct observation and experimentation. Sociology will become more objective and realistic as our understanding of human behavior improves.

McDougall and Sigmund Freud felt that social life could be reduced to psychological forces. In such a situation, sociology would be relegated to a subdiscipline of psychology. However, this view cannot be accepted as the causes affecting social behavior are other than psychological, also like economic, geographical, political, etc. Therefore, social life cannot be studied exclusively with the methods of psychologists. The fact that social psychology and sociology are mutually dependent should not be taken to imply that one is identical to or a branch of the other. There are some key differences between these two closely related fields of study.

i. **The difference in subject matter:** To begin with, sociology is the study of society as a whole, whereas social psychology is the study of individuals interacting in groups and their impact on them. Because sociology studies the organization of social groups, their central values, and the various forms of institutional behavior that arise as a result of them, and social psychology is concerned with individuals as members of the group, they have been aptly compared to the science of mechanics, which considers masses of matter and properties of matter in mass, and molecular physics, which deals with molecules and their invocation.

   In social psychology, the individual is the unit of analysis. "The primary concern of the sociologist is group behavior, and the primary concern of the social psychologist is individual behavior in a group situation," writes Klineberg, while Bogardus writes, "as psychology analyses mental processes, sociology analyses social processes."

ii. **The difference in attitudes:** Furthermore, sociology and social psychology approach social life from several perspectives. The former looks at society from the community's perspective, while the latter looks at the psychological forces at play.

■ SOCIOLOGY AND PSYCHOLOGY

Psychology is the science that studies the internal mechanisms of human behavior. It is clear that studying human behavior thoroughly is essential to study internal aspects. Almost all our actions overtly express our motives, desires, instincts, impulses, and emotions. Our activities are also regulated or modified through external conditions and stimuli. Sociologists study these external conditions, and this knowledge is helpful to psychologists in their analysis of human behavior. Psychologists must depend on sociologists to learn about the changing aspects of social life, which affect our thinking, attitudes, and values.

Sociology is a social science that deals with group life, whereas psychology only deals with the human being as an individual. Sociology is mainly concerned with the external aspects of behavior, while psychology deals with the internal elements. The two sciences' methods are different—psychology uses experimental methods and testing, whereas sociologists use surveys and statistical methods.

■ SOCIOLOGY AND ETHICS

Ethics is the science that discusses the good or evil of human conduct, which is not possible without society studied by sociology. There is a relationship between the individual and society, ethics and sociology related. Man cannot even be imagined outside society. He acquires his concepts of good and evil, duty or nonduty, virtue, vice, and convention from society.

Man undertakes good deeds not because God desires them or because they are required for survival in society but because society recognizes them as good individuals, and the ethical considerations accompanying such behavior are inherent in social structures. As a result, goodness is a social issue. On the other hand, the evolution of society depends on the people's ethos because, at its core, society is nothing more than a web of social ties.

Due to this reason, again, ethics and sociology are closely related. Ethics concerns ethical ideals, the right and wrong of actions, moral development, and the individual's character. Sociology studies the nature of human society, its origin, and its development.

Ethics relies on sociology to express man's ultimate good about society. We only know an individual man as a member of society; what we call his virtues are most prominently displayed in his dealings with his fellows, and his most prominent pleasures are derived from intercourse with them; thus, maintaining that man's highest good is independent of his social relations, or the constitution and condition of the community of which he is a part, is a paradox.

As he is an integral member of society, the ultimate good of the individual is founded on the ultimate good of society. Individual and social good, selfishness, and altruism are all purposes of ethics. Social science studies men's social habits, conversions, and institutions. As a result, ethics is influenced by sociology. Sociology, on the other hand, is reliant on ethics.

The differences between ethics and sociology are the following:
1. Normative science studies ideals and positive sciences study facts.
   Sociology gives factual knowledge of social relations while ethics

ideals. It decides the good and evil in social conventions, habits, traditions, etc. In this way, sociology and ethics are related, but their scopes do not coincide.

2. Sociology is a comparatively theoretical study, while ethics affect our practical life. It seeks the ultimate good and, in its light, makes judgments concerning virtues, duties, good and evil in social institutions, conventions, authority, economic and political laws, etc. In the form of the science of ethical ideals, it is also related to philosophy.

3. Sociology studies man as a member of sociology. Ethics studies man as a responsible individual having freedom of will.

4. Sociology is an objective science, whereas ethics is a normative science. Sociology studies objective processes and conventions, laws, organization, etc. The subject of ethics is internal motives, desires, violation, and man's conduct in the context of intentions.

▚ METHODS AND TECHNIQUES OF SOCIOLOGY

The term *"method"* means an apt way of doing something. As we know, sociology is also a science, so it uses specific methods by which sociological facts can be collected, analyzed, and put into proper form, and certain conclusions can be drawn from them. To qualify as a science, sociology must employ a methodology that eliminates the possibility of personal bias impacting our comprehension and appraisal of social facts.

Sociology is still in its infancy. So, it does not have a specific method for its research. However, it has achieved appreciable success in analyzing social phenomena using other social sciences techniques.

Sociology, like any other science, is an objective study of natural systems, and because social systems, like all systems, evolve, they must be investigated in the process of evolution using methods used in such fields. Because the social phenomenon is so complex and the amount of data to be collected is so large, it is difficult to say which method sociologists should use.

There are many methods in sociology, namely, historical method, observation method, laboratory or experimental method, common-sense method, statistical method, anthropological or comparative method, survey method, detective method, philosophical method, etc.

The following are the most common sociological methods:

Case Study

A case study is "an investigation of an individual or group in which the variables measured and the empirical relations explored are characteristics of the individual or group rather than a subunit of it." It is a type of qualitative analysis that entails a meticulous and thorough observation of a person, a situation, or an institution.

This method is usually employed to study professional criminals and other social deviants and involves an investigation and analysis of all factors entering the case and its examination from as many points of view as possible. Some techniques used in this method are interviews, questionnaires, life histories, documents of all kinds bearing the subject, and all such materials, which may give sociologists a deep insight into the problem. Thoroughness is the keystone of this method.

Acceptance, self-determination, and confidentiality are the guiding concepts of casework. The code of acceptance refers to the worker's attitude and respect for the client as an individual, which gives him a sense of security and encourages him to speak openly about his problems. The principle of self-determination allows the client to make decisions for himself rather than having them made for him, and the principle of confidentiality implies that the caseworker-client relationship is one of trust, and whatever is revealed to the worker is kept confidential.

Casework is used in various settings, including child care and guidance centers, schools, colleges, medical and psychiatric settings, family welfare, marriage counseling centers, institutions for the elderly and handicapped, and people suffering from addiction, character disorders, etc., emotional disturbances.

▆ QUESTIONNAIRE AND INTERVIEW METHOD

A questionnaire is a list of essential and relevant questions about a subject. It is emailed to the individuals and organizations involved, asking them to respond to the questions to their knowledge and capacity. The objective is to acquire knowledge from the informant that the investigator does not possess. Predictions regarding social conduct are made based on responses to specific inquiries. Questions should be carefully crafted; they should not be confusing, excessively numerous or personal, or too difficult to respond to by a man of ordinary intelligence and shared knowledge.

The interview method comprises direct personal contact with persons or groups concerned with the problem under study. Discussion of the problem with the person interviewed goes a long way in clearly understanding his issues and remedying them accordingly.

This method has brought out some outstanding works such as *"A medical study of sex adjustments"* by Dr Dickinson and Dr Beam *"The sexual behavior in the human male and female"* by Dr AC Kinsey et al.

Questionnaires and Interviews can be used to gather a variety of data. The questionnaire has the benefit of anonymity, which allows for more honest responses. It also helps to eliminate uncontrollable personal factors and reduces the chance of bias in response coding. In general, the interview is more adaptable. Because the same questions can mean various things to different people, the interviewer can clear up any confusion. He can elicit genuine responses and assign ratings based on the entire subject's conduct. He can rearrange the questions and prevent the subject from reading the complete list before responding.

■ PUBLIC OPINION POLL METHOD

This method gauges the public's beliefs, sentiments, and attitudes on any proposition. "Public Poll" is very popular in America. Data regarding public opinion about various social, political, and economic situations are frequently collected through this instrument. The public gives its view by answering **'Yes,' 'No,'** or **'Do not know'** to the proposition. The public poll results help the authorities concerned in modifying their policies accordingly.

■ THE SOCIAL SURVEY METHOD

The social survey method collects data about people's living and working conditions in a given area to formulate practical social measures for their betterment and welfare.

Thus, a social survey is concerned with collecting data relating to some problems of social importance to plan a constructive program for its solution. It is conducted within a predefined geographical limit. Social surveys are of various types. These are:

- General or specialized surveys
- Direct or indirect surveys
- Census surveys or sample surveys
- Primary or secondary surveys
- Official, semi-official or private surveys
- Postal or personal surveys, etc.

It involves the following steps:

1. Definition of the purpose or objects
2. Description of the problem to be studied
3. The analysis of this problem in a schedule
4. The Delimitation of the area or scope
5. Examination of all documentary sources
6. Fieldwork
7. The arrangement, tabulation, and statistical analysis of the data
8. The interpretation of the results
9. Deduction
10. Graphic expression

These surveys are useful because they provide detailed accounts of social and economic facts and bring to light various social evils among the people of the area in question, drawing the government's attention to the need to eradicate these evils through appropriate legislation. For a long time, America and England have relied on general and specialized social surveys to solve some of their social problems on a massive scale. India and other developing countries benefit from social surveys in urban and rural areas, which they conduct on their own or with the cooperation and assistance of other developed countries.

IMPORTANCE OF SOCIOLOGY FOR HEALTH CARE PROFESSIONALS

Because it bore many of the problems of the present world, sociology has assumed such great importance that it is considered the best approach to all the healthcare and social sciences. Giddings has rightly pointed out, *'Sociology tells us how to become what we want to be.'*

Sociology is a beneficial science, especially for physiotherapy and nursing professionals, as discussed below:

- **Sociology enlightens man's social nature:** Sociology thoroughly examines man's social character. It explains why man is a social animal who lives in communities, societies, and groupings. It looks at the individual-society relationship, the impact of society on man, and other topics.

  Sociology will help physiotherapists, nurses, and doctors know the patients' culture and social life. In a country like India, where people have affiliations with different religions, castes, tribes, and communities, it is essential to know the culture of these groups. The patients' customs, traditions, folkways, mores, and values must be known before treating them to make the medical, physiotherapy, and nursing services more effective. For this, sociology is necessary.

- **Sociology studies society scientifically:** Before the emergence of sociology, there was no systematic and scientific attempt to study human society with its complexities. Sociology has made it possible to conduct scientific research on society. This scientific understanding of human society is required for advancement in various fields.

  Technological progress has successfully eliminated many diseases, bringing new problems and challenges to physiotherapists/ nurses. The issues of the aged, patients suffering from AIDS or persons suffering from permanent disabilities due to industrial or other accidents are all examples. A deep understanding of human behavior, relationships, and psychology can be beneficial in handling such situations.

- Treatment of mental or physical diseases is a cooperative venture in which a united effort of various medical, paramedical and even nonmedical personnel is required. Knowledge of sociology helps the physiotherapist/nurse maintain cordial relationships between personnel at different levels.

- The patient himself is the most significant person who can aid in rehabilitation. Treatment and physiotherapy care becomes difficult unless he wants to be healed and cooperate. As a result, the ability of the physiotherapist to earn entire confidence in the patient is critical. Her understanding of the social system and social interactions is crucial in this process.

- To meet the needs of her patient adequately, the physiotherapist/nurse must develop self-understanding. She must constantly strive to become emotionally, mentally, morally, and socially mature. The study of sociology and psychological training is beneficial in this process.

- **Sociology investigates the influence of institutions in people's development:** The scientific study of the great social institutions and the individual's relationship to them is done through sociology. Institutions through which society functions include the home and family, the school and education, industry and work, the church and religion, the state and government, and the community and association. Sociology investigates these institutions and their role in the development of individuals and recommends ways to strengthen them so that they can better serve the individual.

- **Healthcare professionals** are required to act as behavioral scientists. A holistic approach is needed to understand health and illness comprehensively. Culture influences the roles and status of physiotherapists and affects institutional networks, which directly or indirectly helps in the health improvement process and helps identify cross-cultural similarities and variations in such behavior patterns of patients.

- **Sociology has drawn our attention to man's intrinsic worth and dignity:** Sociology has helped to change our attitude towards human beings. In a technological society, we are all limited to the amount of the whole organization and culture that we can directly experience. We can hardly know the people of other areas intimately. To have insight into and appreciate the motives by which others live and the conditions under which they exist, the knowledge of sociology is essential.

- **Social problems are to be solved with the help of sociology:** Social issues can be solved only when society and the individuals living in the community are analyzed scientifically. The behavior of human beings is to be scientifically studied to understand social problems and find solutions. Knowing what leads to the problem and the causes would only help them find the answers.

- Today physiotherapy is not simply an effort to cure illness. Preventive services and health promotion are also equally important aspects of physiotherapy. To be an effective agent of health promotion, knowledge of the community and the facilities and resources available therein are essential. Sociology, called the science of human society, can play a crucial role in understanding and improving community life.
- **Sociology increases the influence of social action:** The study of society can help a person better understand himself, his abilities, capabilities, and limitations. It enables him to adjust to his surroundings. Culture, social groups, social institutions, associations, functions, and so on, all assist us in living a useful social life.
- **The study of sociology is crucial for understanding and planning society:** Society is a complicated entity with numerous complexities. Without sociology's help, it is impossible to comprehend and solve the country's myriad problems. Indeed, we cannot comprehend and repair society until we understand its mechanisms and construction. Without sociology's examination, no true effective social planning could be accomplished. It assists us in determining the most effective means of achieving the agreed-upon objectives. Before any social policies can be implemented, a certain level of information about the society is required.
- Many physiotherapists are working outside the hospital nowadays. In programs like public health, industrial health, school health, and so on, the physiotherapist must work closely to different sections of society. The knowledge she has about culture is helpful.
- **Sociology is of great importance in solving social problems:** The present world is suffering from many issues that can be solved through the scientific study of society. It is the task of sociology to study social problems through the methods of scientific research and to find out solutions to them. The scientific study of human affairs will eventually supply us with the knowledge and principles that will allow us to manage and enhance the conditions of social life.
- **Sociology has changed our outlook on the problems of crime:** Our whole perspective on various aspects of crime has changed through the study of sociology. The criminals are now treated as human beings suffering from mental deficiencies, making efforts to rehabilitate them as valuable members of society.

- **Sociology has significantly contributed to enriching human culture:** Sociology has contributed to the enrichment of human civilization. In the light of scientific knowledge and study, the social phenomenon is now comprehended. According to Lowie, most of us believe that our manner of doing things is the only rational, if not the only feasible, way of doing things. Sociology has prepared us to tackle concerns about ourselves, our religion, culture, values, and institutions rationally. It has also taught us to be objective, critical, and detached. It enables man to have a better understanding of both himself and others. By comparing societies and groups other than his existence, his life becomes richer and fuller than it would otherwise be. Sociology also impresses us with overcoming narrow personal prejudices, ambitions, and class hatred.

- **Sociology is of great importance in solving global problems:** The progress made by physical sciences has brought world nations nearer to each other. However, in the social field, the world has been left behind by the revolutionary progress of science. Political divisions exist over the world, causing stress and conflict. Men have failed to bring peace to the world. Sociology can assist us in gaining a better understanding of the underlying causes and conflicts.

- **The value of sociology lies in keeping us updated on current situations:** It aids in developing good citizens and resolving community issues. It contributes to society's knowledge. It assists the individual in determining his place in society. One of the most pressing demands of modern society is the study of social phenomena and the ways and means of creating what Giddens calls "social adequacy." Because of its direct influence on many of the world's initial problems, sociology greatly appeals to many types of minds.

- **The study of society has helped governments to promote the welfare of the tribal and marginalized communities:** Many socioeconomic and cultural issues confront tribal and marginalized populations. Sociologists and anthropologists have studied tribal societies and issues, which have aided governments in implementing social welfare and healthcare programs for welfare objectives.

- **Role of institutions in developing individuals:** Sociology is a scientific subject determining the relationship between institutes and individuals. The relations such as family and house, work and workplace, education and schools or colleges, and so on are examples of institutions and individuals. These institutions affect individuals present in society. These institutions help strengthen human resources and make the conditions in the community better.

2

Social Factors in Health and Disease

LEARNING OBJECTIVES

☞ Define 'health' and 'social health'.
☞ Describe the social determinants of health.
☞ Explain the role of social factors in health and disease.
☞ Describe health and illness in the social context.
☞ What is a social construction?

INTRODUCTION

A variety of factors influence individuals' and communities' health. Their situations and surroundings affect people's health. Where we live, the status of our environment, genetics, our income, education level, and our relationships with friends and family all have a substantial impact on our health, although more commonly recognized aspects like availability and usage of healthcare services generally have less of an impact.

DEFINE HEALTH

A living organism's functional and metabolic efficiency level is defined as health. Individuals or communities can adapt and self-manage when facing physical, mental, or social changes in humans.

The concept of health has undergone significant transformation. Initially, health was defined as the body's ability to function normally, with occasional disruption caused by illnesses. According to one definition, it was described as "a state defined by anatomical, physiological, and psychological integrity, the capability to perform tasks valued by the individual, family, job and community, and the capacity to handle physical, biological, psychological, and social stress".

WHO defines health as *"Health is a state of complete physical, mental and social wellbeing and not merely the absence of disease or infirmity."* This definition has been subject to dispute, primarily as its lacking operational usefulness, the ambiguity in building coherent health strategies, and the dilemma posed by using the word "complete." Although some praised this description as the novel, it was condemned as being too broad, imprecise, and not quantitative.

■ DEFINING SOCIAL HEALTH

The ability to develop meaningful personal interactions with others is referred to as social health. It demonstrates one's capacity to handle social circumstances and act appropriately. Stress, e.g., might harm a person's social health. "Social wellbeing" is another term for social health. Developing assertiveness, having a circle of supporting friends and family, and the capacity to manage time with friends and alone are all examples of social health. Trust, respect, and acceptance components can determine if a relationship is socially healthy.

Social health involves one's ability to form satisfying interpersonal relationships with others. It also relates to one's ability to adapt comfortably to different social situations and act appropriately in various settings. Spouses, co-workers, and acquaintances can all have healthy relationships. These relationships should include strong communication skills, empathy for others, and a sense of accountability. In contrast, traits like being withdrawn, vindictive, or selfish can harm one's social health.

Overall, stress can be one of the most significant threats to a healthy relationship. Stress should be managed through proven techniques, such as regular physical activity, deep breathing, and positive self-talk.

■ DEVELOPING RELATIONSHIPS

Individuals must be willing to do the following to create relationships and maintain excellent social health effectively:

1. **Give of oneself:** This could include sacrificing time, effort, energy, or money for sustaining relationships.
2. **Have adequate levels of self-esteem:** Being mentally and emotionally secure with oneself can help an individual maintain healthy relationships.

3. **Establish a sense of identity:** Sacrificing personal characteristics often results in less satisfying relationships, while acting as a true self will strengthen social bonds.

All relationships will have emotional involvement, also known as **intimacy**. Determining how intimate a relationship will become is critical to long-term social health. While acquaintances or co-workers may have very little intimacy, family members and spouses often have intimacy levels high enough to be considered love. Characteristics of a healthy relationship include:

- **Trust**—those involved have faith in each other and will do what is best for the relationship.
- **Compassion**—the physical and emotional well-being of others in the relationship is considered necessary.
- **Respect**—sacrifices made for the relationship such as time, effort, and money are acknowledged and valued.
- **Acceptance**—changing individual characteristics and personality traits is not an expectation.
- **Reciprocity**—the give and take of the relationship are relatively equal.

■ CHALLENGES IN RELATIONSHIPS

Relationships can be compromised due to a multitude of factors. Relationships can be pushed to an unhealthy condition by a lack of honesty or transparency, unreasonable expectations, and jealousy. For example, a spouse who expects his or her husband/wife to do most of the housework with no display of appreciation may experience a low-quality relationship. Conflict resolution methods that attempt to solve relationship problems, such as empathy and negotiation, may be needed to help the situation. If attempts to improve the situation fail, an unhealthy relationship may need to end. Being honest, tactful, and compassionate is the healthiest way to maintain relationships.

■ SOCIAL DETERMINANTS OF HEALTH

The social determinants of health (SDOH) are the economic and social factors and their distribution throughout the population that influence individual and group disparities in health status. Individual risk factors (behavioral risk factors or genetics) influence disease risk or vulnerability to illness or injury. Health-promoting factors are found in one's living and working conditions (such as the distribution of income, wealth, influence, and power) rather than individual risk factors (such as behavioral risk factors or genetics). According to certain opinions, governmental policies that reflect the influence of prevalent political beliefs of those in power shape the distributions of socioeconomic determinants.

The WHO says, *"This unequal distribution of health-damaging experiences is not in any sense a 'natural' phenomenon but is the result of a toxic combination of poor social policies, unfair economic arrangements (where the already well-off and healthy become even richer and the poor who are already more likely to be ill become even poorer), and bad politics."*

COMMONLY ACCEPTED SOCIAL DETERMINANTS

In 2003, the WHO recommended that the social determinants of health include:
- Social gradients (inequalities in social status)
- Stress (including stress in the workplace)
- Early childhood development
- Social exclusion
- Unemployment
- Social support networks
- Addiction
- Availability of healthy foods
- Availability of healthy active transport/travel
- Religion, caste, and all the social diversities

ROLE OF SOCIAL FACTORS IN HEALTH AND DISEASE

Income

Income—alone or in concert with other factors–contributes to health and health inequalities. Poverty rates are significantly higher than average among certain groups—lone parents, work-limited persons, recent immigrants, and tribal peoples. Lower-income families and individuals at the lowest income levels are concentrated in lower-income neighborhoods. As a result, they not only deal with individual poverty but with the effects of living in the economically disadvantaged community around them. The concentration of poverty adds to the total impact of individual poverty on health when this results in neighborhoods with fewer resources and services, more crime, and less social support.

Employment and Working Conditions

People with jobs have more economic opportunities, which can have an impact on their personal and family health. The sort of employment and working conditions, on the other hand, can have a substantial impact on physical and mental health.

For many Indians, job-related stress manifests itself in job strain, satisfaction, the impression of physical risk, and job security concerns. More women than men report work-related stress. On the other hand, those in low-income homes report significant levels of worry, which coincides with job uncertainty and discontent. Longer and less predictable working hours might affect the home/family environment.

Food Security

Healthy eating requires being 'food secure' (i.e., having physical and economic access to sufficient, safe, and nutritious foods to meet the needs of a healthy life). Individuals with a higher social and economic status consume more nutritious foods (fruits and vegetables, dairy products, lean meats, and whole grains) than individuals with lower social and economic status.

When children go to school hungry or poorly nourished, their energy levels, memory, problem-solving skills, creativity, concentration, and behavior are negatively affected. Because of being hungry at school, these children may not reach their full developmental potential—an outcome that can have a health impact throughout their entire lives.

Environment and Housing

Where a person lives is very important because both natural and built environments influence health. It creates the context for determinants of health such as income, employment, social networks, and personal behaviors.

Physical Environment

Inequalities in health can also be influenced by the physical environment (e.g., adequacy of housing, indoor air quality, and water supply). Environmental challenges, notably climate change, are likely to inflict increased health burdens on society and infrastructure today and in the foreseeable future.

Outdoor air pollution causes health problems that include coughing, aggravation of asthma, other respiratory diseases, and the exacerbation of cardiovascular disease. This air pollution increases emergency room visits, hospital admissions, and premature death as air quality degrades. Also, for the majority of Indians, water quality is not considered to be safe.

Built Environment

The built environments can influence physical and mental health through community design, adequate housing, access to safe water, good sanitation, safe neighborhoods, fair access to education, recreational services, public transit, and childcare. The built structure provides the setting for many social determinants of health.

Through various social networks and institutions, the built environment can provide chances for social engagement. The larger the city, the more social networks there are and the more complicated they are. Community social involvement—fosters trust, efficacy, and a sense of belonging, linked to more excellent mental and immunological health. Urban centers tend to be less culturally and socially homogeneous and have diverse populations. Within these cities, communities comprising close networks of people of similar cultural and social perspectives offer the benefits to the community, such as social support.

Although cities offer numerous chances for social interaction, they can also foster anonymity and isolation. Regardless of neighborhood density, many urban dwellers say that they do not know their neighbors, many elderly residents live alone, and those not connected with the greater community can experience isolation.

Housing

The availability of housing or lack of it, is a critical component of an individual's environment. In India, majority of people do not have acceptable housing. Acceptable housing refers to affordable housing that does not require significant repairs and is not overcrowded.

Housing has a complex impact on health, as it can affect health directly or indirectly. In harsh conditions, insufficient housing may have immediate consequences. Mold allergies and respiratory disease/poor lung function can develop in cold, damp, or poorly ventilated homes. Other health problems can result from exposure to harmful compounds such as lead and asbestos, which can be found in inadequate plumbing and insulation and tobacco smoke in the environment.

Overcrowding and poorly ventilated houses can also increase susceptibility to disease. The number of people per dwelling has significantly impacted inhabitants' physical and mental health, including raising the risk of acquiring tuberculosis. This situation is especially true for many Indian tribal populations and for immigrants from some countries where older generations infected with tuberculosis in childhood may experience disease reactivation later in life that can infect others in the home.

Homelessness is also a health issue. It is difficult to measure how many people in India are homeless, as homelessness is a continuum with various short- and long-term experiences. Some of these people become homeless due to inadequate income, living in a community with inadequate housing, or having a mental illness, which may hinder opportunities for employment and income.

People living on streets/roadsides report trading sex for shelter, money, and substances and have higher rates of STIs and blood-borne infections than people in the general population.

Early Childhood Development

The first few years of a child's life are critical for their growth and development. Nurturing caretakers, great learning environments, appropriate nutrition, and social engagement with other children all contribute to children's early physical and social development in ways that can positively impact their health and well-being. A bad start in life—frequently leads to issues that affect one's health and long-term prospects.

There are three key areas important to healthy child development:

1. **Adequate income**—family income should not be a barrier to excellent early development, and support systems should be in place to ensure that all children get a decent start in life;

2. **Effective parenting and family functioning**—effective parenting skills are essential to child development. However, parents may also require employer support for flexible work hours and maternity/parental leaves, as well as broader social support for family-based opportunities and resources; and

3. **Supportive community environments**—all community members are responsible for the healthy development of children. Communities must provide accessible health and social programs and resources for families with children.

According to social and economic circumstances, there is evidence of a health gradient in childhood development. Throughout childhood, children from lower-income and less-educated households have poorer overall health and increased incidence of cognitive challenges, behavioral issues, hyperactivity, and obesity. The benefits of happy early experiences are indicated by children's readiness to learn, which measures their early success in terms of abilities, attitudes, and behaviors once they begin school.

Tribal and immigrant children may experience additional barriers if local child programming is not culturally relevant or delivered in a familiar language. The consequences of these disadvantages include children growing into adults with lower educational attainment, weaker literacy and communication skills, fewer employment opportunities, and poorer overall physical and mental health.

Education and Literacy

In general, having a good education leads to a better employment, higher income, improved health literacy, a better knowledge of the consequences of unhealthy behavior, and a better understanding of how to navigate the healthcare system—all of which lead to better health.

High school completion can help young people improve their quality of life by giving them the resources and confidence they need to live healthier, more productive, and prosperous lives that benefit them as individuals and, in turn, benefit their communities. In terms of their effects on health, education and income are frequently linked. Median earnings by level of education gained show that the higher the amount of education, the higher the average earnings.

In general, there is a link between education and literacy, with the more educated a person being, the more likely he or she is to be able to read and comprehend written material at a similar level. The capacity to read, write, compute, understand, and use learnt information in everyday life activities and decisions is now considered literacy. Illiteracy can directly impact one's health, such as inappropriate medicine use or the dangers of misusing potentially harmful materials in the home or workplace.

■ SOCIAL SUPPORT AND CONNECTEDNESS

People have a sense of belonging to something larger than themselves when they have family, friends, and a sense of belonging to a community. Satisfaction with oneself and others, problem-solving skills, and managing life challenges can all lead to improved health. People's long-term physical and mental health can be influenced by how much they participate in their community and feel like they belong.

Most Indians report that they rely on someone (e.g., friends, family members) as a confidante for advice and care in times of crisis. Depending on individuals or communities, assistance from communities or individuals is essential for good mental health and coping skills.

Social cohesiveness is a metric of social connectivity that considers how much people interact in their communities and how content they are with their life there. How safe a person feels and the level of violence to which they are exposed or perceive a danger influence the level of social connectivity, which can impact mental and physical health.

Violence and maltreatment frequently occur in situations where people should expect to feel safe. The distressing problem of family violence persists, involving a variety of abusive acts directed towards someone in a trusting and/or dependent relationship. Children are also victims of abuse and violence. Negative behaviors, physical aggression, hyperactivity, emotional disorders, and destructive behaviors are common in children who experience parental violence.

Many Indians, particularly elderly, suffer from loneliness and isolation, which can be harmful to their health. Seniors who said they did not have any friends were less likely to say they were in excellent or perfect health. When some persons or groups have limited control and access to social, economic, political, and cultural resources, they are said to be socially excluded. Tribal Peoples and marginal groups of people have a long history of unequal access to and control over education and health care and lands and natural resources, which has resulted in social disconnection. High rates of suicide among migrants, particularly among youth, are linked to social exclusion and disconnection from their traditions and culture.

HEALTH BEHAVIORS

Individual behaviors, such as staying physically active and eating well, can contribute to good health. Other behaviors, such as smoking, heavy drinking, and illicit drug use, can negatively affect health. Ultimately, health behaviors are individual choices that people make. However, these behaviors are influenced by the social and economic environments where individuals work, live, and learn. **Figure 2.1** depicts the inter-relationship of various components of 'social determinants of health.'

Smoking

High rates of disease and death are linked to smoking. Lung cancer, head, neck, and throat malignancies, heart disease, stroke, chronic respiratory disease, and other disorders are all linked to it. The majority of smokers admit to starting in their teens. Most people, on the other hand, do not stop smoking until later in life. For some people, being exposed to smoke is unavoidable. Most children under 12 and 15 in Indian households are regularly exposed to environmental tobacco smoke–often called 'second-hand smoke.' Smoking during pregnancy is a known risk factor for unhealthy fetal growth and development.

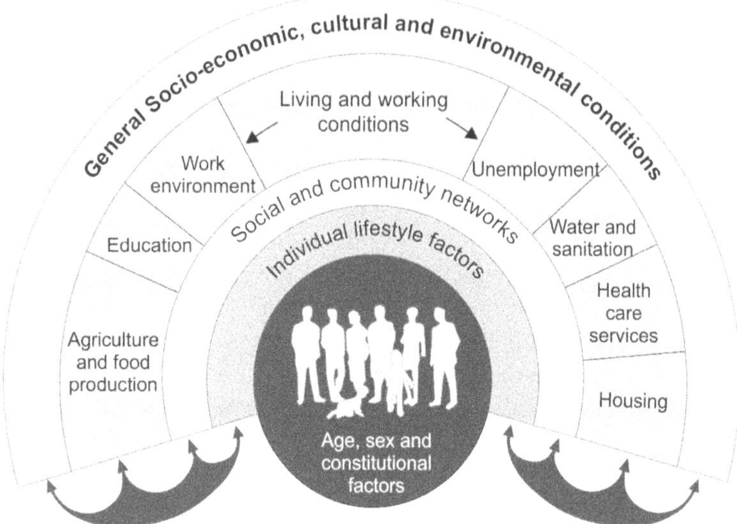

Fig. 2.1: Social determinants of health.

Physical Activity

According to research studies, there is a direct link between physical exercise and health, with the most physically active people having the lowest chance of illness. Many chronic diseases, such as cardiovascular disease, diabetes mellitus, cancer, and depression, have a modifiable risk factor—physical inactivity. Those who report being physically inactive are more likely to rate their mental health as fair or poor than those who report being physically active.

Healthy Eating

The variety, quantity, and quality of food consumed also have an impact on one's health. Aside from nutritional value, healthful food availability and affordability, as well as individual dietary choices, are critical. Body weight can be increased by a combination of poor eating habits and insufficient physical activity. Obesity is linked to a number of chronic conditions in adults, including hypertension, type 2 diabetes, gallbladder disease, coronary artery disease, osteoarthritis, and some cancers.

Eating healthy foods such as fresh fruits and vegetables, fiber-rich foods, and those with a lower fat content–is related to accessibility and affordability. A further challenge to healthy eating is the availability of fast, less expensive, and less healthy foods. Parental practices such as breastfeeding can positively influence an infant's start in life.

Alcohol Consumption

Excess alcohol consumption over both the short and long-term can negatively influence health. Alcohol abuse also has high economic and social costs. Excessive alcohol consumption may lead to alcohol-related acute-care hospitalizations, deaths due to liver cirrhosis, motor vehicle crashes, and suicides.

Drinking during pregnancy can cause severe health and development problems for children because of Fetal Alcohol Spectrum Disorder (FASD)—a preventable lifelong disability.

Illicit Drug Use

Drug use-related deaths are primarily due to overdose, drug-attributable suicide, and infectious diseases (hepatitis C and HIV infections) acquired due to drug use activities.

Sexual Health

Unsafe sexual habits, such as early initiation, infrequent condom usage, and multiple partners, raise the risk of sexually transmitted infections (STIs) and unintended pregnancies.

Access to Health Care

Access to health care is fundamental to health. Not only do people seek treatment through the government-funded health care system, but they also benefit from many disease prevention and health promotion services. These services are integrated into 'primary care' and range from childhood vaccinations to disease screening to advice on healthy living and mental health counseling.

Unfortunately, some people face barriers to health care services, including physical inaccessibility, socio-cultural issues, or the cost of health services (e.g., eye and dental care, mental health counseling, and prescription drugs). Access to health care is also an issue for rural or tribal populations who live in remote places.

Health and Illness

Health and sickness definitions are complicated by cultural differences in how societies identify health and illness, as well as the causes and treatments. However, because the disease manifests itself in patterns, social factors have a role in determining health outcomes. Because we are accustomed to believing the opinions of the medical profession, the way we think about health and illness is socially constructed.

In modern medicine, our bodies are viewed as machines, and doctors as mechanics. Sociological studies, on the other hand, reveal that a variety of environmental, political, and behavioral factors have a role in the formation of health and illness. What appears odd or inappropriate in society is frequently characterized as a disease; disagreements emerge because the causes of illness vary from place to location and time to time. Many studies also suggest that a person's social class has a significant impact on their health and longevity, and that poverty and social class are the most significant determinants of health. The lower one's social status, the more likely one is to die young.

The wealth and health of different social strata followed a pattern; the report indicated health inequality by occupation and suggested that professionals fared better than managers, managers fared better than skilled workers, and so on.

According to the social selection explanation, it is not social class that affects health, but health that affects social class; people with poor health stay at the bottom of the occupational scale because they are not healthy enough to advance, and it is not the lower class that is responsible for their poor health. However, because sick people skip school and work, their chances of succeeding are lower than those who are well and only miss school or work on rare occasions.

Because of their social strata, their living conditions often have an impact on their health and illness. For example, the lower classes' high child death rate can be attributed to poverty, damp housing, low income, poor diet, and unemployment, all of which lead to stress and despair, as the lower classes are locked in a never-ending cycle in which each problem feeds into the next. As a result, lifestyles remain unchanged. This circumstance reduces hope and limits options, posing a health risk. The lowest classes also have the worst health-care facilities.

◼ GENDER DIFFERENCES IN HEALTH PROBLEMS

Our ideas in society construct gender differences in health problems. There appears to be some evidence that men take more risks than women, such as dangerous sports, violent activities, and hazardous occupations. Also, women consult doctors more often, yet statistics suggest women have more ill health, but this could be because women in their socially produced gender roles are more acceptable to show weakness and seek medical help. Women's lives are more often medicalized than men's. In childbirth, reproduction, and mental health, women are more likely to be given prescriptions for antidepressants or tranquilizers; men, however, are more likely to have alcohol-related problems, a more socially acceptable response to stress than it is for women.

Women are typically expected to take care of everyone in the family, and as a result of the additional stress that comes with this responsibility, they may be vulnerable to physical and mental health problems. Women often suffer from "housewife syndrome", which is a condition brought on by social and economic circumstances. The constant decision-making and isolation that come with housework, as well as the responsibility of caring for young children, can be extremely stressful for women.

◼ SOCIAL CONSTRUCTION

There is substantial evidence that illness is socially constructed through the medical profession's intervention in creating iatrogenic diseases; most times, the treatment causes more damage than the illness ever would. For example, the use of thalidomide drug were the effects on the unborn children outweighed the advantages to pregnant women. People suffering from depression are often given tranquillizers, which will cause addiction. There is also much evidence to suggest that the contraceptive pill has many unpleasant side effects as it can cause cancer or thrombosis, and intrauterine devices can cause many infections.

The environment socially constructs health and illness. Technological changes over time have brought improvements in sanitary systems ending the risks of significant epidemics; however, this industrial engineering has also brought about high levels of dangerous chemicals. The major killers in modern industrial societies are heart diseases and cancers.

The world's most profitable drug firms help define the pattern of medicine; medications are designed to make money, therefore there is a link between doctors and drug companies that is designed to boost drug sales.

Many elderly people are admitted to hospitals not because they are sick, but because they have no one to look after them at home, and because health and welfare services fail to provide enough care in the community.

The social construction of health and illness is a multifactorial interaction of gender, age, class, and other social characteristics; however, vast social divisions in health outcomes and social class divisions in mortality and morbidity are almost certainly the result of material factors; what is defined as disease frequently occurs in patterns that are best understood sociologically. The increase in life expectancy over time is due to the reduction of epidemic diseases due to improved sanitary conditions. From this perspective, modern medicine has been less relevant than environmental changes.

Socialization

☞ Describe the meaning and nature of socialization.
☞ Write the goals of socialization and their importance.
☞ Describe types of the socialization process.
☞ What are the stages of socialization?
☞ Which are the agencies of socialization?

▍ MEANING AND NATURE OF SOCIALIZATION

According to McIver, socialization is the process by which social beings form broader and deeper bonds. They become more entwined with and sensitive to their own and others' personalities, forming a complex structure of closer and wider association.

By the term 'socialization,' we mean the process by which an individual develops into a functioning member of the group according to its standards, conforms to its modes, observes its traditions, and adjusts himself to social situations, Gillin and Gillin.

HT Majumdar defines socialization as "the process whereby original nature is transformed into human nature and the individual into a person."

Every man tries to adjust to the condition and environment predominantly determined by the society in which he is a member. If he cannot do so, he becomes a social deviant and is brought back into line by the group's efforts. This process of adjustment may be termed socialization. It is the opposite of individualization. The extension of the self is the process that develops in him the community's feelings.

Socialization is a lifelong process during which we learn about social expectations and how to interact with other people. Almost all the behavior we consider 'human nature' is understood through socialization. During socialization, we learn how to walk, talk, and feed ourselves, about behavioral norms that help us fit into our society, and much more.

Socialization is a learning process whereby a person gains the patterns of social action, and the culture of a society is transmitted to the new generation through socialization.

■ GOALS

- The teaching of essential discipline through controls and rewards.
- The instilling of fundamental values, goals, and aspirations into the individual.
- The transmission of skills.
- The ability to play social roles.

The Importance of Socialization

The process of learning how to fit into society is known as socialization. One learns the culture's language, role in life, and what is expected of them through socialization. Socialization is a crucial step in the development of a person's personality. When people engage with one another, they develop very similar values, norms, and beliefs, which allows everyone in a society to develop very similar values, norms, and ideas. In the long run, the early phases of socialization are critical. A person's physical and mental problems will worsen if they are not socialized. Socialization is an essential aspect of existence.

The importance of early childhood socialization cannot be overstated. Children only interact with a few distinct people during their first few years, usually family. Children are influenced by everything they see and hear. Children learn to walk, communicate, gain the ability to form relationships and begin to build their personalities throughout this time. Role-playing is an essential aspect of socialization. The first step in role-taking is *the preparatory stage*, also known as an imitation. This stage begins shortly after the first year of life. In this stage, children imitate things around them, including sounds and physical movement, but do not understand what they are imitating.

Children enter the play stage around the age of three or four. Stage children begin to take on the roles of one person at a time in the play. Children pretend to be a mother, father, teacher, police officer, firefighter, doctor, or someone else they know or see, most often a role model. Children simulate being someone else during this period by doing activities they think that person would do.

The third and final stage of developing role-taking is ***the game stage.*** The game stage starts around age six. In the game, stage children imitate the roles of several others at the same time. In the game stage, the children learn to play sports and participate in group activities that require them to know what other people expect from them. In this stage, the children understand the roles of multiple people simultaneously. Role taking permits people to be part of a group.

Cognitive development is another aspect of the socialization process. The growth of thinking, knowing, seeing, judging, and reasoning is called cognitive development. Children acquire these skills due to events that occur in their environment. Cognitive intelligence develops in phases, according to Piaget's hypothesis. There are four stages, according to Piaget:

a. ***The sensorimotor stage,***
b. ***The preoperational stage,***
c. ***The concrete operational stage, and***
d. ***The formal operational stage.***

The sensorimotor stage begins at birth and ends around the age of two. During this stage, the children learn to coordinate body movements with thoughts. They understand that they are separate from other objects and can cause things to happen.

The second stage is the preoperational stage. This stage starts around age two and ends around age seven. In this stage, the children associate symbols and language with objects. Children see everything from their viewpoint. During this stage, children are very self-centered.

The third stage, concrete operations, begins at the age of eight and concludes around twelve. Children learn to solve issues and reason using tangible items during this period.

The formal operational stage is the fourth and final stage. This period starts around the age of thirteen and lasts into adulthood. Individuals at this stage reason without the use of real things or symbols. They learn how to formulate a hypothesis to solve a problem. Cognitive growth is made up of several stages.

TYPES OF SOCIALIZATION PROCESS

- **Primary socialization:** Learning from primary groups like family, peers, and neighborhood.

- **Secondary socialization:** Learning from secondary groups like schools, organizations, clubs, books, and mass media.
- **Anticipatory socialization:** Learning in preparation for future roles.
- **Developmental socialization:** The process of learning and adapting to social roles and expectations during different stages of life.
- **Resocialization:** The process of unlearning old behaviors and learning new ones in response to a dramatic change in one's social environment, such as entering the military or a religious order.

Primary Socialization

The socialization process that occurs in the family ever since the birth of a child is known as primary socialization. Whatever one learns in the family from the formative period of one's personality affects how one feels and acts throughout life. Primary socialization is usually carried out through tender care, emotional support, and rewards in informal ways.

Similarly, peer groups and neighborhoods are equally significant primary socialization agencies. Cooley, an American Sociologist, called the primary groups.—*The nurseries of human nature.*

Secondary Socialization

The process of secondary socialization starts at a later stage than the process of primary socialization. Adolescents are also exposed to school, mass media, organizations, clubs, etc. These are also agents of socialization. What one learns in these secondary groups is known as secondary socialization. This learning process is **'task-oriented'** and not **an 'emotional'** one with family, peer group, or neighborhood. The strategy of the secondary organization is geared through secondary agencies more formally.

Anticipatory Socialization

This means socialization before actually entering a position. One learns many roles by playing the roles as play. For example, one takes over imaginatively the status of a doctor or a judge. The educational process provides much of the anticipatory socialization. Similarly, anticipatory socialization takes place through imitation.

Here, the person copies their role model's attitudes and behavior patterns, anticipating appearing like a role model. Anticipatory socialization thus relates to the learning of future positions and roles.

Developmental Socialization

Developmental socialization occurs during adulthood. This type of socialization depends on primary and anticipatory socialization. In the early two stages, an individual has acquired the skills, developed his attitude, and established the goals for the future, which have prepared him for the position he is likely to hold as an adult. An adult individual encounters new situations and roles such as marriage, job, husband, and employee or employer, which will require new expectations and obligations. In this stage, new learning combines with old to continue the process of developmental or professional socialization.

Re-Socialization

Whenever an individual changes his group and becomes a part of a new group, he must abandon his old way of life. Such situations compel an individual to leave the old values, norms, and beliefs. To adjust to a new group, he must learn the new group's values, norms, and beliefs. Learning a new lifestyle is called re-socialization.

STAGES OF SOCIALIZATION

The Oral Stage

During this stage, the child depends upon oral signals for pressing needs. The child is a 'possession' in the family. Freud called this stage a stage of 'primary identification.'

The Anal Stage

It continues from the first year to three years of age. During this stage, the child internalizes two roles—his own and that of his mother, now clearly separate.

The child receives care, but he also receives love and gives love in return. The child, during this stage, is encouraged for correct performances and punished or discouraged for incorrect behavior.

The Third Stage

This stage extends from the fourth year to puberty, i.e., to roughly twelve or thirteen years. A child learns to get along without his family's immediate guidance and support. The child experiences the *'Oedipus Complex'* or *'Electra complex.'* In the Oedipus complex, the boy is attracted to the 'mother,' and in the Electra complex, the girl is drawn to the 'Father' in the family. Many social pressures are brought on the child to identify with the sex during this stage. The socializing agent grants rewards. Boys play with boys, and girls play with girls. Thus, *'identification'* with *'Sex-Roles'* takes place. The mother plays *'Expressive Roles'* whereas the father plays *'Instrumental Roles'* towards the child.

The Adolescence Stage: This Stage begins after puberty or 12 years. At this stage, young boys or girls move away from their parents' control. There is a greater demand for independence in the behavior of the boy or girl. A phase of psychological pressure starts at this stage. A child puts a good deal of his sentiments into a playgroup or gang of boys or girls of his or her age. The adolescent stage finally culminates in *adulthood.*

■ AGENCIES OF SOCIALIZATION

The socialization process is operative not only in childhood but also throughout life. It is a process that begins at birth and continues unceasingly until the individual's death. It is an ongoing process.

Since socialization is essential for society, a child's socialization should not be left to mere accidents but managed through institutional channels. What a child is going to be is more important than what he is. Socialization turns the child into a valuable member of society and gives him social maturity. Therefore, it is of utmost importance to see who socializes the child.

There are two types of socializing for children. Those who have authority over him fall into the first category, while those with equal power fall into the second. The first group could include parents, teachers, the elderly, and the government. The second group consists of the club's playmates, friends, and members. His education differs in content and importance depending on which source he received it.

In one category is the relationship of the constraint; in the other, it is that of cooperation. The relationship of constraint is based on unilateral respect for persons in authority, while the relationship of cooperation is based on mutual understanding between equals. Under the first category, the rules of behavior are felt as superior, absolute, and external, but regulations in the second category have no superiority or absoluteness in themselves but are the working principles of association. Persons having authority over the child are older than he, while persons sharing equality with him are apt to be of similar age.

The chief agencies of socialization are mentioned here:

The Family

A child's 'first world' is his family. It's a separate universe where the youngster learns to live, move, and exist. Within it, the biological functions of birth, protection, and feeding take place and the formation of the child's first and most intimate relationships with people of various ages and sexes, which create the foundation of the child's personality development.

The family is the primary socialization agent. The infant develops an early sense of self and habit-training (feeding, sleeping, etc.) during this time. Whether in a primitive or modern sophisticated civilization, the primary family group is responsible for a large part of the child's indoctrination. The immediate members of the child's family—mother or nurse, siblings, father, and other close relatives—are the child's first human relationships.

He experiences love, cooperation, authority, direction, and protection here. Language (a particular dialect) is also learned from the family in childhood. People's perceptions of behavior appropriate to their sex result from socialization, and a significant part of this is understood in the family.

As the primary agents of childhood socialization, parents play a vital role in steering children into gender roles that society considers suitable. They continue to instill gender roles in children, whether intentionally or unwittingly. Families also instill values that they will carry with them throughout their lives. They frequently absorb their parents' perspectives on labor, education, patriotism, and religion.

The child's socialization begins with his or her parents or family. They have a strong bond with the child and are closer to him than others. He picks up his speech and language from his parents. He is instilled with societal morality. He learns to respect people in positions of authority. He learns several civic virtues from his family. The family is rightfully referred to as the "cradle of social virtues," as it is in the family that a child learns cooperation, tolerance, self-sacrifice, love, and affection. A family's environment has an impact on a child's development.

Psychologists have discovered that a person's personality is shaped by his family. In a terrible family, a child picks up harmful behaviors, but he picks up positive ones in a good family. A dysfunctional family environment is a significant contributor to adolescent criminality. When choosing a mate, parents look into the boy's and girl's family histories to learn about their strengths and weaknesses.

The relationships between parents and children are of constraints. His parents are older than he is and have the authority to compel him to obey. The child may be coerced if he does not follow the rules. The mother is the one who initiates the socialization process among the parents. The family's effect lasts for the rest of one's life.

The School

After family, the educational institutions take charge of socialization. Socialization occurs almost entirely within the family in some societies (simple non-literate societies), but the educational system also socializes children in highly complex societies. Schools teach reading, writing, and other essential skills; they also introduce students to develop themselves, discipline themselves, cooperate with others, obey rules, and test their achievements through competition.

Schools teach expectations about employment, professions, and occupations, which they will follow as they grow older. In contemporary society, schools have the statutory task of conveying knowledge in the most important fields to adult functioning. Some

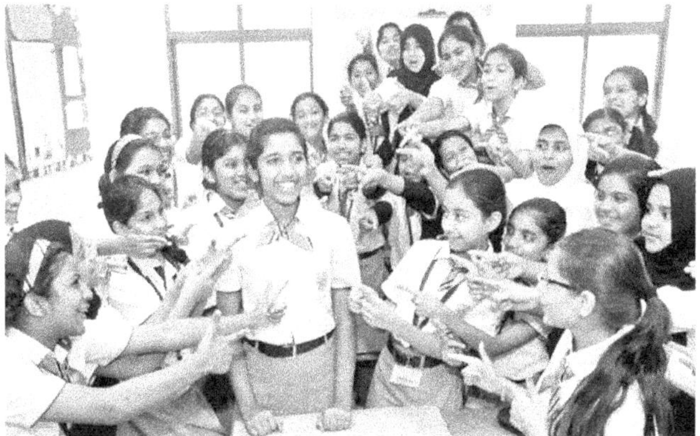

Fig. 3.1: Socialization in school.

argue that learning at home is more personal and emotional than learning at school.

The school is the second agency of socialization. The child gets his education in school, which molds his ideas and attitudes. A good education makes the child a good citizen, while a lousy education can turn him into a criminal. Education is of great importance in socialization. A well-planned system of education can produce civilized persons **(Fig. 3.1)**.

The Playmates or Friends

Besides the world of family and schoolfellows, the peer group (the people of their age and similar social status) and playmates highly influence the process of socialization. In the peer group, the young child learns to conform to a group's accepted ways and appreciates that social life is based on rules. The Peer group becomes significant others for the young child. Peer group socialization has been increasing day by day these days.

Young people nowadays spend much time with one other outside of the home and with their families. Young people with access to automobiles who live in cities or suburbs spend much time together away from their families. According to studies, they establish their subcultures—college campus culture, drug culture, motorcycle cults, athletic group culture, etc. Peer groups play an essential role in assisting the transition to adult duties.

Teenagers emulate their peers partly because the peer group has a significant incentive and punishment structure in place. The group may inspire a young person to pursue activities that society values.

The group may encourage someone to violate the culture's norms and values by driving recklessly, shoplifting, stealing automobiles, and vandalism. Some studies of deviant behavior show that the peer group's influence on cultivating behavior patterns is more than the family.

Why do some youths choose peer groups that embrace socially acceptable adult beliefs while others choose peer groups that oppose adult society? The decision appears to be linked to one's self-image. Perhaps the axiom "seeing-is-behaving" is true. How we see ourselves determines how we act.

Unloved, unworthy, unable, unaccepted, and unappreciated is how the persistent delinquent views himself. He forms a delinquent peer group with other similarly impoverished youngsters, promoting and sanctioning his resentful and aggressive behaviour. The law-abiding adolescent perceives himself as loved, deserving, capable, accepted, and valued. He forms a conforming peer group with other like-minded young people, reinforcing socially acceptable behavior.

Playmates and friends are also important socializing agents. The child's relationship with his playmates is one of equality. Because they are mostly of the same age, it is based on cooperation and mutual understanding. Friends and playmates provide something to the child that he cannot get from his parents. He gains collective morality and some key aspects of culture from them, such as fashions, fads, crazes, modes of gratification, and forbidden knowledge.

From a social standpoint, knowledge of such things is required. For example, we consider our society's understanding of sexual relations to be unsuitable for youth until they marry. If such knowledge is strictly prohibited until marriage, many aspects of sex life may become complicated after marriage. This child gains knowledge from his peers and playmates.

Books

In literate societies, another essential agency of socialization is the printed word in books and magazines. Our cultural world—experiences and knowledge, values and beliefs, superstitions, and prejudices—is expressed in words.

"Words rush at us in torrent and cascade; they leap into our vision as in newspapers, magazines, and textbooks. Someone always writes the words, and these people too—authors, editors, and advertisers — join the teachers, peers, and parents in the socialization process".

Temple/Church/Mosques, etc.

Religion has been an important factor in society. In ancient civilization, religion provided a bond of unity. Though the importance of religion has diminished in modern society, it continues to mold our beliefs and ways of life. In every family, some religious practices are observed on one occasion. The child sees his parents going to the temple and carrying out religious ceremonies. He listens to the holy sermons, which may determine his life course and shape his ideas.

Mass Media and Technology

The means of delivering impersonal communications to a large audience is known as mass media. The name "media" comes from the Latin word "media," which means "middle," implying that the purpose of the media is to link people. Because the media has such a significant influence on our views and behavior, especially regarding violence, it helps with the socialization process **(Fig. 3.2)**.

The media, from early forms of print technology to electronic communication (radio, TV, internet, and so on), plays an integral part in forming people's personalities. Technological advancements such as radio, motion pictures, recorded music, television, and the Internet have been crucial socializing agents throughout the previous century.

Television and the Internet, in particular, are critical forces in the socialization of children almost all over the new world. Apart from sleeping, watching television and the Internet is the most time-consuming activity for young people.

Relative to other agents of socialization discussed above, such as family, peer group, and school, TV and internet have specific distinctive characteristics. It permits imitation and role-playing but does not encourage more complex forms of learning. Watching TV and internet is a passive experience. The role of television and the Internet are very significant. It communicates directly to our ears and eyes, thus leaving a powerful impression.

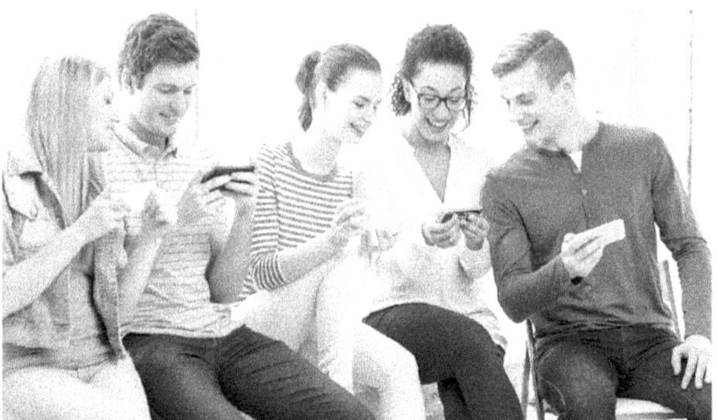

Fig. 3.2: Influence of mass media and technology.

Workplace

A fundamental aspect of human socialization involves learning to behave appropriately within an occupation. Occupational socialization cannot be separated from the socialization experience during childhood and adolescence. We are mostly exposed to occupational roles by observing our parents' work, people we meet while performing their duties, and people portrayed in the media.

The State

The state is an controlling agency. It makes laws for the people and lays down the expected modes of conduct. The people have compulsorily to follow these laws. If they cannot adjust their behavior by the state's laws, they may be punished for such failure. Thus, the state also molds our behavior.

Because of its rising impact on the life cycle, social scientists have increasingly recognized the state's role as a socialization agent. Outside entities such as hospitals, health clinics, and insurance firms have increasingly taken over the protective functions that family members formerly fulfilled. As a result, the government has taken on the function of a child care provider, giving it a new and direct involvement in the socialization of newborns and young children.

The failure of socializing agencies to properly and adequately socialize the child is one of the reasons for the rise in crime in society. The modern family is in crisis, and parental maladjustments are having a negative impact on the socialization process. There are numerous flaws in the educational system. The school is no longer regarded as a place of learning. It is a place where young people learn more about drugs and alcohol than about their cultural heritage. The onslaught of urbanization has obliterated the neighborhood system and snatched playmates from children who now spend more time playing video games than playing with their peers. Similarly, in urban society, religion has a weaker hold, and state authority is more disobeyed than obeyed.

It need not be said that these agencies should function efficiently to have socialized beings. Modern society has to solve several socialization problems, and for that purpose, it has to make these agencies more active and influential.

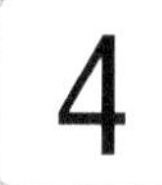

4   Social Groups

LEARNING OBJECTIVES

☞ What is the meaning of social groups?
☞ Define social group.
☞ Describe characteristics of social groups.
☞ Why are social groups formed?
☞ Discuss essential conditions for the formation of social groups.
☞ What are the functions of a social group?
☞ Describe the classification of social groups.
☞ What is group cycle? What are the features of group cycles?
☞ Learn about Ingroup and outgroup.
☞ What are tribe and its characteristic features?

■ INTRODUCTION

Humans are sociable creatures by nature. They dislike living in isolation. They live in families, clans, tribal communities, and so on. These groups are known as natural groups. The reason why human beings are social is that they are gregarious by nature. They are fond of group life. Apart from this, they form groups consciously to satisfy their various needs. Thus, they live in groups. They deliberately and regularly establish these artificial organizations with the assistance of other beings. They have always lived in groups due to their circumstances and nature.

Social groups are universal. All societies in the world have some type of group. Men and women are born and brought up in groups, spending their lives in them. Man can only fulfill his biological, physical, and emotional needs by being in groups.

The simple meaning of the social group is the individuals in mutual relationships. The social group is a collection of interrelated individuals engaged with each other in social processes.

It is a social unit that consists of several individuals who are more or less of the same definite status and role relationships and possess a set of values or norms of its own, which regulate the behavior of individual members in matters of the group.

MEANING OF SOCIAL GROUPS

A group means different things to different people. Some say a group is several units of anything close to one another. Thus, many persons working together or sitting face-to-face in a single room or bus or railway compartment may be regarded as an example of groups. Likewise, several houses on the street, several planes in an airport, several buses in a bus stand, or many trees in a forest may be accepted as other examples.

Others define a group as a collection of persons who do not know each other; a group can also refer to any collection of human beings. However, judging from the strict sociological point of view, the different versions of groups we have already mentioned do not give us an accurate idea of what a social group means.

DEFINITION OF SOCIAL GROUP

Many scholars have attempted to define the social group in different ways. Some of the crucial definitions are mentioned below:

"A group is an aggregate of individuals which persists in time, which has one or more interests and activities in common and which is organized."   —*Arnold W Green*

"A social group grows out of and requires a situation that permits meaningful inter-stimulation and response between the individuals involved, common focusing of attention, common stimuli and interest, and the development of certain common drives, motivations, or emotions."   —*JL Gillin and JP Gillin*

"A group is any collection of human beings who are brought into a social relationship with one another."   —*MacIver and Page*

"Whenever two or more individuals come together and influence one another, they may be said to constitute a social group."   —*Ogburn and Nimkoff*

"A social group is a given aggregate of people playing interrelated roles are reorganized by themselves or others as a unit of interaction."   —*Williams*

A social group may be defined as several persons whose relationships are based upon a set of inter-related roles and statuses, who share certain beliefs and values, and who are sufficiently aware of their shared or similar values and their relations to one another to be able to differentiate themselves from others.   *—Ely Chinoy*

Considering the definition given above, we conclude that a social group consists of such members who have reciprocal relations. A sense of unity binds the members. The 'we' feeling dominates them. Their interests and ideals are common, and their behavior is similar. Two or more persons in interaction constitute a social group bound by the shared consciousness of interaction. Examples of social groups include a family, husband, wife, friends, political parties, caste community, village, cricket club, trade union, social class, etc.

■ CHARACTERISTICS OF SOCIAL GROUPS

Following are the essential characteristics of the social group:
- **Collection of individuals:** Social group consists of people. There can be no group without people. We can't have a group without people, just as we can't have a college or university without students and teachers.
- **Interaction among members:** Social interaction is the foundation of group life. As a result, a collection of individuals does not constitute a group. Interaction between the members is required. In reality, a social group is a system of social interaction. The boundaries of social interaction delineate the boundaries of social groups.
- **Mutual awareness:** Group life involves mutual awareness. Group members are aware of one another, and this mutual recognition determines their behavior. This awareness may be due to what Giddings calls, 'Consciousness of kind.'
- **We-feeling:** We-feeling refers to the tendency of the members to identify themselves with the groups. It represents group unity. Our feeling creates sympathy and fosters cooperation among members.
- **Group unity and solidarity:** Group members are tied by a sense of unity. The solidarity or integration of a group largely depends upon the frequency, variety, and emotional quality of the interactions of its members.

- **Common interests:** The interests and ideals of groups are common. Men not only join groups but also form groups to realize their objectives or interests. Forms of the groups differ depending upon the common interests of the group. Hence, political groups, religious groups, economic groups, etc.
- **Group norms:** Every group has its rules and norms, which the members should follow. These norms may be in the form of customs, folkways, mores, traditions, conventions, laws, etc. They may be written or unwritten norms or standards.
- **Similar behavior:** The group members behave more or less similar to pursue common interests. Social groups represent collective behavior.
- **Size of the group:** Every group involves an idea of size. A group may be as small as a 'two-member group,' e.g., husband and wife, or as big as a political party with millions of members. The size will have an impact on the character of the group.
- **Groups are dynamic:** Social groups are dynamic rather than static. They are subject to change, whether it be gradual or sudden. Old members pass away, and new ones are born. Groups alter as a result of external or internal factors.

Social groups are formed when the following conditions are fulfilled:

- Two or more individuals get together at a place
- Interactions develop among these people
- These individuals come to a specific understanding among themselves due to shared goals and interests
- There is mutual awareness among members
- Because of interactions, a definite structure of the group is formed.

WHY ARE GROUPS FORMED?

One who lives in a group feels that he is a part of something larger than himself and is involved in a whole, which often acts independently of the individual's wishes. However, we cannot forget the fact that individuals form groups. Neither the individual nor the group is a good exhibit of all aspects of social life.

In socialization, the individuals are taught the values of group living. The group's customs, traditions, habits, beliefs, folkways, mores, and ideals are oriented and aim at maintaining and improving group life. In the family group, an individual is taught the fundamental lessons of group living, cooperation, and coordination. Later, the individual becomes a member of many other groups.

Essential Conditions for the Formation of Social Groups

Several conditions are essential for the formation of social groups. Some of them are mentioned below:

- **Social relations:** Without people establishing contacts and relationships with each other, social groups cannot be formed. Social interaction is thus essential for a group.
- **Common aims:** There should be a similarity in aims for forming a group.
- **Ability to influence each other:** This comes from the interaction of interrelationship. Interaction or interrelationship involves mutual influence. As soon as a teacher enters the class, the students stand up; and as he starts teaching, the students open their notebooks and start writing.
- **Physical presence:** People should be present physically to form a social group.

FUNCTIONS OF A SOCIAL GROUP

While some communities and societies are relatively large, small groups are formed by people to fulfil specific basic social needs. They may be summarized as follows:

- **To ensure the continuity of society:** The family group is actually entrusted with this essential function.
- **To maintain and perpetuate culture**, one group maintains the culture and transmits it to the coming generation.
- Groups enhance the progress of culture and civilization.
- Groups promote the 'we' feeling.
- Groups function as basic units of the human social system.

CLASSIFICATION OF SOCIAL GROUP

According to Charles H Cooley, the group is classified into two types:
1. Primary group
2. Secondary group

Primary Group

Cooley defined the primary group as, "By primary group, I mean those characterized by intimate face-to-face association and cooperation. They are primary in several senses, but chiefly in that, they are fundamental in forming the social nature and ideals of individual".

According to Lundberg and others, the primary group means, "Two or more persons behaving to each other in an intimate, cohesive and personal way."

Primary groups are:
- The family
- Playgroup of children
- Neighborhood
- Small village community
- Work team.

Characteristics of Primary Groups

The characteristics may be classified into two types:
1. Physical conditions
2. Internal characteristics.

Physical conditions

The physical conditions of the primary group are:
- **Physical proximity:** The primary group members should be found nearby. This proximity of group members is required to develop intimate relationships.
- **The group's small size:** A primary group has to be small, i.e., 50–60 people at the most. Intimate interaction is possible only when the group is small.
- **Durable relationship:** The relationship in the primary group has to exist for a long time. For example, a family relationship is lifelong.

Internal characteristics

- Identity of ends: In a primary group, the aims, objectives, and ambitions of the members are identical to a great extent. Everyone is interested in the personal well-being of others in the group.
- A relationship is an end in itself. The relationship is not for attaining any particular end, but only for the relationship's sake. It cannot

be termed a primary relationship if it achieves specific personal purposes. For example, if a person marries to get a considerable dowry, the marital relationship cannot be primary.

- The relationship is personal. The parent-child relationship, the husband-wife relationship, etc., are examples of relationships and are pretty personal. All others know a member's ideals, desires, ambitions, likes and dislikes, weaknesses, and strong points.
- The primary group relationship is spontaneous. Such a relationship is not made, but it develops spontaneously without effort from the side of any person. According to his innermost wishes, a person enters a primary group relationship out of his free will.
- Relationship possesses the power to control the individual. The control in the primary group is not because of external pressure, but it is voluntary. A person may please another or even undergo hardship and adverse conditions out of the freewill. A mother or father may sacrifice her/his comforts and interests for the child's sake. In extreme cases, a person is even willing to sacrifice his life for others in the primary group.

Functions of Primary Groups

Primary groups fulfill very vital functions for the members of society. Some of these functions are given below:

- Individuals are born and brought up in primary groups.
- Socialization of the individual takes place in the primary group.
- Primary groups maintain social order. The social organization depends on the members of the primary groups.
- All essential functions of society, such as reproduction, sex satisfaction, emotional security, and social control, are fulfilled in primary groups.
- Primary groups teach individuals high ideals like freedom, loyalty, love, sacrifice, patriotism, justice, etc.

Secondary Group

Definition

Secondary group means "Two or more persons behaving toward each other in an impersonal way, concerned with specialized interests and guided by consideration of efficiency."   —*Lundberg*

Most social groups we see in the contemporary world are secondary groups, e.g., trade unions, political parties, clubs, occupational associations, etc.

Characteristics of Secondary Groups

- **Large size:** Most secondary groups are large in size. The membership of some of the secondary groups might be in lakhs or even crores.
- **Spatial distance:** Members of the second group are dispersed and may not even meet each other personally.
- **Relationship duration may be short:** Secondary group relationships may not be long-lasting. Some secondary groups, like the audience or crowd, may last only for a short while, while others, like a nation or an association, may last longer than the individual.
- **The disparity in ends:** In secondary groups, members have different goals. Because of a lack of close interpersonal relationships, one person's plans may not be known to others.
- **Extrinsic valuation of relations:** The relationship is valued only for gain. It is unusually discontinued when there is no utility out of a relationship.
- **Extrinsic valuation of other persons:** The other persons are evaluated not as a person but by the function he is performing. For example, a teacher is considered on how well he can teach. All his other personal qualities are often forgotten.
- **Specialized and limited knowledge regarding the other persons:** In secondary groups, people have minimal knowledge regarding the other persons. Usually, a person is known only as a functionary, e.g., shopkeeper, driver, newspaper vendor, vegetable dealer, etc. Even the name of the other person may not be known.
- Secondary groups are usually formed for specific, definite purposes. The group may even get dissolved once the purpose is served.
- The relationship is formal and superficial. There is no depth in the secondary group relationship.
- The control in the secondary group is formal and through external forces. Rules, regulations, bylaws, legislation, constitution, etc., form the courts of behavior in the secondary group.

In short, we may say that the secondary groups are the opposite of the primary groups. They are increasing daily because of the improved means of transportation and communication, urbanization, and increased population. The modern man prefers superficial relations of 'giving and taking nature.' Persons and relationships are often discarded as soon as their purposes are served.

Group Cycle

Group cycle or group dynamics help understand the nature of groups, their development, and their inter-relations with individuals and other groups. Group dynamics aim at studying the mental and social forces associated with groups. It makes us understand the principles of group life and group activities. When the head of the family dies, the family changes. When a new political party comes into power, changes take place. So the fundamental problems are studied in group dynamics.

Essential Features of Group Cycle

Throughout one's life, a person remains a member of social groups. The characteristics and objectives of these groups may be different. At birth, a person is a family member, but he establishes his own family after marriage. Even after launching his new group, his membership in the old group continues. Like this, a person can simultaneously be a member of several primary groups. On being dissociated from one group, he gets associated with another group. Hence, a person keeps forming or dissolving the groups based on age, objectives, culture, professional interests, and family interests. This cycle continues all his life. Because of man's social nature, the utility and the absolute necessity of the group cycle for man are undisputed.

■ INGROUP AND OUTGROUP

In their work, The Science of Society, WG Sumner and AG Keller first presented the idea of ingroup and outgroup.

An ingroup is any group or social category to which a person feels they belong to the family, people of the same age group, students of a class, workers in a factory, etc. There is a sense of unity, friendship, commitment, sacrifice, and so on in an ingroup. Though, the attitudes toward the outsiders are animosity, contempt, and hate.

According to Horton and Hunt, there are some groups to which I belong to—my family, my church, my profession, my race, my sex, my nation—any group which starts with the pronoun 'my.' These are in-groups because one feels that *I belong to them.*

The outgroup is any group or social category to which a person feels they do not belong from other families, people of different castes, or other religions; outgroups include both people an individual rejects or ignores and those who reject or ignore that individual.

There are other groups to which one feels that *I do not belong to'*—other families, occupations, races, religions, nationalities, and the other sex. These are outgroups, as one feels that *I am outside them.'*

People feel comfortable and secure with a member of their ingroups because they know their specific experiences and beliefs. 'We go to church every Sunday.' 'My school is the best in the city.' Those statements denote the feeling of being a member of an ingroup.

Often people are hostile towards outgroups. Lack of contact with other groups can lead to misunderstanding and suspicion. Hence, members of an ingroup assume they would feel uncomfortable with members of outgroups. Strangeness and ignorance of other people's ways set the stage for prejudice, avoidance, hostility, and outright aggression. Negative impressions harden into stereotypes; the ingroup is glorified; the outgroup dehumanized. Intense competition and frustration also promote hostility toward outgroups and the formation of negative stereotypes. The same forces that create solidarity within a group create hostilities between groups.

Ingroups and outgroups are present in all societies, while the interests they develop vary from society to society. Since there are thousands of tribes, castes, sub-castes, sects, and races in India, there may be conflict between individuals and groups. The ingroup members believe their welfare is tied up with the other group members.

The attitudes of both the in- and out-groups are very striking. One must make changes and cultivate a sense of tolerance and coexistence; otherwise, disputes, tensions, and disruptions will occur. Ingroups and outgroups are vital because they affect behavior.

They deserve appreciation, loyalty, and helpfulness from fellow members of an ingroup. There is also great solidarity between them. They show goodwill, mutual support, and respect for each other's rights in their relationships.

The relation between comradeship and peace in the **we-group** and hostility and war towards other groups correlate. Loyalty to the group, sacrifice for it, hatred and contempt for outsiders, brotherhood within, and war likeness without all grow together, products of the same situation.

According to Federico, "Sumner meant that when an individual develops a sense of belonging with one group of people, he automatically feels that he does not belong with others. There is no 'we' without a corresponding 'they,' ingroups and outgroups are two sides of the same coin."

◼ TRIBE

A tribe is a community inhabiting a common geographical area and having a similar language and culture.

Characteristics of Tribe

- **Definite common geography:** The tribe inhabits and remains within common geography. Without shared geography, the tribe would lose its other characteristic features, such as community sentiments, common language, etc. For this reason, a common habitat is essential for a tribe.
- **Sense of unity:** Any group of people living in a particular geographical area is not enough to be called a tribe. Also, a mutual understanding of unity among its members must be there in the tribe.
- **Common language:** The members of a tribe speak a common language. This common language also helps develop a sense of communal unity among them.
- **Endogamous group:** The members of a tribe generally marry into their tribe. However, this scenario is now changing, thanks to increased contact with other tribes due to an increase in the means of transportation.
- **Ties of blood relations:** The sense of communal unity in a tribe is primarily because of the ties of blood relations between its members. The members believe in having descended from a common ancestor, real or mythical, and hence in blood relations with the other members.

- **Experience of the need for protection:** The members of a tribe always feel the need for security. With this need in mind, the political body of the tribe is established, and all authority for administration is vested in one person. This person becomes the leader and employs his intellectual power and skills to protect the entire tribe.
- **Political organization:** Each tribe has its own political body, maintaining harmony and avoiding conflict among its members. Thus, it acts as a canopy of protection for its members.
- **Common name:** A tribe has a common name.
- **Importance of religion:** Religion has great significance in a tribe. The political and social body of a tribe is based on its religion. Social and political laws become unbreakable once granted religious sanctity and recognition.
- **Common culture:** A tribe has a common culture. This shared culture develops from a sense of unity; common language, religion, a standard political body, etc.
- **Organization of clans:** A tribe makes up several clans. There is the law of mutual reciprocity among its members.

5

Marriage

LEARNING OBJECTIVES

☞ What are the functions of marriage?
☞ Describe different forms of marriage.
☞ Describe inter-caste marriage.
☞ Discuss marriage legislation and family problems in India.
☞ Describe the marriage-health connection.
☞ What are the effects of marital status on health?

■ INTRODUCTION

Marriages are usually arranged within recognized social units consistent with customs and traditions. Also, societies have formulated rules for that purpose throughout history. Across every society, it is found that men and women are aware of the husband and wife's rights and duties well before they enter into any relationship, and these rights and duties are part and parcel of the entire marriage complex in every society.

Marriage implies social sanction, generally in the form of civil or religious ceremonies, authorizing persons of the opposite sex to engage in sexual union and other consequent or correlated socio-economic relationships **(Fig. 5.1)**.

It is a family life institution that accepts both men and women. It is a stable relationship in which a man and a woman have the social right to have children, implying the right to sexual relations. All living things, including humans, satisfy their instincts and desires for survival and continuity. The essential desires are hunger and sexual instinct in the natural environment. Human beings accomplish them according to their society's established norms. An institutionalized pattern called Marriage regulates the human sex instinct.

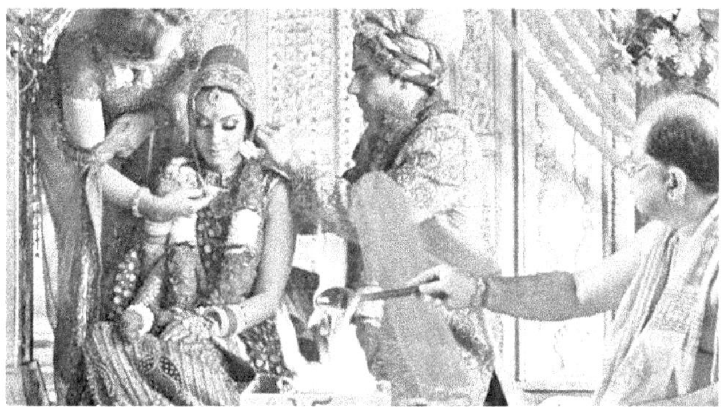
Fig. 5.1: Indian marriage ceremony.

FUNCTIONS OF MARRIAGE

Marriage is an institution that initiates a man and a woman to establish a family life and play the role of husband and wife **(Fig. 5.2)**.

a. It makes arrangements for permanent human interactions and lifelong relationships between men and women.
b. Husband and wife are allowed to have children in a social context. The right to have children requires the right to sexual intercourse.
c. Marriage provides adequate control, order, and stability of relationships by regulating sexual relations.
d. Marriage and the family are responsible for the survival of society through procreation and the provision of descendants.

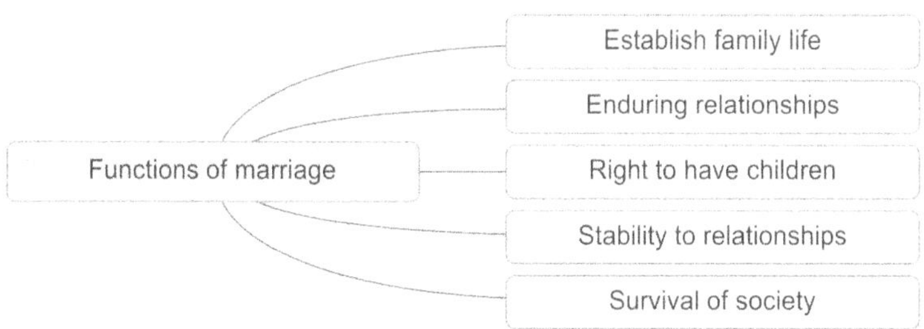

Fig. 5.2: Functions of marriage.

▨ RULES OF MARRIAGE

- Marriage is a social, legal, or religious agreement between one or more males and one or more females for procreation, sex gratification, and psycho-physical satisfaction.
- In some communities, people have to avoid seven degrees from the father's side and five degrees from the mother's side. Each society has got its prohibited degree of relations.
- The prohibition of incest forbids Marriage among those close relatives. Universal incest consists of sexual relations between parent and child, father-in-law and daughter-in-law, and mother-in-law and son-in-law.
- Virginity is usually considered among orthodox and conservative people worldwide as an absolute precondition for Marriage.
- Modern societies have statutory legislation to prevent child marriage and ensure the spouses are mature enough to enter into Marriage for which a minimum age is recommended.

Definitions of Marriage

Marriage, according to **Edward Westermarck**, is a more or less durable bond between a male and a female that lasts beyond the act of reproduction until the birth of offspring.

Ernest R Groves: Marriage is a public confession and legal registration of a fellowship adventure.

B Malinowski: Marriage is a contract for the birth and upkeep of children.

George A Lundberg: Marriage consists of the rules and regulations that define the rights, duties, and privileges of husband and wife to each other.

PB Horton and CL Hunt: Marriage is the accepted social pattern in which two or more people form a family.

HT Mazumdar: Marriage is a socially sanctioned union of male and female, or a secondary institution devised by society to sanction the union and mating of male and female for (1) establishing a household, (2) engaging in sexual relations, and (3) providing care for the offspring.

Anderson and Parker: Marriage as a society's sanctioning of a long-term bond between one or more males and one or more females established to allow sexual intercourse for the implied purpose of parenthood.

Harry M Johnson: Marriage creates a stable relationship in which a man and a woman are socially permitted to have children.

Robert H Lowie: Marriage is a relatively permanent bond between permissible mates.

■ FORMS OF MARRIAGE

Following are forms of marriage **(Fig. 5.3)**:

Monogamy: When a male marries a single female, the Marriage is called the monogamous type. Monogamy appears to be the most popular form of Marriage in all societies.

Polygamy: Polygamy is a Marriage that permits a man to marry two or more wives at a time. The principle followed in polygamy is 'one husband, several wives.' A plurality of wives is more frequent and generally practiced among the pastorals and agriculturalists.

Polyandry: Polyandry is similar to polygamy. In this kind of Marriage, a woman is permitted to have two or more husbands. It is found among the Todas of the Nilgiri Hills of Tamil Nadu, in the inhabitants of the Jaunsar region in the Siwalik Hills of Uttarakhand, the Tibetans, and the people of Sikkim.

Endogamy: Endogamy means Marriage within one's group. The best example of this is caste endogamy. The basic rule in caste is to marry within the caste group and the sub-groups.

Exogamy: Exogamy means to marry outside the group. It is the process through which group ties are expanded. People also believe that marrying their near kin is not a healthy practice. Exogamy is

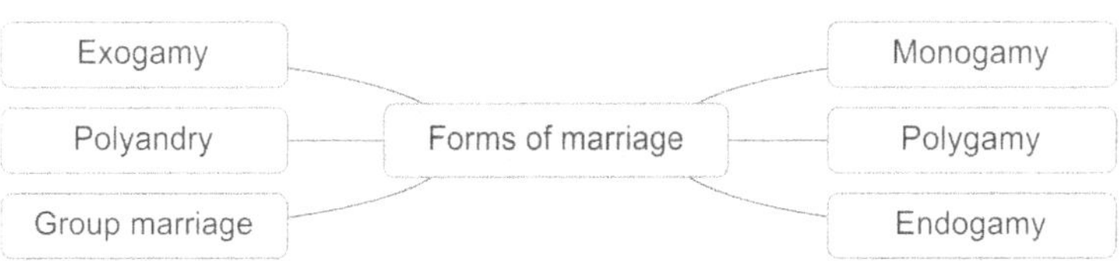

Fig. 5.3: Forms of marriage.

advantageous from a biological point of view. This is beneficial in the reproduction of healthy and intelligent offspring.

Group marriage: Group marriage implies two or more women married to the same two or more men, but this arrangement is rare. This type of Marriage is found only in polyandrous societies. Group marriage is not a marriage but a kind of sexual communism.

ENDOGAMY

According to **Joseph K Folsom**, endogamy is the rule of marrying within one's caste or other groups. Following are forms of Endogamy **(Fig. 5.4)**.

Race: In race endogamy, Marriage outside the race is prohibited—for example, people of the Veddah race practice endogamy.

Divisional or tribal: In divisional or tribal endogamy, Marriage is contracted within the tribe or division.

Caste: In caste endogamy, no individual can marry outside his caste.

Sub-caste: In sub-caste endogamy, Marriage can only occur between the members of a particular sub-caste.

Class: In class endogamy, the choice for Marriage is restricted to people of only one class or special status.

Causes of Endogamy

The separation policy: An endogamous group often has the will to separate from others.

To keep the group strong: When any woman of a group marries another, her children belong to the other group. This leads to the numerical weakening of the first group.

Religious difference: Generally, Marriage between people of different religions is not considered good.

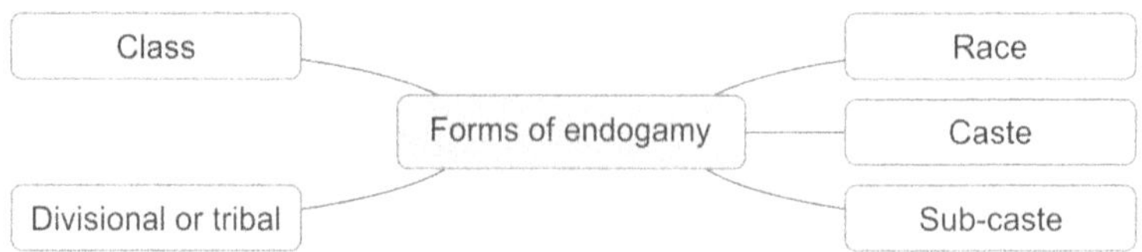

Fig. 5.4: Forms of endogamy.

Sense of superiority or inferiority: At the root of caste endogamy and racial endogamy is the sense of superiority or inferiority.

Long-distance: Those who live long distances naturally prefer not to marry one another.

Racial and cultural differences: Racial and cultural differences act as barriers to marrying outside.

Advantages of Endogamy

Endogamy leads to a sense of unity within the group. It helps maintain the purity of a group. People outside the group do not gain authority over the group's wealth. The group manages to keep its business secrets intact. Marrying within their group makes women happy.

Disadvantages of Endogamy

The scope for choice of a life partner is limited in an endogamous marriage. This leads to malpractices such as unsuitable marriages, polygamy, dowry system, bride price, and so on. Endogamy breeds hatred and jealousy for groups other than one's own. Marrying within one's caste has been responsible for the rigid casteism in India. Endogamy, therefore, gives a blow to national unity.

▨ EXOGAMY

Exogamy means to marry outside the group. It is the process utilizing which group ties are expanded. People also believe that to marry in their near kin is not a healthy practice.

According to Sumner and Keller, endogamy is conservative while exogamy is progressive; exogamy is approved from the biological viewpoint.

Forms of Exogamy

Following are forms of Exogamy **(Fig. 5.5)**.

Gotra exogamy is a practice among the Brahmins to marry outside the gotra. If a man marries within the gotra, he must repent and treat the woman like a sister or a mother.

Gotra exogamy among the Kshatriyas and Vaishyas: Among the Kshatriyas and Vaishyas, it is the gotra of the purohit which is taken

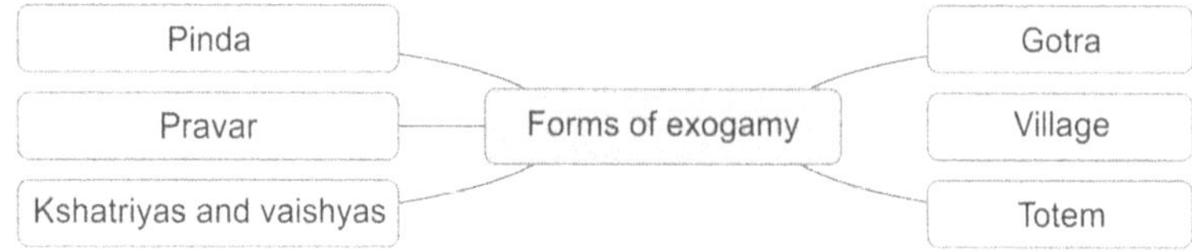

Fig. 5.5: Forms of exogamy.

into account. In their case, the ancestry is carried on not through the saint but by some followers of the saint.

Pravar exogamy: Let us first define the term "privacy." People who say the name of a common saint at religious functions are thought to be members of the same pravar. It is a religious and spiritual relationship. Marriage between people from the same pravar is forbidden by the Brahmins. This is in addition to the previously mentioned gotra restrictions.

Pinda exogamy: In Hindu society, Marriage within the pinda is prohibited. Pinda means common parentage. According to **Brahaspati**, offspring from five maternal and seven paternal generations are sapinda and cannot inter-marry.

Totem exogamy: In most tribes of India, it is customary to marry outside the totem. Totem is the name given to any specific vegetation or animals with which a tribe believes it has some specific relation.

Village exogamy: Among many Indian tribes, people marry outside their village. The Mundas and other tribes of Chhota Nagpur of central India practice village exogamy.

Causes of Exogamy

According to **Westermarck**, the absence of erotic feelings or the presence of sexual indifference between close relatives is the most crucial cause of exogamy. Incest taboos exist because they are necessary for the survival of the family structure. In their absence, the family's various statuses and relationships would become confused, resulting in a loss of organizational and functional efficiency. Sagotra marriages were considered invalid in India until recently. They were only declared legal in 1948. In ancient times, people living in the same household were not allowed to intermarry; however, when the household broke up, the prohibited range of Marriage also contracted.

▣ POLYGAMY

Following are causes of Polygamy **(Fig. 5.6)**.

Enforced celibacy: In uncivilized tribes, men did not approach the women during their pregnancy and while the child was being breastfed. Thus, the need for another marriage was felt due to this long period of enforced celibacy.

Earlier aging of the female: In the uncivilized tribes, men remarried several times because the women aged earlier.

Variety: Upon questioning why polygamy should be practiced, a Muslim from Morocco replied that a person could not live forever on a fish diet. The above incident may be apocryphal, but it is crucial to the point it drives home. The desire for variety is a cause of polygamy.

More children: A son has much utility in an uncivilized society. In agriculture, war, conflicts, and so on, numerical superiority is essential. Second, in these tribes, the birth rate is low, while the infant mortality rate is high.

Social prestige: The leaders of uncivilized tribes in Congo exaggerate the number of their wives to prove their superiority. A single marriage is considered a sign of poverty. In this way, where the number of spouses is flaunted as a sign of prestige and prosperity, polygamy is natural.

Economic necessity: In *the History of Human Marriage*, Westermarck writes that when a Zulu is asked why he has married a second time, he is apt to reply that who would cook when his only wife, if she were the only one, fell ill.

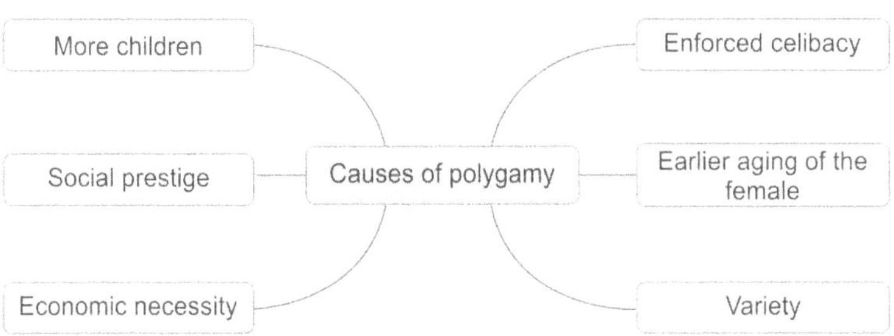

Fig. 5.6: Causes of polygamy.

In this way, one cause of polygamy is an economic necessity. In the Himalayan tribes of India, men often marry to increase their property and obtain help in their agricultural activities. Thus, they get a cheap and reliable laborer as a wife.

Forms of Polygamy (Fig. 5.7)

Polygamy: In this form, one man marries several women. The causes mentioned earlier pertain to this form of polygamy.

Bigamy: In this form, one man marries two women.

Polyandry: In this form, one woman marries several men and lives as their wife.

Group marriages: In this form, several young men and women gather on special occasions and marry collectively.

Advantages of Polygamy

Superfluous and powerful offspring: The practice gives a more significant number of strong children because powerful men can beget children from more than one woman.

Less corruption: Cases of sexual infidelity are few because the husband finds the desired variety in his numerous wives.

Disadvantages of Polygamy

The disadvantages of polygamy outnumber its advantages. For this reason, it is not considered good in civilized societies.

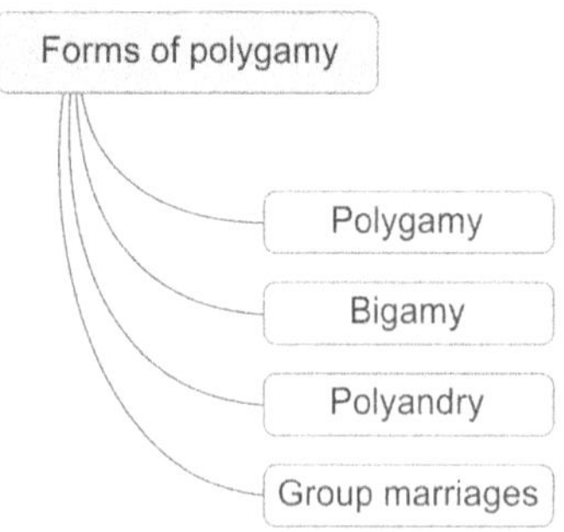

Fig. 5.7: Forms of polygamy.

The disadvantages are as follows:

a. The status of women suffers.
b. Jealousy, and hatred, increase among the women
c. The financial burden is much increased, and the children cannot be raised well.

■ POLYANDRY

Polyandry is the Marriage of a single woman to multiple men. It is much rarer than polygamy. The practice of polyandry is seen in many parts of the world. In India, tribes such as Tyan, Toda, Khasi, and Bota of Ladakh are polyandrous. The Nairs of Kerala were polyandrous previously.

Types of Polyandry

Fraternal Polyandry

In this type, one woman is regarded as the wife of all brothers, and all have sexual relations with her. The resulting children are treated as the offspring of the eldest. This practice is found in Punjab, Malabar, Nilgiri, Ladakh, Sikkim, and Assam. It also exists in Tibet.

Non-fraternal Polyandry

In this type, one woman has many husbands with whom she cohabits. These husbands don't need to be brothers. Social parents are elected through a special ritual if a child is born. This practice once prevailed among the Nairs of Malabar, but it is not seen nowadays.

Causes of Polyandry

Although polyandry depends to a large extent upon local conditions, its causes can be generalized to an extent. The following are the causes:

- Shortage of women as compared with the number of men.
- Extreme poverty due to which one man alone cannot support one wife.
- Desire to limit the population.
- Disutility in society from an economic viewpoint.

- Desire to maintain the strength of the joint family.
- Being situated far away from the centers of culture and progress.
- The bride price is high on account of the lesser number of women.

POLYGYNY

Polygyny is a form of marriage in which one man marries more than one woman at a given time. It is more popular than polyandry. It is not as universal as monogamy. It is practiced among the Nagas, Gonds, and Baigas in India. It is permitted among the Muslims and various tribal communities of the world.

Causes of Polygyny

Enforced celibacy: Men did not approach the women during pregnancy, and while the child was being breastfed. Due to this long-enforced celibacy, a second marriage was considered.

Earlier aging of the female: In the uncivilized tribes, men remarried several times because women aged earlier.

Variety: The desire for variety is also the cause of polygyny.

More children: Polygyny is also a practice to obtain more children.

Social prestige: In some tribes, the leaders have more wives to prove their superiority. A single marriage is considered a sign of poverty.

Advantages of Polygyny

Polygyny checks prostitution because men can satisfy their sexual desire in a better way by keeping themselves within the confines of Marriage. It gives healthy children to society because only the rich can afford to maintain several wives. Children are better looked after because there are several women to look after them.

Disadvantages of Polygyny

Polygyny increases the economic burden on the head of the family because he has to support many women and children. The children cannot be looked after properly because too many are there to be looked after. Polygyny can create jealousy among wives and their children. It can destroy family happiness. The women are given a lower position.

Types of Polygyny

Sororal polygyny: A type of Marriage in which the wives are almost always sisters. It is commonly referred to as a sorority. The Latin word soror means "sister."

Non-sororal polygyny: A marriage in which the wives are not related as sisters. Some people practice this polygyny for social, economic, political, and other reasons.

■ MONOGAMY

Monogamy is a type of Marriage in which one man marries only one woman. This is the most common type of Marriage in both primitive and civilized societies.

Advantages of Monogamy

Universally practicable: In almost all societies, only monogamy can provide marital opportunity and satisfaction to all individuals.

Economically better suited: No man of ordinary income can think of practicing polygyny. But monogamy can adjust itself to poverty.

Promotes a better understanding between husband and wife: Monogamy fosters the most intense love and affection between husband and wife. It promotes family peace, unity, and happiness.

Contributes to a suitable family and sex life: A monogamous family is more stable and long-lasting. It lacks the conflicts that are common in polyandrous and polygynous families. There is no scope for sexual jealousy, either.

Helps in better socialization: Since husband and wife have a better understanding, they can give greater attention to the socialization of their children.

Aged parents are not neglected: It is only in monogamy that old parents are protected and looked after properly.

Provides better status to women: In monogamy, women enjoy better social status. In modern families, women enjoy almost equal social status with men.

Reasons for Monogamy

The sex ratio in most societies is almost equal; hence, monogamy is the natural form. Everywhere, there is a set of rules governing the division of labor among the sexes, so for practice and economic reasons, monogamy is often the best form. Strong feelings of affection and loyalty often develop between one man and one woman, even if they are not present at the beginning.

Monogamy probably offers the best environment for the rearing of children. Due to the influence of Christian and Jewish teaching, monogamy has been widely accepted. The economic conditions of many societies forced people to be monogamous.

■ INTER-CASTE MARRIAGE

When a man from a particular caste marries a woman from another caste, we call it inter-caste marriage. Sociologists believe that inter-caste marriage was not alien to people living in ancient India.

However, with the Varna system transforming into a rigid caste system, strict endogamy laws came into force. This led to difficulties in finding a bridegroom and made him a scarce commodity. As a result, such malpractices as dowry, unsuitable marriages, and bride prices came into being. Encouraging inter-caste marriages will undoubtedly put an end to such malpractices.

MARRIAGE LEGISLATION AND FAMILY PROBLEMS IN INDIA

According to traditional Hindu law, marriage is a sacrament in India, not a civil contract. It is a *samskara* or purification ritual obligatory for every Hindu.

The Hindu religious books upheld Marriage as an obligation since some of the most important religious rituals cannot be performed by an unmarried man. Thus, Marriage in India is a holy performance of religious duties. Among Hindus, Marriage is considered compulsory. This is a sacred and indestructible association. Second marriages aren't often tolerated, especially for women.

Hindu Marriage Act of 1955

The Hindu Marriage Act of 1955 has now regulated Marriage among Hindus. Section 5 of the Act lays down that a marriage may be solemnized between any two Hindus if the following conditions are fulfilled:

a. Neither party has a living spouse at the time of Marriage.
b. Neither party is an idiot or a lunatic at the time of Marriage.
c. The bridegroom has completed the age of 18 years, and the bride has completed the age of 15 years at the time of Marriage, which has now been raised to 21 and 18 years, respectively.
d. The parties are not in a prohibited relationship unless the custom or usage that governs each of them allows Marriage between the two.
e. The parties are not sapindas unless the custom or usage governing each of them permits their Marriage. Where the bride has not reached the age of 18, the consent of her guardians in Marriage, if any, has been obtained.

Divorce in India

In the Hindu scriptures, Marriage was viewed as an inseparable bond in life. There was no such thing as divorce, according to Hindu law. The custom of divorce existed only among the lower castes.

The Hindu Marriage Act of 1955 recognized the Hindu woman's right to divorce her husband. According to Section 13 of the Act, any marriage solemnized before or after the commencement of this act can be dissolved on a petition presented by either the husband or the wife, by a divorce decree on the ground that the other party:

- Is living in adultery.
- Has abandoned Hinduism in favor of another religion. Has been incurable of unsound mind for a continuous period of not less than three years immediately preceding the presentation of the petition.
- Has been suffering from a contagious and incurable form of leprosy for at least three years before filing the petition.
- Has, for not less than three years immediately preceding the presentation of the petition, been suffering from a disease in a communicable form.
- Has given up the world by joining any religious order.
- Has not been heard of in seven years by those who would have naturally heard of it had that party been alive. Has not resumed

cohabitation for two years or upwards after passing a course for judicial separation against that party.

- Has failed to comply with a decree for restitution of conjugal rights for two years or upwards after passing the degree.

■ MARRIAGE LEGISLATIONS RELATED TO INDIA

The Hindu Widow Re-marriage Act of 1856

The Hindu institution of Marriage was established on the ethical foundations provided by religion. Therefore, the wife was not permitted to contract the second marriage after the death of her husband. The Hindu widows' plight drew the attention of many social reformers, such as Iswarachandra Vidyasagar and Raja Ram Mohan Roy.

The Hindu Widow Re-marriage Act was passed in 1856 due to the efforts of these social reformers, and from that day onwards, widow remarriage gained legal legitimacy.

The Special Marriage Act of 1872

In 1872 the British Government enacted the Special Marriage Act to abolish the endogamous restrictions on selecting mates for Marriage. This act allowed a man to contract lawful Marriage with a woman not part of his endogamous community.

The Child Marriage Restraint Act of 1929

The British Government and the Indian social reformers made great efforts to end child marriage. In 1929 Harvilas Sharda submitted a bill in this direction, and the Child Marriage Restraint Act was passed. This act is also called the Sharda Act of 1929. According to it, the minimum age for Marriage between boys and girls was fixed at 18 and 15 years, respectively.

The Hindu Women's Right to Property Act of 1937

The 1937 Hindu Women's Right to Property Act recognized a deceased person's widow as his surviving personality, having the same right as his in the joint family property.

The Special Marriage Act of 1954

The Government of India passed the Special Marriage Act in 1954. This act is also known as the Civil Marriage Act. This act is an amended form of the Special Marriage Act of 1872. It fixed the minimum age of Marriage at 21 years and 18 years for boys and girls, respectively.

The Hindu Marriage Act of 1955

The Hindu Marriage Act of 1955 applies to all members of Hindu society. According to this Act, the word *Hindu* includes a Jain, Buddhist, or Sikh by religion and any person who is not a Christian, Muslim, Parsi, or Jew. This Act has recognized the equal right of a woman and a man to divorce. Section 13 of this Act has laid down the grounds for divorce.

The Hindu Succession Act of 1956

The legislation which has affected our property and family relations very much is the Hindu Succession Act of 1956. This Act was passed to recognize equal rights for women in property inheritance. Before this Act's enactment, under Hindu law, a woman had no right to inherit property. According to this Act, a man's property after his death is divided equally among his widow, sons, and unmarried daughters.

The Dowry Prohibition Act of 1961

The main object of this act is to abolish giving and taking dowry at the time of Marriage. The provision of this Act was enforced on 1 July 1961. The Dowry Prohibition Act of 1961 extends to India except for the state of Jammu and Kashmir. According to this Act, giving and taking dowry before, during, and after Marriage is a crime. This act prescribes punishment for the persons who are giving and accepting dowry. The punishment is imprisonment for six months or a fine of ₹ 5000. In exceptional circumstances, both types of punishment can be imposed.

Marriage and Family Problems in India

Present Lower Status of Women

When considering marriage and family issues in India, we must first consider the status of women in Hindu families. Critics of the Indian family system claim that Indian women do not have equal rights with men in social, political, religious, and economic fields, that they are mistreated, and that they cannot claim any share of family property. A woman depends on her father before marriage, her husband after marriage, and her sons in old age.

Reform Movements

Women began to take part in the freedom movement in the 1920s. The part they played amazed the world. The Hindu Marriage Act of 1955, the Hindu Succession Act of 1956, the Dowry Prohibition Act of 1961, and the Commission of Sati (Prevention) Act of 1987 are new efforts to remove most of the disabilities from which Indian women are suffering. The Department of Women and Child Development in the Government of India has been primarily responsible for coordinating and executing the welfare program for women in India. A national commission of self-employed women has also been appointed. However, there is much to be done, especially for the womenfolk of the villages, where old prejudices and customs still hold deep roots in family life.

Dowry System

Another issue to consider when it comes to marriage problems in India is the commercial aspect of Marriage, i.e., the dowry system. It is unnecessary to dwell on the system's flaws. The girl's father commits suicide because he cannot pay the dowry demanded by the groom's parents. On occasion, the girl herself commits suicide as a result of this. To manage dowry money, the parents frequently commit theft, forgery, or misappropriation.

■ MARRIAGE–HEALTH CONNECTION

All married couples are considered to be healthy. However, it is only the selection of a healthy life partner that leads to a healthy life. Various attributes are desirable for the marriage partners, such as good physical status, attractiveness, earning potential, mental well-being, and a certain degree of self-sufficiency.

Social scientists, who do in-depth research in these areas, describe that married people tend to select a healthy partner to marry. Health has multidimensional concepts with an extensive collection of measures that include behavioral, physical, social, spiritual, and emotional outcomes.

Here, health outcomes from five broad areas are selected and discussed:

1. **Health behavior:** There are certain healthy behaviors observed after Marriage, such as performing regular exercise, eating a balanced diet, avoiding risky behaviors, such as smoking and drinking, and so on, in the initial period of marriage life. Many families evidence alcoholism and smoking prevalence as an effect of poor married life.

2. **Healthcare access and use:** Marriage is the holding between two families where two new persons are bonded to start a new life. Certain factors will affect the health of the couples; therefore, there is a need to access health care and understand people's usage of its facilities, for example, health insurance and its status; pre-conceptional counseling sessions, cancer screening for couples; total health cost, and so on. Healthcare services are opted for couples to strengthen their healthcare needs and improve quality care.

3. **Mental health:** Marriage can affect mental health. As two new people get bonded, there are many expectations and predictions about each life. Literature proves that most couples quickly drop their life and go into depression, which debilitates physical health. Counseling cells should be established to solve the conflicts among the couples, and mental assessment should be done to solve the problems at the earliest in each community.

4. **Physical health and longevity:** Health is an essential concern for everyone. After Marriage, every person is concerned about health and longevity; some illnesses arise due to family problems that predispose many cardiovascular illness risk factors. There are many studies done on Marriage, health status, and longevity; though there are other causes for the illness, particular illnesses can be specified due to family conflicts. To earn longevity, there is always a need to preserve health. Marriage life should be directed so that longevity is prolonged, and risk factors for the illness should

be analyzed and assessed to prevent illness. Approaching a health center with counseling cells for couples to treat the illness at the earliest prolongs longevity.

5. **Intergenerational health effects:** Couples' marital status affects the children's health. Also, long-term consequences are experienced by the child once they reach later adulthood. Many studies represent that a couple's health status is important to strengthen their child's health and longevity. Many factors intervene in marriage life while bringing up the children. Many couples may be unable to afford healthcare for their children's illnesses, which affects their children's longevity.

■ EFFECTS OF MARITAL STATUS ON HEALTH

Analysis of the health status of couples before and after Marriage shows that health status was affected more and improved after Marriage; for example, in divorce, older Marriages, or never-married men, health status is affected and deteriorates early.

Remarriage improves their health level because the health benefits are more after a remarkable married life since a person is cared for in times of illness, improved nutrition is available, a homely atmosphere is without stress, healthy behavior is encouraged, and unhealthy behavior is discouraged. Good married life encourages a healthy life and longevity.

6

The Family

LEARNING OBJECTIVES

☞ Define family and describe the characteristics of a family.
☞ What are the types of families and essential features of the family?
☞ Describe the joint family.
☞ What is a modern family? Describe the characteristics of a modern family.
☞ What is a nuclear family? Describe the characteristics of the nuclear family.
☞ Describe the blended family and extended family.
☞ What is the sociological significance of the family?
☞ Describe the social functions of the family.
☞ Discuss the influence of family on health and illness.

INTRODUCTION

Family is known as a primary group, social institution, and fundamental unit of the society, and a strong association of human society. There is no society where a family is not found—primitive society, rural society, and urban society. The family fulfills the basic needs of society. Family is the cradle of socialization of the child. It is here where the child learns health habits.

DEFINITION

According to **ME Jones**, the family is *'The social institution based on the fact of sex which has the production and nurture of children for its function.'*

McIver and Page have defined a family as a "Group defined by a sex relationship precise and long enough to provide for childbearing and upbringing." Sex satisfaction, procreation, and the upbringing of children are the essential functions of the family as a primary group.

The early and classical definitions stressed that the family was a social unit based on marriage, common residence, emotional ties, and stipulation of domestic services. Some sociologists feel that a family is a social group characterized by common residence, economic cooperation, and reproduction.

Recently, the concept of a family has been viewed in terms of specific criteria applicable to all societies. For example, it is felt that the family is a primary kinship unit that carries out reproductive, economic, and educational functions. Considering these definitions, we picture a family as a durable association of man and woman and children. As a result, family members live together, combine their resources, collaborate, and have children.

A family is also seen as an adult male and female living together with children in a more or less permanent relationship called marriage.

These definitions highlight the fundamentals or bare necessities of the family as a social grouping:

- It entails a sexual relationship between adults of opposite sexes;
- It involves their cohabitation or living together ;
- It requires at least the expectation of relative permanence of the relationship between them; and
- The relationship is culturally defined and has societal sanction-it is a marriage.

Marriage and family life are not something that people choose on their own. Some of how they must relate to each other are decided by their society. It is a well-known and recognized fact that marriage is the basis for the family. Marriage is recognized as a special relationship since it is the one in which families are created and perpetuated, and the family is the ultimate basis of human society.

CHARACTERISTICS

Some important characteristics are:

- A mating relationship between the husband and wife in a family results in the procreation of children.
- There are many forms of marriage in the family, such as monogamy, polygyny, and polyandry.
- There is also a nomenclature system in the family, such as father, mother, brother, sister, uncle, aunt, etc. The family's nomenclature system also involves a mode of reckoning descent. The children take the family name of either father or mother, and the transfer of property usually follows the nomenclature pattern.

- In the family, there is an economic provision, too, so that the economic needs of the family members, such as food, clothing, and housing, are met.
- A typical home or household is also a characteristic of the family.
- There is close interaction between members of the family. An interpersonal relationship is the keynote of any family.
- The maintenance of culture is also a characteristic of the family. The merging of cultural patterns transmitted from the two sides of the family in interaction with outside cultural influence creates the distinctive cultural patterns of every new family.
- The family has certain essential functions as well as status. Functions relating to sex, procreation, and the upbringing of children are crucial. Family is one of the status-giving agents of society **(Fig. 6.1)**.

Essential Features of Indian Family

In a family in India, certain striking features are noted below:
- There are different types and forms of family and marriage in India, such as nuclear family, joint family, monogamy, polygyny, polyandry, etc. While most society has monogamous families, polygyny is prevalent among some tribes like **Bhils** and **Nagas**. It is also found among some Muslims and Hindus. There is polyandry among some people in the Himalayan hilly areas and the **Todas**

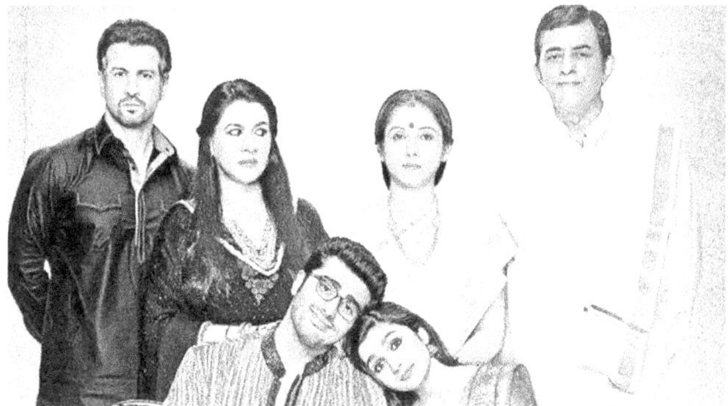

Fig. 6.1: A family.

of Nilgiris. While most families are nuclear, there are joint families in villages and cities.

- The traditional family in India, especially the joint family, is changing its structure and functions.
- Rules of endogamy and exogamy are practiced. However, intercaste, inter-religious, and inter-community unions are taking place in India, facilitated by certain factors such as education, urban life, social legislation, and government programs.
- Family planning and welfare measures are being adopted by Indian families more and more, especially among educated people.
- Marriage still has religious significance to most people in India, e.g., Hindus, Christians, and Jains.
- Child marriage is still prevalent in villages, especially in Northern and Central parts like Madhya Pradesh, Uttar Pradesh, Rajasthan, Bihar, and orissa.
- The status of women in India is still poor. However, women's status is steadily improving, facilitated by education, employment outside the home, and economic independence.
- Child-rearing practices are still traditional in India.
- Parents and elders still arrange most marriages.
- Dowry and bride prices are still practiced.

TYPES

Family can be divided into:

Family of orientation—the family into which one is born.

Family of procreation—the family one enters into as an adult.

Matrilocal arrangement—a married couple living near or with the bride's parents.

Patrilocal arrangement—a married couple living near or with the groom's parents.

JOINT FAMILY

The joint family comprises males with a common male ancestor, female offspring not yet married, and females brought by marriage into the family. These people may live next to each other in a common household or several households. In a joint family, the members must contribute to the entire family's support and receive a share of its overall product as long as the joint family remains together.

Characteristics of the Joint Family

Large size: The joint family consists of parents, children, grandchildren, and other near relatives along with their women. It is a group in which, at the same time, many primary families live together.

Combined habitation: The most striking characteristic of the joint family is living in a single house with many families. It allows for shared accommodation.

Depth of generation: The joint family comprises members of three or more generations, including at least grandparents, parents, and children. Certain kith and kin, including uncles, aunts, cousins, and grandsons, often live in the same household.

Common roof: Joint family members usually live under the same roof. Nonetheless, due to the scarcity of accommodation or problems relating to education and jobs, members of the joint family may reside separately.

Joint property: Within a joint family, wealth ownership, production, and consumption occur jointly. This arrangement is a cooperative body. This arrangement is like a joint-stock company in which common property exists. The family's head acts as a trustee, managing the family's assets for the family's monetary and spiritual well-being.

Cooperative organization: Cooperation is the cornerstone of the joint family system. A joint family consists of many members, and if they do not cooperate, the unity and function of the joint family cannot be sustained.

Common religion: The members of a joint family usually believe in the same religion and worship similar deities. They jointly perform religious rituals and duties.

Exercise of authority: The eldest male member generally exercises authority within the patriarchal joint family. The eldest member's superordination and the subordination of all other members to him is a fundamental feature of the joint family.

Identification with an obligation towards the family: The members associate themselves with their family. Every member has his or her duties and obligation toward the family. The family, in turn, defends the interest and promotes the well-being of all. The family's senior-most member acts as a guide to other members.

A productive unit: This feature of a joint family is found among agricultural families. All the members work in the same agricultural field.

Self-sufficiency: There was a time the joint family was primarily self-sufficient. It helped fulfil the family's economic, recreational, medical, educational, and other needs. Agricultural joint families were self-reliant, primarily in rural areas.

■ MODERN FAMILY

Since the 18th and 19th centuries, the traditional patriarchal family has started collapsing. New social, cultural, and technological forces influenced the character of the patriarchal family. The social value of the family was influenced by industrialization, urbanization, democratic values of independence and equality, and the fall of authoritarian mores. All this gave rise to what we may call the modern family.

The modern family is more individualized and democratic, where women enjoy high prestige and position. About a century ago, the family was more of a community. Nowadays, it has become an association. It has accomplished the transition from an institution to an association. The role and statuses of men and women have changed very much. The economic liberalization of women has resulted in equal status for them. The changing equation of women in the family has changed the family into a new kind of partnership and created new problems for the present and future families.

Characteristics of the Modern Family

The modern family is small. It is not a joint family. There is a tendency to have a smaller family and the growing use of contraceptives. Women are employed in factories and offices. They are economically independent. The family moved from the unit of output to the unit of consumption. Various home appliances for cooking, baking, washing, and ready-made food provide women with plenty of leisure time. Young people choose life partners freely, and marriage is based on individual romantic love. Parental control and authority have diminished.

The modern woman in the family is not inferior to the man but is considered an equal partner with equal rights in life. Both men and women have ample opportunities for frequent contact outside, which may lead to the leniency of sex relationships, resulting in pre-marital and extra-marital relationships. In character, the modern family is secular. There is little religious control. Religion's influence over marriage and divorce has diminished dramatically.

■ NUCLEAR FAMILY

Typically, a nuclear family consists of a father, mother, and children, whether adopted or biological. The nuclear family has traditionally been the fundamental unit of the larger family structure. Various values are learned from the nuclear family, such as love, tolerance, and coexistence. However, the increasing divorce rates, delayed marriages, and childbirth affect the nuclear family.

The parents and children living in the same household best define a nuclear family. *Nuclear families are named for being the nucleus, or core structure, in which other family members can be anchored.* An example of other relatives anchored to the nuclear family is the extended family, meaning aunts, grandparents, etc.

According to some philosophers, the nuclear family could include an adopted sibling, stepchildren, stepmother, or stepfather. However, others limit *nuclear families* to pure bloodline children with biological mothers and fathers. Around three decades ago, the nuclear family started as a concept. In the initial times, it was more of a compulsion. The husband had a job outside the hometown and had to carry the wife and children along.

Now, it is more of a choice. The reason behind this is the need for autonomy and independence in decision-making. It began with the male siblings separating after marriage. The split was a relief from the quarrels of daily family life.

Characteristics of Nuclear Family

Monogamous: A nuclear family's core is the union between one mother and one father. An existing marriage or legal union between the father and the mother is also a defining aspect of a nuclear family. Additionally, the father and mother in a nuclear family generally tend to stay together under one roof, despite occasional travel for work, unlike a single family where a child's father and mother stay separately and are not within an existing marriage or legal union.

Responsibilities: The duties of running a nuclear family are solely on man and wife of the home. Both parents work outside the home in some nuclear families, while the man works outside the home while the wife stays at home in others, and the man stays at home while the wife works in a small minority. In contrast, additional family members such as grandparents and uncles may take on some of the family's obligations in joint or extended families.

Small and intimate: Modern nuclear families are typically small and tend to be close. However, some slight variations in that some families have a mother, father, and many biological or adopted children. These are nuclear families, even though they are not modeled from the basic modern family.

Emotional component: The emotional unit of the family structure is the nuclear family. Children's emotional and cognitive senses are developed by the mother and father, who are the core of the nuclear family. The father and mother gain the ability to handle emotions such as fear, wrath, and disappointment between themselves and their offspring inside the nuclear family. The emotional component is then passed down to the children's family, continuing the cycle.

Not permanent: The nuclear family is not permanent because, at some point, the children of that family stop living with their parents. These children move away to create their own families, and the strong ties between their original family and their family of procreation (the family where you marry and have children) tend to erode. This is unlike the joint or extended family, which increases in size as offspring grow up and create their own families.

Blended Family

The successful integration of step-family members into the family unit is a blended family. In other words, when a step-family joins another family unit, there is a tendency on the part of parents or grandparents to put the families together socially. Even if the head of the family has a positive attitude toward joining together distinct families, there are advantages and disadvantages to this type of family cohesion.

The remarriage of a divorced or widowed parent creates a mixed family. It includes the new husband and wife and some or all of their former marriages' children. A blended family is a word that was recently coined to describe families with parents and children who are not all blood *relatives. Step-parents and stepchildren* are the outcomes of mixing a family. Those living in blended family households are aware of the pressures and challenges that impact blended families. The more participants there in any family, the more difficult the task is to relate.

Extended Family

The word *extended family* describes the family that expands beyond the nuclear family consisting of grandparents, aunts, uncles, and cousins all living in the same household.

Living in an extended family can have many advantages, but many issues can also be. Among the benefits of the extended family is that many more adults are present to help raise the children.

This takes much pressure off the parents to be the only role models and sources of discipline at home. Grandparents are also a substantial source of information for their grandchildren about the past.

This is important at a time when change is constantly occurring throughout the world. Grandparents are a link to that bygone era that is part of family lore, glory, history, culture, and ways of life of their time.

Changes in Family Patterns Worldwide

Changes in family patterns are generated by such factors as the development of a centralized government, the expansion of towns and cities, and employment within organizations outside family influence. These changes are producing a worldwide movement toward nuclear-family systems, eroding extended-family forms and other types of kinship groups.

The most significant changes occurring worldwide are the following:
- Clans and other kin groups are declining in influence.
- There is a widespread trend toward a spouse's freedom of choice.
- Women's rights are becoming more widely recognized for initiating marriage and making decisions within the family.
- Kin marriages are becoming less common.
- In relatively restrictive societies, higher levels of sexual freedom are emerging.
- There is a growing movement in favour of expanding children's rights.

Sociological Significance

Stressing the sociological significance of the family, **McIver and Page** have written that *".... of all the organizations large or small, which society unfolds, none transcends the family in the intensity of its sociological significance. It influences the whole life of society in innumerable ways and its changes, as we shall see, reverberate through the whole social structure."*

Eight distinctive features of a family suggest its sociological significance:

1. **Universality:** Family is found in all societies, primitive and modern, rural and urban, and everywhere. Family is found even among animals.
2. **Emotional basis:** The love, affection, sense of belonging, and intimate relationship and concern show the emotional basis of the family. Everybody is fond of the home, and there is an eagerness to return home.
3. **Formative influence:** The family molds the character and personality of the individual by the impression both of organic and mental habits. It is the most vital agency of socialization of the child. The family is the first and the best school.
4. **Limited size:** Family is a small group. The smallness of the group affords intimate and intensive relationships. It is the smallest of all

the organizations that make up the social structure. It is the most significant primary group.

5. **Nuclear position in the social structure:** The family has a central place in the entire social system. It is the nucleus of other social organizations. The whole social system is built of family units. The family is the basis of all classes, castes, and communities. The community itself is a union of families.

6. **Responsibility of the members:** The sense of responsibility between the family members is unique. Men may work, fight, and even die for their country in times of crisis, but they toil for their families their whole lives. The first responsibility is towards his family, and after that, only his duty toward his community and nation. The loyalty, cooperation, and sacrifice of family members are very striking.

7. **Social regulation:** Family is a significant agency of social control. Socialization and personality development takes place right in the family. The discipline learned and followed in the family is the foundation of control.

8. **Permanent and temporary nature:** The family is both permanent and changing. As an institution, the family has existed ever since the creation of human society, but then the form of a family, the pattern of interpersonal relationships, and the functions of the family have been changing from time to time. For example, a family had different forms like polyandrous, polygynous, and finally monogamous. Likewise, the size of the family was large previously, but now, it has become small. A small family is the norm now **(Fig. 6.2)**.

Functions

The family is the most vital social institution as it fulfills essential functions such as Affection, Sex, Procreation, Upbringing of the children, Religion, and Socialization.

To meet these functions, the family should have several facilities. A healthy family requires the following:

- Healthy parents
- Healthy children
- Good house
- Employment of parents

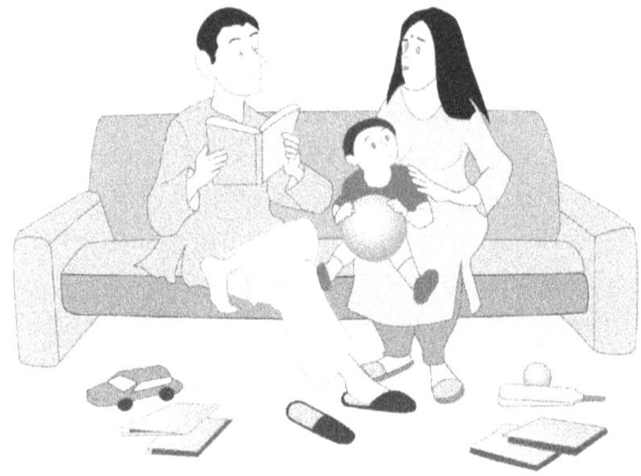

Fig. 6.2: A nuclear family.

- Education of children
- Healthy neighborhood
- Good recreation
- Good standard of life.

Nutrition, environment, and interpersonal relations are necessary for a good family. Family welfare needs family planning and family education. The family should meet the needs of children, adolescents, youth, adults, and the aged. This was so in the traditional joint family of India.

If we divide the needs of a family, two major types of needs may be pointed out, namely, **(i) physical needs** and **(ii) sociocultural and psychological needs**.

The physical needs are included health, food, housing, and household amenities. The sociocultural and psychological needs may consist of education, socialization, recreation, and moral and spiritual needs.

The family must be called the *'sweet home'* where all members should be eager to go and spend their life. This is called a centripetal tendency. On the contrary, if the family does not meet essential needs, there will be a centrifugal tendency; members will be eager to go out. Concerning juvenile delinquency, it is said that the absence of meaningful relations inside the family is very much responsible for it.

The family functions may be broadly classified into two, i.e., Essential functions and non-essential functions.

Essential Functions

- Stable satisfaction of sex urge.
- Procreation and upbringing of children.
- Affection function.

Non-Essential Functions

- Economic function
- Educational function
- Religious function
- Recreational function
- Medical function
- Protective function
- Governmental function
- Status giving function
- Transmission of culture

As the name indicates, the essential functions of the family are the most basic functions which no other agency/ institution can perform. Though extra-marital and pre-marital sex relations might occur, stable and socially approved satisfaction of sex urge is possible only within the family. Similarly, children born in wedlock only receive social and even legal recognition. Human childhood extends for many years, and the presence of both parents is essential for the children's entire physical, mental, and emotional development. Love, affection, and concern exist between the family members, and the same cannot be found in other groups. Family is considered a center of emotional and psychological tension release in the family. A person can share all his problems and worries and expect full sympathy and understanding.

The non-essential functions are those that the family used to perform in the past, but they are now transferred to other institutions. The economic function was and is still an essential function of the family. The family provides for its member, especially the children and the aged. Educating and training the children was done earlier within the family. The mothers trained the girls, and the fathers trained the boys. Even formal education was offered within the home with the help of private tuition.

Now, the role of the family in educating children has become very insignificant, as we have specialized institutions, right from nursery schools to highly developed technical institutes. Religious education and training were an essential part of training in traditional; societies. With the decline of the impact of religion, this part is losing its significance in many societies. Recreational facilities were minimal in earlier times, and people had to look for whatever entertainment possible within the family.

With the advent of mass media, especially movies and television, commercial recreation has taken over above all earlier simple forms. Unlike the traditional joint family, the modern nuclear family has no role in providing recreation to its members. However, it may be mentioned that the radio and the TV provide recreation for the family.

Elderly family members, with the help of household remedies and indigenous herbs, did look after the sick and ailing. Childbirth also took place within the family with the assistance of older women or a local maid. With the development of medical science and specialized medical and paramedical personnel, hospitals, nursing homes, clinics, and many other facilities, families have hardly any role in caring for the sick.

The role of the family in controlling its members is limited to childhood years. In maintaining and administering justice, secondary agencies like the state, laws, regulations, legislation, police, court, etc., are the primary agencies. A person's status depended on the family to which he belonged.

This was doubly so in India due to the caste system. However, education, occupation, economic condition, possessions, political affiliation, and several other matters determine a person's social status in modern times. Transmission of culture was an essential function of any family group. In our country, care was taken to teach all the elaborate norms of one's caste. However, the modern youth is more influenced by the ideals they see on the screen or television and peer group culture.

Thus, we find that the functions of the family have undergone drastic changes. With industrialization, urbanization, modernization, and the spread of education, science, and technology, more and more family functions are transferred to other institutions and agencies. Even the essential functions of the family-like, sex and reproduction, are fulfilled outside the family. With such changes, the very existence of a family is threatened. Unless we revert to some of our old values and patterns, the family is in danger of becoming obsolete.

From the previous discussion, we can deduce that the family remains an important institution in human society. Emotional support from the family is particularly significant during sickness. To a great extent, physical recovery depends upon the state of mind.

A physiotherapist/nurse should understand the role of family members in providing emotional support to the patient, even when they cannot provide physical care. Similarly, family members will be anxious and concerned about the patient's condition. A sympathetic understanding of them is essential, and they should be reassured and comforted wherever possible—a healthy rapport between the physiotherapist, patient, and family results in better care and speedy recovery.

Social Functions of Family

The functions that the family fulfills for individuals and society are the primary reasons for the family's endurance and universality. The significant functions the family accomplishes are discussed below:

- **Member replacement and physical maintenance:** To survive, every society must replace members who die and keep the survivors alive. The regulation of reproduction is centered on the family, cooking and eating, and caring for the sick.
- Children shall be nourished and protected within the family after birth. They are fed, clothed, and housed by their family.
- **Regulation of sexual behavior:** The family regulates sexual behavior. Every member's sexual behavior is influenced by what is learned in the family setting. The sexual attitudes and behavior patterns we know in the family reflect societal norms and regulate our sexual behavior. The sociological notion of sexual regulation should not be confused with repression. On the other hand, the norms specify under what conditions and with what partners sexual needs may be satisfied.

- **Socialization of children:** The family carries out the responsibility of socializing with each child. Their families primarily teach children to conform to socially approved behavior patterns. If the family serves society as a vehicle for cultural transmission, it also helps the individual as a vehicle for socialization. A family educates its children to participate in the more fantastic world by introducing them to different cultures.

- **Status transmission:** An individual's social identity is initially fixed by family membership by being born to parents of a given status and characteristics. Children adopt their parents' socioeconomic status and the culture of the social class into which they are born, including their beliefs, behavior patterns, and concepts of reality. Others characterize children as an extension of their parent's social identities and internalizing family attitudes and values. In other words, the family serves as a vehicle for passing down culture from generation to generation.

- **Economic activity:** Until recently, the family was a fundamental unit of production and consumption. The family produced most of the goods. It consumes most of the goods that are made. However, today, modern families mainly earn incomes. Thus, their principal function is consuming the goods and services they purchase. Because of the production of income, they are providing economic support for family members is a significant function of the modern family.

- **Social-emotional support:** The primary group, the family, is an essential source of affection and social interaction. The responsibility of caring for family members does not end with childhood. Humans naturally form social interdependencies to meet physical requirements and satisfy psychological needs for response and attachment.

- **Inter-institutional linkage:** Each child has the potential to participate in society's communal life. Individuals who belong to religious, political, economic, recreational, or other organizations as a family are often able to participate in activities that would otherwise be unavailable to them. The family then helps the individual fill social roles, achieve social standing, and participate in community activities. Some institutions rely on the functioning of families to ensure their survival and continuance.

■ CHANGING FAMILY PATTERNS IN INDIA

The family system's strengths and weaknesses often determine a society's cohesion and disintegration. Family is the foundation stone of society. It teaches us to be social. It teaches us to recognize that shared interests may be more significant than personal ones. As a result, it may be necessary to forego it in favor of family interests. It modifies individual behavior and cultivates tolerance, patience, respect for others, love and affection, dedication, care, and sacrifice. It checks selfishness and restrains rigidity.

The family is the first institution to instill societal norms and behavior in people. Social values can be deduced from family values. Concepts like nationalism would never have emerged if the family had not been present. Traditional Asian societies have endured for thousands of years thanks to a persistent emphasis on family values. The dissolution of society accompanies the breakdown of the family structure. There has been a noticeable increase in criminal activity and violence. The individual's ability to tolerate individuals who are different from him deteriorates.

A large joint family was the norm in traditional Indian families. Three to four generations could live together in the same house vertically. Many brothers and their families lived in one house horizontally. Rural landholding or a traditional enterprise was the foundation of such a joint family.

Women were usually uneducated but well-versed in Indian epics such as Ramayana and Mahabharata. These epics are encyclopedias of family values and societal behavior, and they provide clear rules for what to do in specific situations that a family or a nation may face. At the same time, these women were well-versed in the stories of famous warriors from each society. Every kid was educated by the epics mixed with a frequent recital of hero stories, from which they learned social rules. The child was well-versed in such ideals by the time they reached adulthood. As a result, generations have continued to follow them.

These norms and values are so comprehensive that no other example of such comprehensiveness can be found in modern literature. The Mahabharata, for example, provides thorough social etiquette guidelines. When it came to most matters, such as marriage or business decisions, such a family structure required joint decision-making.

As the modern age dawned and urbanization took over, the structure of the Indian family system witnessed a transformation. People began to adopt non-agricultural activities as a livelihood, which naturally required moving from their traditional joint family into an urban center. In the beginning, these urban breakaway families behaved as satellites of their parent families, which still lived in the village. Their dependence on their parent family for decision-making declined, and they began to act as independent units. Nevertheless, the structure continued more or less the same pattern. The patriarch made decisions based on his experience, and others learned from him until they attained the same position. Family values and norms of social behavior were still derived primarily from epics and hero stories.

The Indian family system has changed dramatically during the last decade. The family has dropped drastically in size. Three to four persons make up the average metropolitan household. There are just two of them without children. Both the husband and the wife work to support themselves. The practice of reciting epics has dwindled.

It is frequently misconstrued as a sign of backwardness. The reciting of the Ramayana or Hanuman Chalisa has been replaced by television. Children pick up on what the media tells them. Instead of mythical heroes, children today discuss movie heroes. On social media, boys chat about gorgeous girls, and girls talk about handsome boys. Pop music albums have displaced folklore. As a result, the epics' family values and societal conventions are not being passed along to the next generation. They are becoming obsolete.

Modern man's commercialization and globalization have ensured that he only runs after money, status, and consumer goods. Everyone is ***insecure*** because there is none to fall back. If their parents leave a rural or semi-urban joint family, their children break away further, searching for employment and livelihood. They make their own life decisions, which their parents may or may not comprehend. Due to a lack of understanding, such decisions are frequently rejected, resulting in a split between parents and children. Insecurity has come from the dissolution of the joint family arrangement.

Modern education has increased our understanding of modern concepts. However, the family values and social conventions that have held us together as a homogeneous society for the past 5000 years are rapidly dissolving due to commercialization, globalization, a mania for profit, and the influence of glossy media.

INFLUENCE OF FAMILY ON HEALTH AND ILLNESS

Chronic illness denotes a chronic, progressive, and degenerative disease. It is found that treatment of chronically ill-related affective disorders is the most neglected area of research, despite both the seriousness and the prevalence of emotional disturbances among patients and their families with chronic illness.

Rodgers and Calder highlighted the importance of marital adjustment as a critical factor influencing emotional adjustment in a couple relating when there is a chronically ill member. Referring chronically ill patients and their families to psychiatrists, psychologists, social workers, marriage and family therapists, or psychiatric nurses "may benefit patients with adjustment issues and marital and family dysfunction."

The Meaning of the Illness

Chronic illness is more than just an individual's subjective experience; It is also a social and interpersonal issue. How a person defines or interprets sickness is heavily influenced by his or her social environment. The individual's experiences shape social culture and social networks. In everyday contact, the meaning of the illness is shared and negotiated, firmly embedded in the social world. It is inextricably linked to the structures and processes that make up the social world. Health-related life events unexpectedly create many issues for therapists and other healthcare providers, such as:

- What factors determine the onset of severe, chronic, and degenerative diseases, and how does illness progression affect families?
- To what extent do gender, life cycle stage of the players at the time of illness onset (childhood/adulthood), roles, couple relationships, social support systems, and finances influence how families cope?

- In the face of health issues, can family systems be strengthened rather than weakened?
- How do members' physical well-being and ability to adapt to physical health problems depend on marriage and family relationships, belief systems, rules, and boundaries?

Family Life Cycle Considerations

In response to developmental stages, biopsychosocial variables change systematically. For example, the biological functioning of elderly people is challenged by many more chronic diseases than that of middle-aged adults or children simply because their bodies have been subjected to more prolonged normal wear and tear.

Rolland (1989) offered a model that stresses the intertwining of evolutionary threads: sickness and the life cycles of particular families. He provides a typology that distinguishes between (1) beginning, (2) course, (3) outcome, and (4) degree of incapacitation.

Rolland creates a typology of 32 potential psychosocial illness types by combining the types of onset (acute versus chronic), course (progressive versus constant versus relapsing/episodic), outcome (fatal versus shortened lifespan versus nonfatal), and incapacity (present versus absent) into a grid format.

Besides the core themes, he also utilizes the context of three major disease phases: (1) crisis, (2) chronic, and (3) terminal, to follow the history of the disease process. This allows for a better understanding of the patient's, couple's, and family system's ever-changing needs and requirements throughout the family life cycle. In addition, he integrates family, individual, and sickness development by incorporating the notions of centrifugal (forces that drive members apart) and centripetal (forces that push members together) family types and phases in the family life cycle.

Illness as a Life Event

Being diagnosed with a chronic illness is a life-changing event. A life event is an assortment of experiences that necessitate significant adjustments in the individual's life pattern. There are three life events: normative age-graded events like marriage, childbirth, or menopause; normative history-graded events like wars, economic depressions, and so on; and non-normative events like disease, disability, or job loss. The chronic disease comes into the last group, and as a result, all family members must redefine their roles.

This redefinition process involves incorporating the idea that a family member is ill. It primarily consists of constructing a reality centered on the concepts of sickness and disease, often involving isolation and control. The "sick" family member becomes more isolated as healthy people take on more controlling attributes. Life events can be roughly defined as situations that need a *"major change in the individual's ongoing life pattern."*

Hultsch and Deutsch classified events into three categories:
The first, normative age-graded events, are dictated mainly by physical capabilities or social norms, and as a result, many people's timing and duration are similar. Marriage, childbirth, menopause, and retirement are all excellent examples.

The second category, normative historically graded events, is something that most cohort members have gone through. War, political upheavals, economic depressions, and significant immigration are good examples.

Non-normative events fall into the third group. These are sporadic in frequency, limited to a tiny percentage of the population, and weakly connected with life stages or historical time. Illness, disability, and job loss are examples.

The sociological impact of a family or cultural membership affects belief systems, family rituals, and how people use the healthcare system at different times during the life cycle. The response to a child's illness, the role of sick family members, and the respect for or willingness to use health professionals have roots in family-of-origin dynamics.

As a result, interventions that improve people's ability to delay or cope with the onset of severe illness must include knowledge of disease entities, expected physical prognoses, and psychosocial implications, particularly interpersonal relationships, coping styles, and current and past family dynamics, when chronic illness strikes at critical junctures in an individual's or family's life cycle, complications increase. *"A progressive disease's extra centripetal pull raises the possibility of reversing normal family disengagement (i.e., a child leaving for college) and freezing a family into a permanent state of fusion.*" Frank's conversations about what they regard as realistic alternatives and options are an essential part of couples therapy in overcoming such centripetal overreactions.

Reactions to a Diagnosis of a Serious Illness

A diagnosis of a severe illness provides medical practitioners with a label and frame of reference with which to approach patients. While the diagnosis speaks to the bio-physiological factor, it does not begin to suggest the psychosocial demands that the diagnosed individual, couple, and family may face.

The disease label itself frequently addresses the beliefs and past experiences of those affected by the illness. When a person is diagnosed with cancer, they may have several expectations. If a person believes that cancer is not *"treatable"* or *"beatable"* and is physiologically devastating, compensations may begin before severe symptoms appear. Under the diagnosis alone, the person may develop a *"sick"* role. People here relinquish their responsibilities to others. This can lead to a shift in family power and encourage the diagnosed person to define himself or herself as incapable. This sick role may have some advantages; for example, it is a disease that has a specific course, and it may allow the diagnosed person to rest and recover while being relieved of their normal responsibilities. On the other hand, it may deter the individual from maximizing their coping abilities.

Even when the disease requires the ill person's constant self-monitoring, people who have taken on the sick role relinquish their decision-making rights and caretaking to health providers or significant others. Some people may believe that cancer is not a death sentence but an opportunity to deepen their lives, bring new meanings to their relationships, increase their religious affiliations, or take control and "be strong," perhaps for the first time. As a result, these responses can result in many positive changes in family systems.

Shontz (1975) describes a typical sequence of reactions people have when they are diagnosed with a serious illness. Bewilderment characterizes the first reaction, shock. The person acts in an automated manner, displaying feelings of disconnection from the current situation. People use avoidance behaviors to detach themselves from overwhelming emotions.

During the second phase, a person may exhibit disorganized thinking and feelings of loss, grief, and despair. This is more common when a seemingly healthy person receives an unexpected diagnosis.

The third stage is distinguished by denial of the circumstances and acceptance of the existence of the health problem.

However, when a person's ability to cope improves, the reality of the circumstance gradually returns. If avoidance and denial are continued for an extended period, a person's ability to obtain information about the problem may become immobilized. This may make it difficult for them to make timely decisions about their treatment or care requirements. Another family member may step in to make decisions, evaluate treatment choices, and provide daily care. Power shifts, role reversals, and conflicting triangulations occur in this situation. Alternatively, as the family surrounds the ill member, it can result in bonding more closely, strengthening each member into a support system. These increases in family bonding and support also may increase healing and promote coping.

While the shock is a relatively consistent initial response, some persons who become ill do not become disorganized or show avoidance behaviors. They seem much more in control, accept the illness, and begin to structure their lives around the accommodations. People's beliefs about the identity of an illness, the cause, the duration, and the consequences of their conditions are significant predictors of their ability to adjust.

Implications for the Family

When a chronic illness enters a family, individuals and their families face many issues. Issues can range from pre-existing problems to fear of abandonment, fear of death, spiritual beliefs, and exhaustion from caring for others and interacting with the medical community. Although a severe illness manifests itself in one family member, other family members perceive it as an intruder. The illness eventually becomes an independent functioning system member with its own identity. It is demanding because it necessitates readjusting schedules, roles, finances, and so on. It arouses rage because it is frequently uncontrollable and causes pain and fear. It is selfish in the sense that it must be attended to whenever it so desires, regardless of other activities or interests. It is isolating because it frequently alters intimacy and friendship patterns.

While the family's task is to meet the ill person's medical and other caregiving needs, the entire system's emotional well-being is compromised. This may lead to a couple or family discord that continues to decrease health status, negatively affecting family dynamics. Family scripts and experiences with the illness have implications for the functioning of the system and its ability to adapt. If, for example, the family believes that the disease could have been avoided or that they or another family member caused it, a point of blame is sought, such as the family's diet being unhealthy because it was not a priority for the meal preparer, the ill person working too many hours at his or her job, or the children causing "too much stress." These mental processes try to explain or provide some control over what appears to be an uncontrollable event. As the family system is endangered, hostility, low self-esteem, and other negative tendencies may emerge.

These patterns establish distance from the problem or between family members, effectively shutting off dialogue and providing little room for adjustment to the new situation. Outside of the family system, blame is sometimes sought. In this case, it is frequently addressed by the medical profession, i.e., the doctor misdiagnosed the illness or took too long to notice it. There is a lack of faith in the medical system in these circumstances, which causes treatment to be delayed. The disease demands can sap vitality, destroy optimism, and cause sadness. If a chronically unwell person develops depression, it may raise the risk of depression in other family members.

When an illness disrupts a diagnosed member's physical capabilities and personality attributes, the person must constantly fight to maintain homeostasis. As needed shifts in roles, power, and duties emerge, this battle can lead to growth, development, new closeness, and trust in fundamental family relationships.

In some circumstances, however, when a person's self-care abilities diminish, resentment, jealousy, and/or emotions of overburdening may develop as family connections deteriorate. Maintaining family support and intimacy is a never-ending endeavor for all family members. It is beneficial for family members dealing with significant sickness to know the predicted patterns of the disorder or illness and the practical and emotional demands these patterns may place on them to accommodate and achieve equilibrium adequately.

All family members must communicate openly. Fear and guilt can be exacerbated by keeping secrets. Because everyone in the family may be grieving, it's a good idea to talk about health care, living wills, powers of attorney, and finances now.

This may assist the family in keeping their affairs in order while under much pressure. The nature of the typical evolution of a given disease (progressive, steady, or relapsing) and the predicted outcome for survival have consequences for how families will function, as does the commencement of an illness, whether an acute attack or a slow buildup of symptoms. Is it possible to predict a person's course of events once they've been diagnosed, including the degree of handicap and agony they'll experience, or is the future ambiguous and uncertain? What medical treatments are available, and how do people get them?

Enmeshment/Disengagement

Family members who cannot cope or care in acceptable ways to themselves or the system may become disengaged. Others may become so engrossed with the illness symptoms that distinguishing between the sick and healthy members becomes impossible. While the unwell individual can still do parts of their previous functions or tasks with minor changes, the entangled family may usurp that ability and instill a sense of incompetence. When a person with a formerly dependent spouse is assigned the ill role, the spouse may become more assertive and better functioning if supported. However, as they do so, there is a noticeable shift in the power in the relationship away from the ill spouse.

The Roller Coaster

Periods of remission between bouts of severe debilitation can occur with chronic illnesses like cancer, causing a roller-coaster effect. There is a gradual "lulling" during remission away from the immediacy of loss, anxiety, and suffering. Impending loss, helplessness, wrath, perplexity, and dread will likely resurface during the recurrence phases.

Individuals' short-term goals and plans are significantly disturbed under this situation, and life appears to be uncertain.

Finances

There may be worry about the future when an ill spouse plays a primary role, such as providing for the family's income or childcare. Furthermore, guilt can emerge from time to time. An unwell spouse may be forced to make decisions that require them to accept the consequences of their disease. The family's task is to express their feelings and aid the sick individual in keeping as much independence as possible while releasing obligations.

Life-cycle Issues

The life cycle of the sick person and the developmental stages of the other family members have implications for the family's ability to adapt. The influence of disabilities on expectancies and skill mastery varies significantly from one stage to the next, but illness and disability have a tremendous impact on family systems at all stages of life. Chronic sickness, for example, has a different effect on a youngster who has not yet developed independent living abilities than it does on a child later in life. If a specific degree of success is attained in a field that needs abilities that cannot be maintained, it may have a different impact on the individual and his or her family than if it happened towards the end of the career or before that particular career was chosen.

Families, according to Rolland, require assistance in developing "beliefs that sustain hope and empower, rather than those that create blame, shame, or guilt." Independence and the ability to function at a high level within the confines of the illness must be encouraged.

Furthermore, he recognizes the need for families to view health problems as a couple or family problem to avoid aggressive power and control imbalances. Severe chronic sickness might lead to a re-enactment of the past to find significance in the present. People who have remission from a severe illness can achieve a much greater meaning for each life event. This powerful experience of vulnerability can be an opportunity to strengthen marital bonds, emotional intimacy, profound expressions of caring and commitment, open communications, and increased trust.

Chronic Illness and Children

Bronchial asthma, juvenile diabetes, leukemia, and some cancers are among the more severe chronic and debilitating diseases that affect children and young adults. While once fatal, due to medical technology and practical pharmacology, children often live with these illnesses and their related problems for the whole of their lives. The preconceived notion about chronic disease affects a family's ability to cope and adjust.

In early childhood, the parent-child relationship can be interfered with by long in-patient separations where the doctors or nurses meet the child's needs. These have implications for maintaining the family hierarchy where there are physical disabilities that may interfere with attempts at independence; children's self-confidence may be compromised.

Over-compensating parents may inhibit their child's development. Task mastery of the child can become rebellious to push out the boundaries. In later childhood and early adolescence, the peer system provides a yardstick by which children measure themselves and develop their self-image. Peer relationships may become problematic if a child has a chronic illness at this life cycle stage. Peers can be cruel and significantly make it more difficult for the child to develop a social network if the disabilities are severely restricted. When this occurs, the family may overcompensate by becoming overly protective of the child and meeting more of the child's needs than is necessary.

This is important and difficult for families, as adolescents with chronic illnesses try to navigate adolescence through solid friendships and personal beliefs that differ from their families. An unwell child's seclusion and loneliness can sometimes lead to rage and self-recrimination. Adolescent rebellion may manifest in refusal of treatment or medicine if the family is invested in maintaining the adolescent's health without encouraging their full participation. When an ill child needs to adjust to a family's daily routines, other family members, particularly siblings, may get enraged and resentful while feeling guilty for any attention they receive.

Siblings in a family with an ill child adapted best when schedules, visits, and vacations were tailored to the entire family's needs rather than just the disabled child. When the sibling's identities and importance in the family are supported and appreciated, less resentment and anger are felt, where a family's encouragement in maintaining an ill child's involvement in his or her care and decision-making (where developmentally appropriate), the child's confidence and coping ability are maximized.

The interaction patterns, communication, and feelings of the entire family unit are necessary therapeutic materials. External resources (financial, childcare, etc.) can either strengthen or weaken the family's stability and ability to accommodate the illness. Helping families with many support services they might need to survive a severe childhood illness requires a multi-systemic intervention.

The difficulties that young children confront when a parent is seriously unwell are less well-studied in the literature. The youngster may have insecure emotions due to the diagnosed parent's divorce and fragility. When the focus is on the sick parent, the family's protective atmosphere appears to be jeopardized. Children may feel particularly vulnerable because temporary caregivers do not set proper boundaries. Children may feel excluded from family interactions, especially if the system changes or their parents' health status are not explained to them. There have been several cases where a young child's parent was taken to the hospital and died, with no explanation given to the child other than "Mommy/Daddy went to heaven." Later in therapy, the adult explores the child's anger due to feelings of abandonment.

Even during the acute stages of the disease, children may be expected to become caretakers for their ill parents or siblings as they enter puberty. Their ability to develop socially and form peer relationships may be hampered due to their caring. Children, like adults, may be enraged by their sick parent or sibling, silently wishing for their death.

Chronic Illness in Adults

When a significant chronic sickness strikes an adult, it is often in the immediate family or the elderly parents. It can be difficult for people to marry, have children, or advance employment when it hits early adulthood. Illness can disturb the family and job structures in middle adulthood. Mid-life is when most young children's financial and other duties are fulfilled. People have established themselves in their roles, and many couples are preparing for a healthy retirement. Plans that had been put off for a while now appear nearing completion, if not already in place.

Couples in their forties and fifties are always aware of the possibility of disease, but their life scripts have it postponed life. With today's advanced medical technology, the first acute sickness (cancer, heart attack) rarely results in death. A couple will frequently have the opportunity to live with some quality of life for several, if not many, years. Their ability to modify their definition of themselves to suit changes in their physical ability is sometimes linked to their quality of life. Their quality of life determines how well their resources support their medical and caregiver responsibilities.

Couples find transitioning from an intimate romantic relationship to caregiving and receiving care challenging. Sexual and social boundaries may be disrupted if the spousal connection is jeopardized by a loss of ability to do basic hygienic tasks. For example, in sexuality, spousal carers of partners with dementia or Alzheimer's disease have reported feeling particularly distressed when their partners make sexual overtures but have no memory of who they are or that they have engaged at all.

When an illness changes sexual intimacy, the couple or the caregiver may have to redefine their relationship from lovers to companions. Caregiving may also change the family's roles. The marital connection may be replaced by a parent-child dynamic when there is a loss of control over body functions, and the caring partner performs diaper changing and dressing chores. The sick individual gets self-conscious about their limitations, withdraws or reacts aggressively, and/or becomes dejected. Finding new meanings for relationship adjustments requires a conversation between the parties. While physical dependency may occur, the therapist can assist the partners in eliciting the sick partner's maximum participation in family decisions and other ways. Encouraging the ill spouse's full involvement throughout the illness improves the quality of the relationship.

Gender factors have played important parts in how care is given. Because of differing socialization, women accept caregiving roles more readily than men do. Studies on post-cardiac incidents indicate that women can better provide environments for their husbands to rest and recover because they have been responsible for family chores. Men seek caregiving or housekeeping help from others when their wives are recuperating from acute illnesses.

Caregiving obligations are transferred in less demanding situations, such as Alzheimer's disease. Adult daughters are the most frequently requested caretakers, while the healthcare system does provide some nursing and home health aide assistance, which women mainly offer. Caring for others isolates people and puts carers at risk for sickness. If and when one of the members of a mid-life marriage becomes chronically ill, the status of the couple's social system in terms of past experiences with illness can impact their quality of life. Adjustment and support systems may be available if others in their peer group have had similar experiences. Adult children might act as a social support network if they are close.

The easier it is to adjust, the less interruption there will be in social events or family reunions. Families can be encouraged to involve the sick member in social situations as much as feasible but not to take on all of the sick person's obligations.

If these family and friend support networks are not available, medically-based peer organizations (Heart clubs, Partners of People with Parkinson's Disease, etc.) can help families reconnect. These organizations frequently provide a place for couples to meet new people and form new friendships. A physiotherapist or physician can help the family feel less lonely and isolated by providing psycho-education about these support groups.

Chronic Illness in The Elderly

Chronic sickness is frequently referred to as "old age illness." People assume that if they live long enough, they will develop a chronic illness, leading them to believe they will become unwell.

The life circumstances, loss experiences, socioeconomics, and support systems of older people are frequently linked to their stage of old age (65-75; 75-85; 85+) and ability to cope with illness. Belief systems about aging frequently influence how families and the healthcare system respond to chronic disease in later life. If the disease is an expected component of advancing age and older people are not likely to care for themselves, family members or the health system may take over their care. They may relinquish themselves to the caregiving situation if they share this notion. Comments like "I am old" are often synonymous with "I am feeble" or "unable." This self-determination may result in self-fulfilling prophecies often encouraged by well-meaning healthcare providers or children who become parents to their elderly parents.

If it is acceptable for elderly persons to cannot care for themselves and regain health positions after a severe illness, they may not be encouraged to do so. However, many older people do not succumb to these definitions and fight hard to maintain independence and self-sufficiency. They heal and refuse care, much to the displeasure of their families. The willingness to provide care, the style of caregiving, and the subsequent effect are determined by the family's definition of itself as a caregiver for its older relatives. A spouse, siblings, or children may provide for the caregiving needs of the elderly. In long-term relationships, spouses often envision themselves caring for one another in old age and feel most at ease when they can do so. "Till death do us part" is written into their scripts. Children frequently obstruct these efforts, fearing the excellent parent's health would be irreversibly jeopardized. The ideal spouse or caretaker responds to family pressure by giving up the role or keeping the family at a distance, and this interference may undermine the lifetime promise. Older spouses who relinquish responsibilities may feel as if they have abandoned their sick partner, leading to depression and withdrawal. In other instances, the caring spouse or caregiver continues to provide care even though it may jeopardize their health. In certain circumstances, spousal partnerships begin later in life, and the caregiver's role and the families' expectations may already be unbalanced due to the differences in their life scripts. When a severe sickness strikes, boundaries between the "new" well spouse and the birth of children or other relatives of the ill spouse are frequently erected. Who makes the decisions, who provides the care, and where it will take place are all issues that must be addressed.

As they safeguard "their own," reconstituted families are bound to engage in power battles. Wherever possible, environments that promote older people's belief systems and independent decision-making should be supported. Frequently, a couple has never addressed their concerns or fears regarding who would die first or who will look after whom. Couples are going through a difficult period right now.

General Caregiving Issues

Historically, the care of disabled people was the family's responsibility, and where no family existed, the religious institutions. In families, men handled the money to pay for their health needs and women for hands-on care. Love and intimacy, forgiving, demonstrating one's maturity, fulfilling commitments, and so on are all examples of caregiving. Caregivers experience a great deal of aggravation and *"irrational rage, ambivalence, death wishes, or escape fantasies"* on occasion. The caregiver may withdraw and feel guilty due to these powerful sensations. Directing the caregiver's passionate, explosive frustrations at the sickness rather than the ailing partner can help the family feel less guilty and closer together.

7

Community

In sociology, a community is defined as a group that conforms to a social structure within a society (culture, norms, values, status). They may work together to organize social life in a single location or be united by a shared sense of belonging that transcends time and distance.

Communities are as diverse and unique as the people who make them up. People frequently belong to two or more communities. Family, school, business, work, athletics, religion, and culture all involve communities that we take for granted. They appear to be in the backdrop. We only notice things when they are not going the way we want them to.

Most people think of communities as their neighborhood or city. A community is much more. They shape our lives and relationships. We also belong to and associate with other communities. Communities help us understand our surroundings, participate in activities, and share experiences. They provide self-identity, purpose, and belonging.

When people gathered around a common space for mutual benefit, "community" likely emerged. Sharing a language, customs, beliefs, talents, goods, and services, or protection from enemies are group benefits. The community has developed to meet different requirements. A group unites or lives together to share something valuable with the community's members **(Fig. 7.1)**.

MEANING OF COMMUNITY

The type of community in which people reside impacts their social lives. It was defined as a place characterized by a sense of communal life. It includes:

- a group of people,
- within a geographic area,
- with a common culture and a social system,

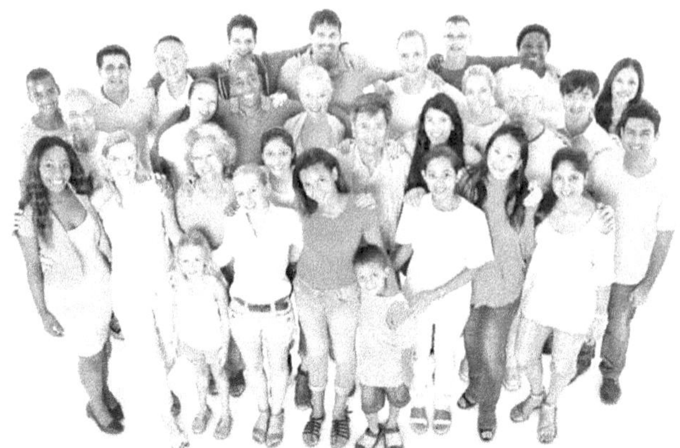

Fig. 7.1: Our community.

- whose members are conscious of their unity, and
- who can collaborate in an organized manner?

The two main aspects of a community's concept are a geographic area and a sentiment of unity.

■ COMMUNITY AS LOCALITY

The community is a geographically defined group of people who share common land and way of life. It's no coincidence that people congregate and focus in one location. Nearness makes it easy to make contact, project ideas, and organize and integrate the group. People who live in the same neighborhood develop a tremendous sense of community.

When a group of people is attacked, space is introduced into social interaction. Local affiliations become more important than blood ties. People who reside in the same neighborhood but of different bloodlines constitute a community. Even if an immigrant does not have blood relations, they can become a local community member.

Unplanned community physical structure deserves consideration. Villages, cities, and regions lack a long-term strategy. Congestion, damaged habitations and buildings, and an uneven increase in living spaces and economic activity have occurred. Appropriate community planning can solve this problem in major cities. The United Kingdom, the United States, and Russia have established community planning programs.

The Punjab town of Chandigarh was built according to a plan that split the city into numerous sectors, each of which was assigned for specific habitations. However, rebuilding a community's physical structure is difficult, fraught with practical difficulties such as a lack of materials, architectural issues, and vested interest opposition. Designing the shape of a new community may be simple, but revamping an existing one is significantly more difficult.

COMMUNITY AS SENTIMENT

"Community" is more than its location. It's sentimental. Living in close quarters and spending time together creates a "we-feeling." They consider their current location their 'home' living together creates shared memories, traditions, practices, and institutions.

Their views and preferences change. In their personalities, community emerges. He adopts the community's values. Individual connects personal interests to group goals. It's "bone of his bone and flesh of his flesh" to him. Physical and psychological community sustain and care for him, meeting his material needs.

Every member of the community has a status and should contribute to its functioning. Community feeling induces the urge to donate. Feeling, dependency, and role-feeling characterize community sentiment. Every group has its own traditions, hobbies, beliefs, superstitions, folktales, and myths.

Community sentiment is dynamic. No one today belongs to a single, all-inclusive community, but many. Today's man has many groups to meet his needs. He's involved with groups that represent community sentiment.

In big cities, the neighborhood as a community may not exist. Transport expansion has weakened community cohesion and intensity. As modern rapid transit increased physical contact between rural and urban populations, ties to the village community and reliance on it weakened. In short, local attachment is waning. Today's man seeks it in groups.

◼ EIGHT BENEFITS OF COMMUNITIES

1. **A network of support:** As a community member, you have access to a peer support network. Having a supportive group in your life can profoundly affect your general well-being, whether you turn to them for commiseration, guidance, or simply to tell your story.

2. **Professional development:** Members of a profession-based community can contribute to the growth and performance of the organization. In particular, Employee Response Group (ERGs) have the potential to produce internal leaders, educate employees, and improve retention for underrepresented groups.

3. **A sense of purpose:** People are increasingly yearning for a sense of purpose due to the pandemic, which comes with a sense of belonging. Belonging and purpose can make people feel more connected and fulfilled, which is beneficial both personally and professionally. Furthermore, having a strong sense of purpose can help you live longer.

4. **Alleviate stress:** Communities may bring joy to people! Coming together in person or virtually, discovering points of connection with people, and sharing moments of celebration and camaraderie can leave us feeling energized. These good emotions may aid in the reduction of stress and anxiety.

5. **New inspiration and ideas:** Immersion in a group of people exposes you to various ideas, perspectives, and personalities. There's likely to be something new to learn or a strange thought to admire from your fellow members.

6. **Empowered decision-making:** Mutual trust and respect create an empowering environment, emphasizing the importance of community growth. People feel more confident and engaged inside the business and on an individual level when they are part of a strong community where they can help each other grow and create trust.

7. **Better communication skills:** Connecting with people, a vital pillar of a community, is required for effective communication. Listening and cultivating a meaningful rapport with fellow community members is an exercise in developing relationships.

8. **Greater resilience:** Resilience is a personality trait that influences how people react to and manage change. Belonging to a community gives a sort of support that protects resilience from the stressors it faces.

7.1 RURAL COMMUNITY

LEARNING OBJECTIVES

- ☞ Define village.
- ☞ Discuss characteristics of the rural community.
- ☞ Describe the rural health problems in India.
- ☞ What are the causes of ill health in rural communities?
- ☞ What are the measures to promote health in rural communities?

INTRODUCTION

Human society has mainly two communities: rural and urban communities. The rural community or the village pre-existed the urban community or the city. The first collective life was in the village, with a sense of 'we' feeling and cooperation. Agriculture is the starting point of human civilization, as it helped man have a settled life in a village. Before that, the man had a nomadic life, as people engaged in hunting or food gathering and tended to the sheep and cattle (pastoral life). Thus, village life is the first significant stage in man's life to have group life.

DEFINITION OF VILLAGE

"The rural community comprises the constellation of institutions and persons grouped about a small center and sharing common primary interests."
—Merrill and Eldridge

"The village is a unit of rural society. It is the theater wherein the quantum of rural life unfolds itself and functions." *—AR Desai*

From these definitions, it is clear that the village is an agricultural settlement, and it comprises the institutions and interactions of the rural people **(Fig. 7.2)**.

CHARACTERISTICS OF THE RURAL COMMUNITY

The essential characteristics of the rural community are as follows:

- **Size of the community:** Village communities are smaller than urban communities in size. The population of the villages is low due to the small size of the communities.

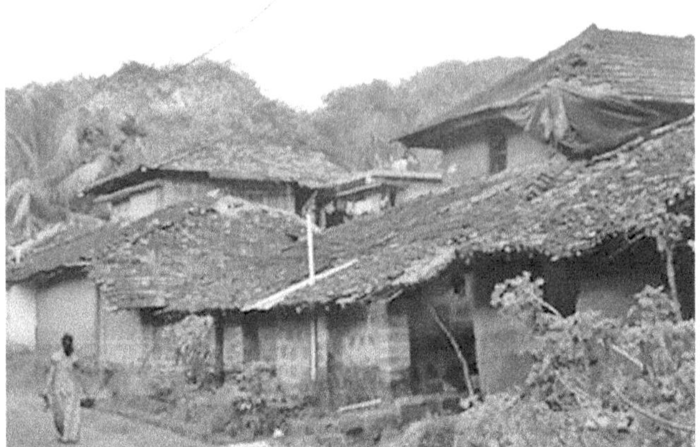

Fig. 7.2: Rural landscape.

- **Density of population:** Because of the low population density, people develop close interactions and face-to-face contact with one another. Everyone in a hamlet knows everyone else.
- **Agriculture is the main occupation:** Agriculture is the mainstay of rural life and the economic backbone of the rural economy. A farmer must perform a variety of agricultural tasks for which he requires the support of others. These individuals are usually members of his family. As a result, the whole family is involved in farm operations. That is why, according to Lowry Nelson, farming is a family business.
- **Close contact with nature:** Rural people are in close contact with nature because the majority of their daily activities center around the natural environment. This is why rural people are more influenced by nature than urban people. The locals see land as their true mother because they rely on her for food, clothes, and shelter.
- **Population homogeneity:** The village communities are homogeneous. The majority of their residents work in agriculture and related occupations, though they come from various castes, faiths, and classes.
- **Social stratification:** Social stratification is a traditional characteristic based on caste in rural society. The rural community is divided into various strata based on caste.

- **Social interaction:** In comparison to urban regions, the frequency of social interaction in rural areas is lower. On the other hand, the interaction level is more stable and consistent. The core groupings have close links and exchanges. The family provides for the members' necessities while also exercising control over them.

  The family is the one that introduces the members to the society's conventions, traditions, and culture. They lack individuality due to their restricted interactions, and their perspectives on the outside world are narrow, causing them to reject any violent change.

- **Social mobility:** Because all occupations are based on caste in rural areas, mobility is restricted. It is tough to change occupations because caste is determined by birth. The social position of rural people is thus determined by the caste hierarchy.

- **Social solidarity:** The degree of social solidarity is greater in villages than in urban areas. Shared experiences, purposes, customs, and traditions form the basis of unity in the villages.

- **Joint family:** Another characteristic feature of rural society is the joint family system. The family controls the behavior of the individuals. The father is the head of the family and is also responsible for maintaining discipline. He manages the affairs of the family.

A rural community is distinguished principally by a small, sparsely inhabited, relatively homogeneous population engaged principally in agriculture (although there are exceptions to this rule, especially in industrial societies). A folk society has existed in the traditional rural community. It would be a mistake to club all rural villages together because they are not the same. Certain aspects, however, have become typical in practically all rural communities.

These are:

- Agriculture was the mainstay of rural society. The land was the principal source of income. Almost everyone in rural areas worked in agriculture, either directly or indirectly. Agriculture provided a significant portion of their income. All faced the same challenges, went about their daily lives, and felt helpless in the face of natural disasters (floods, droughts, and so on) that man cannot control.

- Rural life used to differ significantly from urban life. Thrift was an honored value, and conspicuous consumption was an urban vice. His lands, herds, and crops measured a farmer's status and the inheritance he could pass on to his children.
An expected rural attitude was distrust of city people and dislike urban living. People in rural areas used to be suspicious of intelligence and book study. Their lives used to be basic, with no feeling of enjoyment or fairness in the modern sense. They used to have a strong belief in religion and their responsibilities.
- The social system in rural areas was characterized by a lack of social division and stratification. It was primarily founded on land and property rights. These relationships dictated the proportions of various socioeconomic groupings and the distribution of agricultural wealth among rural populations.
- There was a predominance of primary groups. On the one hand, these groups were important in the personality's development (socialization). They used to exercise direct control over the lives of the rural people.

Rural Health Problems in India

Health is an important factor in providing a higher quality of life. Massive numbers of Indian poor people continue to strive in vain and lose the battle for survival and health. The war begins even before birth, as the mother's malnourishment diminishes the fetus's odds of survival.

Only the toughest survive the onslaught of unsafe and unsanitary birth procedures, contaminated water, inadequate nutrition, subhuman habitats, and degraded and unsanitary settings that follow. The bleak battle continues into adulthood with little or no access to health care until tenuous survival produces a new cycle of birth and suffering.

In rural India, where 50% of families are poor, food security and illness cause great suffering. Even after 50 years of independence, infant mortality is 87 per 1,000, with most babies dying from diarrhea and other water, hygiene, and sanitation-related diseases. Over 25% of villages do not have a reliable source of drinking water for 4–5 months a year, and 75% of water sources are filthy and do not fulfill WHO standards.

Less than 10% of rural people use toilets, and their health suffers due to a lack of sanitary conditions and clean water. While the world is concerned about developing diseases such as AIDS, rural India is still plagued by tuberculosis, malaria, and diarrhea and confronts extra challenges from pollution caused by automobiles, industries, and agrochemicals. Without community health issues, advancement and sustainability are impossible in such environments.

At Uruli Kanchan, Mahatma Gandhi constructed the Nature Cure Ashram. He was worried about rural people's health issues. He expected that guaranteeing drinking-water hygiene-sanitation, sanitation, and nutrition would solve most health problems.

Ashram has worked in this area and demonstrated the therapeutic possibilities for a healthy community. However, we now know that the essential parts of community health are being neglected, and as a result, the villages continue to suffer.

Poor health saps rural residents' energy and desire to earn a living. It is difficult to begin any development initiative without primary healthcare. Despite this, health is not regarded as an intrinsic part of the development program due to the sectoral strategy.

Donors and extension workers must change their mindsets to enhance rural health. Primary healthcare should be considered a basic necessity rather than a separate development component.

Field personnel must be trained to internalize health initiatives, focusing on safe drinking water, sanitation, immunization, and nutrition. Creating a safe drinking water source was the first stage in many programs.

Rural Social Problems

Social problems prevail, such as growing rural population, housing problems, family migration to urban areas, bonded laborers, etc. Higher birth and death rates are troublesome in villages. There is insufficient health knowledge, and communicable diseases and illnesses are prevalent, infant deaths, etc. Many primary health centers (PHCs) are defunct in rural areas.

During sickness or ill health, people tend to go to places of worship or resort to witchcraft than try proper medical support. This leads to poor utilization of health care.

Social status does not change much in a rural community, and there are negligible social differences and stratifications. Also, lack of communication and efficient transport systems are other difficulties. Child marriages are still widespread in Indian villages. Lack of education and the persistence of traditions and values are the main reasons behind child marriage.

Unemployment/underemployment, untouchability, and discrimination are significant problems. Problems of sanitation, like lack of sewage disposal system and insufficient drinking water, are other problems. Casteism, group conflicts, and indebtedness are also significant problems rural peoples face.

Causes of Ill-Health in Rural Communities

The health of the individual or the group affects their work effectiveness. Good health is vital to everyday life, but it is also critical to a happier life. Illiteracy, unemployment, poverty, population growth, lack of education, etc., are some of the main reasons rural communities suffer from ill-health.

The following are some crucial factors which are mentioned here:
- **Bad habits:** Bad habits, such as drinking, smoking, using intoxicating drugs, etc., contribute to ill health in rural communities.
- **Lack of medical services:** Only a few healthcare institutions and services are located in villages because of the lack of development of healthcare facilities. This affects the treatment of the patients, which involves the health status of villagers.
- **Lack of proper housing:** In the villages, semi-built houses, temporary structures, and unhealthy residence places are commonly found. They do not have facilities, such as a toilet and/or bathroom, suitable kitchen, lighting, and ventilation—besides, many people are homeless. Hence, lack of housing or inadequate housing in village areas is a significant cause of ill health.
- **Lack of a clean or hygienic environment:** Lack of safe drinking water or even adequate water for daily needs. People in the villages are not cautious of personal hygiene or public health. There are no

waste treatment facilities and latrines. Because of these reasons, the probability of infection is higher in the village communities, and the villagers consequently face severe health problems.

- **Poor tolerance:** Imbalanced diets and lack of adequate nutrition reduce disease resistance. Less resistant people fall victim to illnesses quickly.
- **Social and cultural beliefs:** Most superstitions, rituals, and practices detrimental to health are found in the villages. Some of them are:
  - There are occupational and social constraints in the rural community. This may include having separate sources of water for different caste people. The rural community feels that sanitary work is the job of a particular caste.
  - Poor status is attributed to women.
  - Purdah system and eating from a shared plate with the bride.
  - Religious restriction on the use of contraceptives.
  - Prevalence of child marriage and prohibition of widow re-marriage.
- **Lack of health education:** Due to illiteracy or deficient education, most villagers in India are unaware of the basic facts about health. This leads to a neglect of their health and community sanitation.

Measures to Promote Health in Rural Communities

The health condition of the rural people can be improved by adopting the following measures:

- By reasonable distribution of medical care services and making health facilities accessible at the grassroots level. Equip and improve the healthcare institutions present in the villages.
- Improve the educational quality of the village communities with particular attention to girl child education. Provide facilities for informal schooling.
- Provide clean drinking water and also enough water for other daily needs.
- Improve housing facilities in villages by using local materials and technologies.
- Accept scientific methods of population control. Promote the use of contraceptives.

- Better cooperation with village panchayats or other local self-government bodies to develop the healthcare facilities in the villages.
- Effective management of PHCs, sub-centers, and community health centers (CHCs).
- Population education by effectively using communication facilities and creating health awareness among villagers.
- Better health care management and information systems should be developed for villages so that health care can be provided effectively in times of emergency (plague, cholera, natural calamities, etc.).
- Must strengthen reproductive and child health and school health services in villages.

Promotion of Health Education in Rural Areas

Health education is all about making individuals aware of the many practices that must be followed to guarantee a healthy personal and community life. Health education must raise public awareness of the community's health issues. It should also assist the community in locating resources to remedy those concerns.

Health education should emphasize the necessity of balanced diets for optimal health. Then a person may plan a balanced diet by knowing which foods contain vital nutrients. The community learns how they spread and how to prevent them. Health education makes people aware of the value of good health and that maintaining it requires collective effort. The government built up community health centers to educate rural residents **(Fig. 7.3)**.

Main Functions of Health Centers

- To educate the people about the common disease and their causes.
- To educate the people about the modes of infection of various common diseases.
- To educate the people about methods of prevention of common diseases. Some simple precautions and remedies for a few common conditions are in charts containing such information that may be displayed in the health centers.

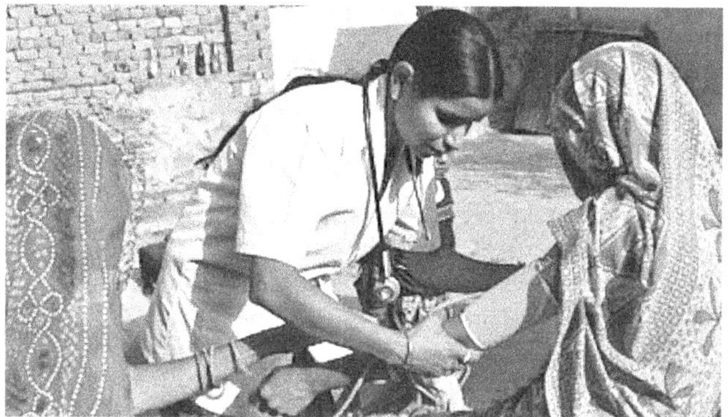

Fig. 7.3: Health education in rural areas.

- Educate people on how to solve health problems with locally available resources. People may be guided to plan a healthy diet from locally available food.
- To educate the people about various precautions to ensure that the food and water they consume are clean and wholesome.
- Community health centers educate the people about the importance of a healthy environment and how it can be maintained.
- Community health centers provide first aid and other courses for emergency handling of situations.

Given our country's large population, it's impossible to expect a doctor to visit every person and educate them on health issues. This education can only spread via the efforts of many. Men and women volunteers should be instructed on health basics. This information can be shared. Health education helps people handle personal and communal health challenges.

Industries release untreated sewage into rivers, ponds, etc. This can make drinking, swimming, and washing clothes unsafe. Polluted water causes GI and skin illnesses. If people know the dangers of contaminated water, they'll take action. Collectively, they may push the industrial unit owner to halt such actions. If people are unaware of the health risks of drinking dirty water, they may continue to do so.

7.2 URBAN COMMUNITY

LEARNING OBJECTIVES

- ☞ Describe urban growth and urbanization.
- ☞ What is urbanism?
- ☞ Describe town and city.
- ☞ What are the features of the industrial city?
- ☞ What are the features of the urban community?
- ☞ What are the problems faced by modern cities in India?
- ☞ What are the impacts of urbanization on health?
- ☞ What are the health hazards of urban people?

▨ INTRODUCTION

The city or the urban community came into being after the development of villages. There were cities in ancient times also, but most were necessary because of religion (pilgrimage), politics (capital), or trade and commerce. Thus, there were cities in ancient Egypt, Rome, Greece, India, and Mexico. However, modern cities are primarily of industrial importance, that is why; the growth of modern cities is due to industrialization.

The study of human interaction and social life in urban regions is known as urban sociology. It is a normative sociological science that investigates a city's structures, processes, changes, and concerns to provide information for planning and policy making. In other terms, urban sociology is the study of cities and their role in societal development.

If one considers the social aspect of the urban community, the city is a way of life. The word 'urbane' suggests this way of life; it indicates a fashionable living, wide acquaintance with things and people and a political manner of speech. However, is the urban way of life-limited only to the urban population? As we know, rural people also have come under the influence of urban ways of life.

▨ URBAN GROWTH AND URBANIZATION

The transfer of people from rural to urban regions, and the accompanying increase in the proportion of people who live in cities rather than rural areas, is known as urbanization. It comes from the Latin word "urbs," meaning "city" in Roman times.

Urban sociology is the sociology of people's urban living in groups and social relationships in urban social circumstances and situations. Thompson Warren has defined it as *'the movement of people from communities concerned chiefly or solely with agriculture to other communities generally larger whose activities are primarily centered in government, trade, manufacture or allied interests.'*

Because it involves transfer from village to city and shifts from agricultural occupation to commerce, trade, service, and profession, urbanization is a two-way process that involves a change in the migrant's attitudes, beliefs, values, and behavior patterns. The global urbanization trend is accelerating. People are drawn to cities for various reasons, including education, healthcare, employment opportunities, civic amenities, and social welfare.

The census of India defines some criteria for urbanization. These are:
- Population is more than 5,000
- The density is over 400 persons per square kilometer
- About 75% of the male population engages in nonagricultural occupations
- Cities are urban areas with a population of more than 1 lakh
- Metropolises are cities with a population of more than 1 million.

Urbanism

Urbanism is a lifestyle. It reflects a social organization characterized by a complex division of labor, high mobility, high levels of technology, the interdependence of its members in carrying out economic functions, and impersonality in social relations. Louis Wirth defined four aspects of urbanism:
- **Transiency:** Urban inhabitants' relations with others last only for a short time; they tend to forget their old acquaintances and develop relations with new people. Since they are not much attached to their neighbor members of the social groups, they do not mind leaving them.
- **Superficiality:** The urban person interacts with a small number of people, and their interactions with them are impersonal and formal. People interact in highly segmented roles. They are more reliant on other people to meet their basic requirements.

- **Anonymity:** Urbanites do not know each other personally. The personal mutual acquaintance between the inhabitants, which ordinarily is found in a neighborhood, is lacking.
- **Individualism:** People prioritize their own vested interests.

Town

The town is located between rural and urban areas. It is too large for everyone to know everyone else, but it is small enough for informal ties to grow. Social conduct resembles the rural pattern more than the metropolitan city pattern. Towns have a population of 5,000 or more people. There are three requirements for a site to be recognized as a town:

- The population is over 5,000
- The density is not less than $400/km^2$
- Not less than 75% of the adult male population is involved in nonagricultural activities.

City

Cities emerge when agricultural surpluses combine with improved transportation, resulting in transit bottlenecks. The metropolitan region, which includes suburbs and accounts for current population expansion, is the most significant current development in city form (**Fig. 7.4**). The city attracts inWdividuals from all around the world to its core. Rural folks facing various economic challenges are drawn to the city and migrate there.

The city offers many prospects for personal growth. It is the epicenter of a flurry of commercial, artistic, literary, political, educational, technological, and other endeavors. Cities are not just the command-and-control centers of their societies but also the incubators of innovation and change. They are sources of new product ideas, consumption pacesetters, cultural guardians, and society's order keepers. In the city cores, society's consensus and continuity are maintained. Control has become legitimized by urban culture.

Walter Christaller defined urban city location in terms of their functions as service centers. The primary idea was that each rural area had an urban center that services the surrounding country

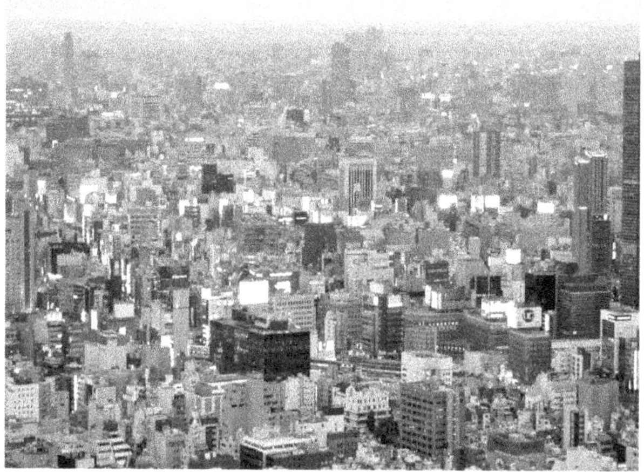

Fig. 7.4: Urban landscape of a modern city.

side. Small towns serve smaller areas, while larger cities serve larger territories.

Christaller was able to construct an interconnected system of cities based on their size thanks to this approach. Edward L Ullman expanded on these ideas, envisioning a city as a central location inside a rural area with significant changes. He concedes the scheme's susceptibility for more prominent positions. In highly industrialized locations, central place designs are often warped by industrial concentration in response to resources and transportation, which may be dismissed as a minor factor for urban location and distribution.

The concentric zone theory given by Park and Burgess suggested that modern cities consisted of a series of concentric zones. There are five such zones:

1. Central business district.
2. Zone in transition.
3. Zone of the working population.
4. Residential zone.
5. Commuters zone.

Gans and Lewis, through compositional theory, hold that the composition of a city's population differs from that of a small town in terms of factors such as class, education, ethnicity, and marital status.

Multiple nuclei theory given by Harris and Ullman discusses that there is not one center but several centers for the city. Each of the centers specializes in a particular kind of activity-retailing, wholesaling, finance, recreation, education, and government. Several centers may have existed from the city's beginning, or many have developed later in a division from one center.

According to Castells, to understand cities and urbanism, one must understand how spatial forms are created and transformed. The architecture of cities expresses the struggles and conflicts between different groups in society. The city is not only a distinct location but also an integral part of the processes of collective consumption.

Features of Industrial City

- A large sprawling open city housing a large percent of the population of the society; relatively low segregation, few outward symbols, segregation based on race, good transportation and communication
- A manufacturing, finance, and coordinating center of an industrial society
- A fluid class structure with an elite of business people, professionals, and scientists
- A sizeable middle class with technologically related jobs
- Wealth by salaries, fees, and investment; high status of business activity; unionization at a national level; specialization of production and marketing; large service sector, fixed price
- Time essential and regular work schedule
- Standardization of process and quality
- Formal public opinion with a bureaucracy based on technical criteria
- A weak religious institution separate from other institutions dominated by the middle class; standardization of religious-experience marked by the disappearance of magic
- Technical and secular education for the masses.

Features of Urban Community

The following are the crucial characteristics of the urban community:
- **Nonagricultural occupations:** The urban man is engaged in many diverse occupations such as industry, trade, commerce,

transportation and communication, education, government, and recreation. There are hundreds and thousands of occupations for the city dwellers.

- **Artificial environment:** The city and its environment are made by man, so it is pretty artificial. The factories, shops, modern roads, railways, buildings, and many other things are created by men **(Fig. 7.5)**.
- **Large community:** Cities are huge communities with populations in the millions or billions. A large number of individuals live in a tiny area. In general, the size of an urban community is substantially larger than that of a rural community in the same country and time period. In other words, urbanity and community size are positively associated.
- **The high density of population:** The population density is very high. There are much overcrowding and congestion. Therefore, slums are also created. Due to such a situation, the health of urbanites is also not satisfactory. The population density in urban areas is more significant than in rural communities. Urbanity and density are positively correlated.
- **Mobility:** An essential feature of the urban community is its social mobility. In urban areas, an individual's social status is determined not by heredity or birth but by merit, intelligence, and perseverance. Urbanity and mobility are positively correlated.

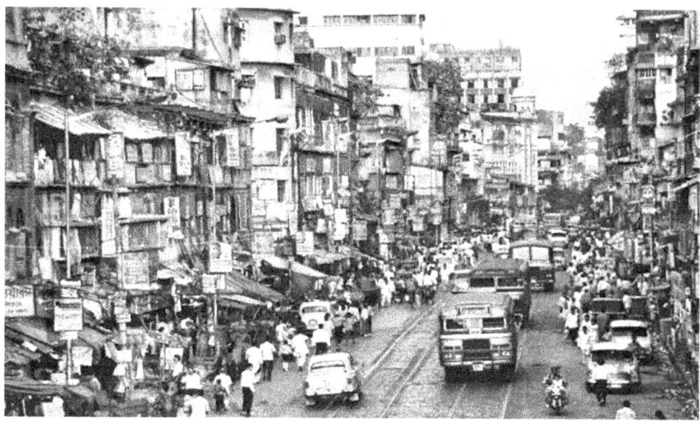

Fig. 7.5: Urban landscape of Kolkata.

- **Heterogeneity of population:** There is no similarity in the life of urban people. There is diversity in occupation, language, religion, and the total culture.
- **High social differences and stratification:** The diversity in various aspects of life and variation in the status of individuals and groups in the city community are striking. For example, while most people in an Indian metropolis may be poor, there are many middle class and a few upper class—similarly, illiterates, semi-educated, and highly educated people in an Indian city. The lifestyle of the people also varies according to religion, occupation, and other socioeconomic status.
- **Occupation:** In the urban areas, the significant occupations are industrial, administrative, and professional. Divisions of labor and occupational specialization are prevalent in towns/cities/metropolises.
- **System of interaction:** According to Georg Simmel, the social structure of urban areas is founded on interest groups. The city's social circles are more extensive than those in the country. Per man and aggregate, there is a larger region of interaction system. This complicates and diversifies metropolitan life. The predominance of secondary interactions and impersonal, casual, and short-lived relationships characterizes city life. In either case, the man on the street effectively loses his identity, being treated as if he were a "number" with a specific "address."
- **Social heterogeneity:** If villages symbolize cultural homogeneity, the cities symbolize cultural heterogeneity. The cities are characterized by diverse peoples, races, and cultures. There is a great variety regarding the food habits, dress habits, living conditions, religious beliefs, cultural outlook, customs, and traditions of the urbanites.
- **Social distance:** Anonymity and heterogeneity cause social distance. In a town or metropolis, the majority of one's everyday social connections are impersonal and segmentary. Social responses in the urban community are insufficient and half-hearted. There is a complete lack of personal involvement in other people's affairs.
- **Class extremes:** According to Bogardus, "class extremes characterize the city." Both a town and a city house both the

wealthy and the indigent. Dirty slums coexist with magnificent bungalows for the wealthy and apartments for middle-class residents in a city. Cities house both the most civilized and the most vicious racketeers.

- **Easy and rapid social mobility:** A city is a location where social mobility is simple and quick. People earn their status; it is not bestowed upon them. The urban man can significantly enhance or lose his status during his lifetime, and the fight for status becomes a constant worry. Social climbing is more widespread in cities than in villages. The development of talent, the attainment of education, and the amassing and display of riches are all paths to a high status in all aspects of urban life. The flexibility and availability of chances in the city enable social mobility, particularly for persons from lower socioeconomic strata.
- **Materialism:** Man's social existence in the urban community depends on riches and material possessions. Today, the value of an urbanite is determined not by who he is but by what he owns. Status symbols such as financial assets, salary, and expensive household goods are significant for urbanites.
- **Individualism:** Urbanites highly value their well-being and happiness. They are hesitant to think or act for the benefit of others.
- **Impersonal human relationships:** Large urban environments hinder all community members from making intimate face-to-face contact. People engage in metropolitan communities for specific and limited purposes, such as buyers and sellers in a store, teachers and students in a classroom, and doctors and patients in clinics. Urbanites rarely get to know each other as a "complete person," that is, they are not interested in all areas of a person's life. Apart from family and friends, they rarely engage with others unless for limited or specialized objectives.

This characteristic is found among city dwellers due to casual, impersonal, shallow, temporary, segmental, and secondary connections. In contrast, people in villages have personal, face-to-face intimacy and long-standing ties with their major contacts. As a result, the city is a secondary location for relationships. Because of its size, the city cannot be considered a leading group. It must instead be a secondary group; people must continuously associate with and be close to strangers. Even friends and acquaintances are likely to be known exclusively in a specific context or sector of life.

- **Rationality:** Because metropolitan interactions are impersonal, urban orientations tend to be utilitarian, i.e., people join into relationships after calculating prospective rewards from these links rather than for the subjective satisfaction of association. Contractual relationships are used here, and profit and loss are meticulously calculated. When the contract expires, the people's partnership ceases. For example, hiring a professional nurse to care for a sick individual, partnering with an advertising agency to promote your goods, etc. This is not to say that all relationships between people in cities are purely utilitarian. Individual connections always have an extensive range of variation. We have highlighted the general nature of urban interactions here. Rationality is valued in the urban community. People are prone to reasoning and arguing. The consideration of benefit or loss mostly governs their interactions with others. A contractual relationship exists. When the contract expires, the human relationship is automatically terminated.

- **Secularism:** The diversity of racial, socioeconomic, and cultural variables in urban living exposes people to a wide range of lifestyles and values. When people become accustomed to seeing others in different ways from their own, they become more accepting of diversity. This accepting and rational worldview leads to secular life orientations. Even if assessing terms like rationalism and secularism is challenging, it is argued that secular, rather than religious, ideas are typically associated with metropolitan social structure. However, this attribute is not always present because communal riots are more common in Indian cities than rural areas. However, secular values are linked to metropolitan settings in a relative sense.

  Ritual and kinship duties are diluted in cities. Economic rationality triumphs over caste and group issues. As a result, the outlook becomes more secular.

- **Anonymity:** "Urban groups have a reputation for namelessness," according to Bogardus. The urban community cannot be called a primary group due to its size and population. Nobody knows anyone here, and no one is interested in anyone. The city dwellers do not care about their neighbors and are uninterested in their pleasures and sufferings.

- **Norm and social role conflict:** Norm and social role conflict define the urban community. Population size, density, heterogeneity, excessive vocational specialization, and the class structure typical of metropolitan areas all contribute to this state of affairs. Individuals or organizations frequently pursue disparate goals in the absence of stable and established societal standards. This greatly leads to social disorder.
- **Rapid social and cultural change:** Urban life is characterized by rapid social and cultural change. The significance of traditional or religious components has been pushed to the margins. The advantages of city life have influenced changes in customs, philosophies, and behavioral tendencies.
- **Voluntary associations:** The urban society is defined by people's impersonal, mechanical, and formal social relationships. Naturally, they have a great need to form meaningful social interactions to satisfy their need for emotional warmth and security. Associations, clubs, societies, and other secondary organizations are formed.
- **Formal social control:** Social control is primarily formal in the metropolitan community. Police, jails, law courts, and other such institutions govern people's behavior.
- **Marriage:** Love and inter-caste marriages predominate in the urban environment. The number of divorces is likewise increasing. Sons and daughters have a lot of freedom in selecting life partners.
- **The loss in family functions:** In the urban social environment, many of the educational, recreational, and other tasks performed within a rural joint family context are taken over by other institutions such as schools, clubs, and other voluntary groups. There is a clear distinction between home and workplace in urban society, which is not necessarily present in rural society. Similarly, metropolitan people's identities are not psychologically connected to their familial roles. Furthermore, frequent communication amongst kin is generally difficult, but not impossible, due to higher geographical mobility in these households. This is not to say that families are not important in urban settings.

In the urban community, the individual is regarded as more important than the family. Nuclear families are frequent among city dwellers.

Problems Faced by Modern Cities in India

The development of urbanization and the rapid population growth places a considerable strain on the surrounding ecosystem. According to one estimate, A million cities require 6,25,000 tons of water each day, 2,000 tons of food grains, and 9,500 tons of fuel. Similarly, it produces over 500,000 tons of dirty water, 2,000 tons of solid trash, and 950 tons of air pollutants every day, providing substantial challenges to municipal authorities. As a result, a city has a double impact on its surroundings.

Thus, uncontrolled, unplanned urbanization may make the city life deplorable and cause severe damage to the surrounding area's physical, social, and economic environment. Urban problems may, therefore, be grouped into two broad categories:

1. Internal problems which affect the city area and its inhabitants.
2. External issues that affect the area and the people who live on its outskirts and in the uplands. Some internal issues include a lack of space and residential housing, transportation bottlenecks, scarcity of pure drinking water, pollution, city trash, sewage disposal, energy and field supply, law and order maintenance, and criminal control.

Problem of Space

Cities are continually in need of more and more space to expand. This space demand is supplied by colonizing the outskirts or rural areas. However, this expansion is occasionally hampered due to physical and other limits. Such issues are caused by Mumbai's island nature and saltwater lakes on the eastern outskirts of Kolkata. Furthermore, city dwellers live closer to their workplaces or commercial premises, particularly in urban areas where internal transportation is expensive and inefficient.

City planners developed a lot of different sectors for industrial, residential, and commercial requirements, which soon became overcrowded and congested. This leads to an enormous increase in land values and rents, making poor people's lives painful. Many people who cannot pay high rent are thus forced to live in slums and squatter settlements, which is a great slur on modern civic society.

Residential Problem

Rising urban populations, especially in emerging countries, are causing a housing shortage. One estimate says Indian cities lack 1.7 million homes per year. This has caused house rent to skyrocket, and many families spend 30–50% of their monthly salary on housing. Low-income people are compelled to live in slums or on sidewalks and roads. In places like Mumbai, Kolkata, Delhi, etc., slum and pavement inhabitants are rising rapidly.

Problem of Transport

Transport bottlenecks and traffic congestion are major problems in Indian cities. Amongst all cities in the country, Delhi is better placed regarding road transport. Here, the average road density is 1,284 km/100 km^2 of area (Chandigarh 1,260 km, Ahmedabad 680 km, and Mumbai 380 km). Most city roads carry higher traffic than their actual capacity. Here, main roads carry 6,000 passenger car units (PCU) per hour, which increased to 12,000 PCU during peak hours.

The International Trade Organization (ITO), built-in 1964–1965, was designed to handle 40,000–50,000 PCU. Capital transit will collapse if vehicle numbers continue to rise without road upgrades. Traffic congestion is increasing in various areas of the old city. Road accident deaths are soaring.

Kolkata's ancient neighborhoods and Howrah Bridge remain congested despite the metro rail and Vivekananda Setu (bridge). Due to congestion, Gandhi Marg and Relief Marg in Ahmedabad have 5 km/h speed limits.

Water Supply Problem

Without water, man cannot live. Water sources are always considered while locating settlements. Modern towns demand a large water supply for home and industrial use. Kolkata residents drink 272 L per day, Mumbai residents 190 L, and Delhi residents 90 L.

Aluminum, cotton textile, rayon, woolen textile, and steel each require 170 m^3 water per ton. Hydel plants need 10,080 m^3/h to generate 3 million kW.

Central Public Health and Environmental Engineering Organization (CPHEEO) has fixed up 125–200 L of water per head per day for cities with over 50,000; 100–125 L for the population between 10,000 and 50,000; and 70–100 L for the population below 10,000.

The Zakaria group recommends 204 L per head per day for cities between 500,000 and 2 million and 272 L for populations over 2 million. This water is utilized for drinking, cooking, bathing, cleaning, and gardening. This shows the dire water situation in four major Indian cities. Despite attempts, the disparity grows.

According to a study, only Nagpur, Pune, Patna, Varanasi, Visakhapatnam, and Ahmedabad can cover their complete population with Delhi municipal water. Mumbai, Kolkata, Delhi, and Chennai have a 10% disparity. Small towns are terrible.

The city is using external water sources to meet demand. Water express trains help Chennai meet demand. Hyderabad gets its water from Nagarjuna Sagar (137 miles) and Bengaluru from the Kaveri (100 km). Delhi also uses water from the Haryana canal. The plan will serve Tehri, Renuka, and Kishau barrages. Transporting water from far away is expensive, time-consuming, and risky, especially in emergencies and insurgencies.

Problem of Urban Pollution

India's cities, industries, and cars are booming. Urban air quality has plummeted. Growing consumerism, luxury lifestyles, and urban environmental ignorance exacerbate the problem. Pollution from air, water, noise, and solid waste harms urban residents' health. Rapid vehicle growth in India causes urban air pollution.

Vehicles pollute entire cities, while industry is localized. Many cities' air is polluted and toxic, according to studies. Air pollution is a problem in cities. Delhi, Kolkata, and Chennai are among the 41 most polluted megacities (SPM).

Mumbai ranks 18th, Delhi 27th, and Kolkata 37th for SO_2 levels. Vehicles cause 52% of Mumbai's pollution. Industries emit 48% of SO_2 and power plants 33%. Fumes from garbage dumps are also a concern in big cities.

Transport causes 60% of Delhi's air pollution. Over 11 lakh registered vehicles produce 250 tons of CO, 400 tons of hydrocarbon, 6 tons of SO_2, and a lot of SPM per day. According to a 1981 report by the National Environmental Engineering Research Institute, Kolkata releases 1,305 tons of pollutants daily. Industrial establishments contribute 600 tons, transportation 360 tons, thermal power plants 195 tons, and kitchens 150 tons.

Mixing sewage with drinking water causes urban water contamination. Most Indian towns allow sewage and wastewater to run into drinking water sources. Slum dwellers without latrines use open spaces. Toxic septic tanks harm urban groundwater. During rains, periphery farmers' pesticides enter the river. Industrial waste pollutes the river.

Noise Pollution

Noise pollution causes discomfort and restlessness from unwanted noise. India's urbanization and industry cause noise pollution. Most of India's cities endure pollution due to a surge in cars, factories, mills, loudspeakers, and crowded markets.Most of India's big cities have noise pollution above 70 dB, including Chennai (89 dB), Delhi (89 dB), Kolkata (87 dB), Mumbai (85 dB), Kochi (80 dB), Madurai (75 dB), Kanpur (75 dB), and Thiruvananthapuram (70 dB). Most of these cities lack adequate noise pollution rules or the will to enforce them.

Deafening sounds of loudspeakers on temples, mosques, gurdwaras, housetops, electric and telephone poles during festivals and rituals, mobile loudspeakers during electioneering, car horns near hospitals, educational institutions, and residential areas are widespread in most Indian towns.

During festivals like Holi, Dussehra, Diwali, Ganesh Chaturthi, Rath Yatra, Id, etc., noise level sometimes becomes intolerable, which causes irreparable damage to the ears and irritation, tension, nervousness, and mental disorder.

Solid Wastes

Solid wastes include worthless household materials. Rusted pins, shattered glass, plastic cans, polythene bags, tins, old newspapers, etc. Refuse garbage, solid debris, etc. Solid wastes are alarming in Indian cities due to population growth, urban youth's attraction to a use-and-throw culture, and urbanites' lack of awareness.

45 Indian cities with over 3 million people generate 50,000 tons of trash per day. Mumbai's 16,000 municipal workers and 270 trucks collect 4,400 tons of rubbish per day. Deonar, Malad, and Bhanwari Mohan Creek are dumping sites.

The Kolkata metropolitan area creates 4,000 tons of solid garbage everyday, but only 70% is disposed of Delhi's trash is disposed of in Jaitpur, Ghazipur, Mandi, and Bhatti.

Kanpur and Lucknow produce 1,000 and 900 tons of waste every day, one-third is uncollected. The previous paragraph describes solid waste contamination. Most cities do not use the scientific garbage disposal. They lack solid waste disposal/treatment plants, or theirs are idle due to exorbitant costs or municipal neglect. Delhi's compost plant also failed.

Hospital trash, including various infectious/communicable diseases, are the most neglected. These are improperly dumped along roadsides, endangering human health and sanitation.

Urban Crime Problem

Increasing urban crime disrupts city peace. Material culture, materialism, greed, competition, lavishness, socioeconomic gaps, unemployment, and loneliness cause this threat. Not only the destitute, deprived, and slum dwellers are prone to such crimes, but also many adolescents from respectable families who want to gain wealth and prosperity quickly or who are discouraged by unemployment and broken homes.

When politicians, bureaucrats, and urban society's elite shield criminals, the problem worsens. Using money and strength, some criminals have gained political positions.

Dutt and Venugopal (1983) analyzed India's urban layout. Rape, murder, kidnapping, robbery, etc., are more prevalent in the north and central Uttar Pradesh. It has two main areas: Moradabad, Bareilly, and Shahjahanpur in Uttar Pradesh and Raipur in Chhattisgarh; and Gaya, Munger, Darbhanga and Ranchi in Bihar and Jharkhand. Theft, cheating, and trust crimes are concentrated in the north-central region.

Dehradun, Meerut, Aligarh, Mathura, Lucknow, Kanpur, Allahabad, and Bareilly in Uttarakhand and Uttar Pradesh; Muzaffarpur, Munger in Bihar. A secondary area connects Amravati to Greater Mumbai via Pune, Maharashtra. Kolar, Karnataka, and Guwahati, Assam, are crucial economic crime hubs.

Crimes are highly connected, and 'crime breeds crime' is true. Poverty-related crimes are frequent and concentrated in Bihar's

Patna, Darbhanga, Gaya, and Munger. This may be due to poverty and caste and class-based riots.

Environmental Pollution and Health Hazards

It is a modern-day contradiction that all development is accompanied by environmental degradation. Man has disobeyed nature's law in his pursuit of money and luxury, disrupting various natural cycles and resulting in environmental damage and health hazards. In short, there is an urgent need to raise public awareness of environmental conservation.

Environmental pollution and health risks have existed since the dawn of human civilization. Previously, pollutants such as gases, smoke, and home wastes gave way to a wide range of industrial waste, ranging from poisonous gases and heavy metallic oxides to various produced chemicals.

Pollution of the Environment

The phrases 'environmental pollution' and 'pollution' are interchangeable. The Dictionary of Biology defines environment as "the entire spectrum of external conditions under which an organism lives, including physical, chemical, and biological elements such as temperature, light, and food and water availability." Pollution, which means to make or make unclean, is an undesired change in the physical, chemical, and biological qualities of land, air, or water that harms human life or valuable species.

Classification of Environmental Pollution

Life requires air, water, and land. Population growth, industrialization, and urbanization have contaminated utilities with dangerous compounds, posing health risks. These 'pollutants' are man-made. Pollutants are degradable or non-degradable. Domestic garbage and sewage are degradable. Inorganic materials, metallic oxides, plastic, radioactive elements, etc., disintegrate slowly or not at all by natural or biological processes.

Pollution includes air, water, land, radiation, and noise. These pose health risks. WHO defines air pollution as hazardous elements in the air. Air, unlike a pond or lake, cannot be contained. This spreads contaminants over large areas, sometimes even across continents, as in the USSR, Chernobyl accident.

Air Pollution

The industrial pollutants emitted into the air through the chimneys of industrial units and powerhouses are the origins of air pollution, including sulfur dioxide, carbon dioxide, carbon monoxide, hydrogen sulfide, chlorine, nitrous oxide, and arsenic. Zone, ash, and an infinite amount of metal particles and gases; residential pollution from human-burned fossil fuels; automotive exhausts and radiation. The following health risks are caused by air pollution:

- Many gases, such as chlorine, sulfuric dioxide, and hydrogen sulfide, have a strong odor and can cause eye irritation, lung congestion, bronchial issues, and other disorders. The chlorine gas that escaped from Shriram Fertilizers in Delhi had the same effect.
- The methyl isocyanate leaked from the in famous Union Carbide plant in Bhopal caused cyanide poisoning in many people and irreversible vision loss, muscular degeneration, lung infection, stillbirths, miscarriages, and newborns with genetic problems.
- Ozone is carcinogenic to the skin and hazardous to the eyes. Carbon monoxide, odorless gas with an affinity for hemoglobin, enters the bloodstream, substitutes oxygen from oxyhemoglobin, and mixes with it, causing headaches, eye irritation, nausea, respiratory difficulty, unconsciousness, and death.
- Fine dust particles generated by industrial units also damage the air. It causes asthma, coughing, and other symptoms. Asbestos, for example, causes lung disease; lead causes mental issues and brain damage.
- Air also includes spores or particles of dangerous weeds, grass, and other plants, such as parthenium. The congress grass, among other things, causes skin irritation and coughing. The list is lengthy, and the consequences are severe.

Water Pollution

Water, another basic necessity, is heavily polluted and poses numerous health risks. Domestic sewage, industrial waste such as caustic soda, miraculous oxide, lignite, sulphuric acid, cyanides, ammonia, and so on, and chemical inputs such as fertilizers and pesticides insects are all examples of water pollutants.

Water pollution causes the following health hazards:

- The health hazards caused by water pollution are the leading cause of the spread of the epidemic diseases such as cholera, jaundice, dysentery, typhoid, gastroenteritis, etc. in the urban areas, the slums are on the rise, and they do not have a safe and separate drinking water sources.
- Human beings and domestic animals inhabit the place and use the same source for all their needs, i.e., drinking, bathing, and washing.
- During the rainy season, water logs in these colonies, and bacteria, viruses, and other parasites breed in that water, as evidenced by the huge number of deaths caused by these epidemic diseases like gastroenteritis in Delhi.
- Mercury, lead, copper, zinc, and other metals and oxides thrown into water sources by industrial units induce nerve problems and even brain damage. When these contaminants are ingested by aquatic species (fish, for example), they pose several health risks to humans.
- The introduction of dyes into water sources by industrial dyeing units results in their use by humans and domestic animals. It disrupts their biological systems.

Land Pollution

Due to industrialization and urbanization, wastes are dumped on vast land areas. Waste from paper mills, oil refineries, power plants, etc., pollutes the land. Fertilizers, pesticides, herbicides, and insecticides boost agricultural output and pollute land and water. Lack of civic sensibility and administrative inspections cause inland contamination. Land contamination causes:

- Agricultural inputs permeate into groundwater. Some gases leak from wells and other water sources and cause dizziness, discomfort, and death. Carbon monoxide has caused deaths in Punjab and other northern regions.
- Insecticides and pesticides applied to crops enter the human system and disrupt its function.
- Industrial units throw ash on land, making it unusable for farming, causing cough, asthma, etc.

Radiation Pollution and Noise Pollution

Nuclear power plants and other nuclear sites emit or leak radiation into the environment.Radiation causes diseases such as skin cancer and leukemia. It also causes mutations, which alter the genetic order and lead to disease. Another important environmental threat is noise pollution. The constant noise produced by industrial equipment and automobiles in cities and towns sickens people physically and mentally.

Noise can permanently harm the eardrum if continuous and of high intensity. It causes weariness, headaches, tension, and nausea.

■ IMPACT OF URBANIZATION ON HEALTH

Nearly 50% of the world population today lives only in an urban area, and by 2050, around 70% of the population will be in towns and cities. Today's world has been rapidly urbanized with many changes in daily living standards, modern lifestyles, and social behaviors.

Health problems are more evident in the urban areas due to polluted water supply to cities; land pollution due to improper sewage disposal; increased violence; the prevalence of noncommunicable diseases, for example, cardiovascular illness, cancer, diabetes, chronic respiratory diseases, and constipation; unhealthy diet; no physical activity due to a sedentary lifestyle; and more prevalence of epidemiological diseases. Urban life has become harmful to humans nowadays due to the availability of unhealthy food; increased pressure of mass marketing directly affects people's health in urban areas.

Even the World Health Organization had chosen the theme of Urbanization and Health for World Health Day on 7th April 2010 to identify the severe effects of urbanization to improve the health quality of every individual. Through this theme, the main goal was to seek worldwide attention and help governments improve urban health. WHO report regarding urban health problems mentions the following:

- More than 50–60% (half) of the world's population resides in cities.
- By the year 2030, it is estimated that 5 out of every ten people will be living in cities, increasing to 7 out of every ten people by 2050. This increase is due to rapid urbanization, where people migrate from villages to cities to earn their livelihood.

- From 1995 till 2005, there was an increase in the urban population of an average of 1.2 million people per week, 1,65,000 people every day.
- Worldwide census reports that one in every three urban dwellers reside in slums amounting to 1 billion people.
- Global statistics report depicts that road accident injury is the ninth leading cause of death. Pedestrians, cyclists, and two-wheeler riders are the most affected by road accidents.
- About 1.2 million people are affected by respiratory tract diseases and die every year due to urban air pollution caused by motor vehicles, industries, electricity generation, etc.
- Tuberculosis is the topmost prevalent communicable disease in urban areas. WHO Report says that the death rate due to tuberculosis is four times the national average. About 83% of people are affected by tuberculosis infection.

Health Hazards of Urbanites

Environmental pollution and health threats are linked; administration and residents must take action. To reduce water and land pollution, we need more river cleaning efforts like the Ganga Action Plan. Industrial units on these rivers should operate only with individual or organized scientific protections and discharge only treated water, which is not the case in most cases.

Residential sewage and animal feces should be used in biogas facilities. Safe cooking fuel and crop manure will reduce health risks. Asthma, eye irritation, and lung infections can be avoided. Fossil fuel combustion is the main source of pollution outside of industrial units, so solar power should be used extensively. Next-generation education is another priority. "Gurukuls" surrounded by nature encouraged students to care for it.

Such courses should be developed to bring the younger generation closer to nature rather than dense literature. Aside from that, illiterate people who cannot attend school or college need awareness. Administrative and volunteer groups can show films and clips about pollution's health risks.

Electronic media is important in this way. Such programs should be in regional and local languages, not jargon. Industrial units should be located in greenbelts and not densely populated areas. Chimneys should be taller, but remember that whatever goes up must come down as particles or acid rain. Smoke must be treated before being released into the upper atmosphere to maintain equilibrium. We are approaching the greenhouse effect. Rapid urbanization has expanded slums. If we cannot stop the growth of slums, we can at least improve their health.

More laws are being drafted, but their proper execution is more important for achieving the desired results. Competent law enforcement requires proper management and resident involvement. Local committees or bodies composed of industrial units, administration, pressure groups, citizens, and other fields should monitor law and pollution control plans. Such bodies need authority. Residents and the administration must work together to control environmental degradation.

Water, the environment, violence and injury, noncommunicable diseases (cardiovascular diseases, malignancies, diabetes, and chronic respiratory diseases), bad diets and inactivity, dangerous alcohol use, and disease outbreaks are major urban health concerns. City living's mass marketing, unhealthy food options, automation, and transportation all impact lifestyle, which impacts health.

The following are some health hazards of urbanites:
- Congested living and unhygienic housing.
- Industrial, transport, and environmental pollution.
- Slums surrounded by dirt, filth, and poor sanitation.
- The high cost of medical facilities.
- Alcoholism, prostitution, drug addiction, etc.
- Stress-related mental problems such as depression, anxiety, neurosis, etc.
- Lack of physical activities and constipation, and obesity usually develop.
- Loneliness for aged people because other family members are working or studying and hence older people become more prone to sickness.

8

Culture and Health

LEARNING OBJECTIVES

☞ Define culture and describe the characteristics of the culture.
☞ Describe seven functions of culture.
☞ Describe the cultural meaning of sickness.
☞ What are the influences of culture on health and illness?

▧ INTRODUCTION

Culture is a fundamental concept in sociology. Culture has a distinct connotation in sociology. Anthropologists believe that the intended behavior is known as Culture. Culture is the behavior that has been passed down to us. A culture is defined by its style of living, talking, eating, dressing, singing, and dancing.

The term culture refers to something beautiful, sophisticated, or appealing. In sociology, the term Culture refers to acquired behavior shared and transmitted among members of society. A culture is a shared system of taught behavior among group members. Simply put, Culture is that element of the human environment that men have formed while living together. Culture is the knowledge, language, values, customs, and material artifacts passed down from generation to generation in a human group or society.

▧ DEFINITIONS OF CULTURE

Sociologists and anthropologists have defined Culture in a variety of ways.

Following are the important definitions of Culture:
- "Culture is that complex whole, which includes knowledge, belief, art, morals, law, customs and any other capabilities and habits acquired by man as a member of society."   —*Taylor EB*
- "Culture is any socially inherited element of the life of man, material and spiritual."   —*Edward Sapir*

- "Culture the handwork of man and conventional understanding manifest in art and artifact, which persisting through which he achieves his ends."   —*Malinowski*
- "Culture is an organized body of conventional understanding manifest in art and artifact, which persisting through, characterizes a human group."   —*Redfield*
- "Culture is the expression of our nature in our modes of living and our thinking, intercourses in our literature, religion, recreation, and enjoyment.   —*MacIver*
- "Culture is all the ways of doing and thinking of a group."   —*Bogardus ES*

Ogburn classifies cultural items into two categories:

a. Material aspects of Culture, such as tools, equipment, arms, etc.

b. Nonmaterial aspects include values, beliefs, customs, norms, law, etc.

Material culture refers to the physical objects ('artifacts') that civilization makes and reflects cultural knowledge, skills, interests, and preoccupations. Nonmaterial Culture is the information and beliefs that shape people's conduct. In our Culture, for example, religious ideas (such as Christianity, Islam, or Buddhism) and/or scientific beliefs—your view of human evolution, for example, has most likely been impacted by Darwin's theories (1859).

While this difference is vital, it is not absolute because physical artifacts (such as mobile phones) have cultural meanings for those who create and use them. A house, for example, is more than just a place to live (although that is its primary or intended purpose). Houses have cultural significance for people who possess them and those who do not. For example, the style of the home someone owns reveals something about them, and this exemplifies a vital concept about the symbolic character of both societies and the artifacts they make. Nothing inherent in the term "house" defines its meaning as distinct from its purpose (or function). It can indicate different things to different people and groups within a society and other things to distinct civilizations.

◼ CHARACTERISTICS

To grasp the concept of Culture, we must first understand its main qualities. Culture has many attributes. The following are the Culture's primary characteristics.

Culture is Learnt

Culture is not inherited biologically but learned socially by man. It is not an inherited trait. Culture is sometimes called acquired habits of conduct because there is no cultural instinct. Some behavior, such as closing one's eyelids while sleeping, the eye blinking reflex, etc., is entirely physiological; Culture includes shaking hands, saying 'namaskar' or gratitude, grooming, and clothing. Wearing clothes, combing hair, wearing jewelry, cooking food, drinking from a glass, eating from a plate or leaf, reading a newspaper, driving a car, performing a role in a drama, singing, worshipping, and so on are all examples of culturally taught behavior.

Cultural is Social

Culture does not exist in isolation; neither is it a unique phenomenon. It is a product of society. It originates and develops through social interaction. The members of society share it. Culture cannot be acquired without interaction with other people. Only among men does a man become a man. Culture helps man develop human qualities in a human environment. Deprivation is nothing but the deprivation of human qualities.

Culture is Shared

In the sociological sense, Culture is something shared. It is not something that a single person can have. For example, people in a community or society share conventions, traditions, beliefs, ideas, values, morality, and so on. Many individuals share the inventions of Aryabhata or Albert Einstein, Charaka or Charles Darwin, Dandi or Dante, the literary works of Kalidas or Keats, the philosophical writings of Confucius or Lao Tse, Shankaracharya or Swami Vivekananda, the creative work of Ravi Varma or Raphael, etc. Culture is something more than one individual uses, adopts, believes, practices, or possesses. Its survival is dependent on group life (Robert Bierstedt).

Culture is Transmissive

Culture can be passed down from one generation to the next. Parents instill cultural features in their children, their children in their offspring, and so on. Language, not genes, is used to convey

Culture. Culture's principal vehicle is language. Language, in its various forms, such as reading, writing, and speaking, allows the current generation to comprehend the accomplishments of previous generations. Language, on the other hand, is a component of Culture. Once a language is learned, it opens up a world of possibilities for the individual. Culture can be transmitted through intuition as much as engagement.

Culture is Continuous and Cumulative

Culture exists as an ongoing process. Its historical expansion tends to become cumulative. Culture is evolving, including past and present achievements and plans for future human achievements. Culture can thus be viewed as a stream that flows through the centuries from one generation to the next. As a result, some sociologists, such as Litton, refer to Culture as man's social heritage. It is not easy to picture what society would be like without this accumulation of Culture and how people would live without it.

Culture is Consistent and Interconnected

Culture has shown a tendency to be constant in its evolution. Different aspects of Culture are interconnected at the same time. For example, a society's value system is inextricably linked to its other characteristics, such as morality, religion, traditions, customs, beliefs, and so on.

Culture is Dynamic and Adaptive

Culture, while relatively stable, is not entirely stagnant. It is changing slowly but steadily. Culture contains the seeds of change and growth. When we compare today's Indian Culture to that of the Vedic period, we see impressive growth. As a result, Culture is dynamic. Culture reacts to the physical world's changing conditions. It's adaptable. It also intervenes in the natural environment to help a man adjust. Just like our house protects us from the elements, our Culture protects us from natural hazards and aids in our survival. Very few of us would be able to survive in the absence of Culture.

Culture is Gratifying

Culture provides excellent chances and specifies methods for satisfying our needs and ambitions. These requirements can be biological or social. Our basic requirements for food, shelter, and clothes are addressed in culturally acceptable ways, as are our cravings for status, notoriety, fame, and money. Culture determines and guides man's various actions. Culture is described as the mechanism through which humans satisfy their desires.

Culture Varies from Society to Society

Every society has its own Culture. It varies according to society. Every society's Culture is distinct from the next. Cultures are not all the same. Customs, traditions, morality, concepts, values, ideologies, ceremonial beliefs, philosophies, institutions, and other cultural elements are not universal.

Eating, speaking, greeting, dressing, entertaining, living, and varied substantially between sects—culture shifts from time to time. No civilization is ever steady or unchanging. If Manu (the first man, according to Hinduism) returned to view Indian society today, he would be astounded by the profound changes that have occurred in our Culture.

Culture is Super Organic and Ideational

Culture is sometimes referred to be hyper organic. Herbert Spencer defined hyperorganic as neither organic nor inorganic but rather something in between. The word suggests the social significance of physical goals and physiological actions. Physiological and physical factors may have little bearing on social meaning. A national flag, for example, is more than just a piece of colored cloth. A nation is represented by its flag. Priests and inmates, academicians and profanity, athletes, engineers and physicians, farmers and soldiers are not simply biological beings. They are viewed differently in their society. Culture is the only way to understand their social standing and role.

■ SIX FUNCTIONS OF CULTURE

Communication

Culture provides the context for developing human communication systems such as language, both verbal and non-verbal (e.g., gestures).

Perception

According to Matsumoto (2007), culture "gives meaning to social situations, establishing social roles and normative behaviors." It impacts how we perceive and comprehend the social and natural worlds. According to Offe (2001), western cultures generally believe that "the future" is not predetermined, whereas "certain African societies" are defined by "the notion of a predetermined future not controllable by individuals."

Identity

Culture influences how people see themselves and others (gender, age, and ethnicity). Durkheim, for example, suggested that societies have a functional requirement to develop two things:

1. **Social solidarity:** The conviction that we are part of a more extensive network of people who share particular values, identities, and obligations to one another. However, for such feelings of solidarity to arise, civilizations must construct social integrating systems.
2. **Social integration:** Individual and cultural purpose and coherence require a commitment to others (such as family and friends). Collective rites (such as royal weddings and burials) and collective identifications, in general, serve as integrating mechanisms. Schools, for example, may aim to integrate pupils through uniforms and competitive sports against other schools to build solidarity through individual identification with the institution. Understanding a society's history, traditions, practices, and so on also shapes identities. In Hofstede's evocative words, Culture is the "collective programming of the mind that distinguishes members of one community from another."

Value Systems

Cultural institutions are a source of values, and people's behavior is influenced by the cultural values they acquire through socialization. Motivation is associated with the notion that cultural values and norms include penalties (rewards and punishments) for specific activities. Cultural values also 'set the behavioral boundaries' in maintaining specified behavioral standards (e.g., laws specify right or wrong behavior, acceptable and unacceptable). This idea is expanded with functionalist stratification concepts.

Stratification

All civilizations distinguish social groupings based on social class (economic divisions), social rank (political divisions incorporating concepts such as aristocracy and peasantry), gender, age, and so on. For writers such as Lenski, social stratification is "inevitable, necessary, and functional" because it creates the "incentive systems" needed to motivate and reward the "best-qualified people" for occupying the "most important positions" within a cultural system. This idea leads to the final function of production and consumption.

Production and Consumption

As part of any society's overall survival mechanism, Culture specifies what individuals "need, use, and value." People must, for example, be organized and motivated to work [thus the necessity for a stratification system that compensates those who occupy social roles that are 'more functionally significant than others,' as Davis and Moore put it] and encouraged to consume workplace products.

■ HIGH AND LOW CULTURE

The contrast between 'high' and 'low' Culture expresses the idea of social distinctions based on the production and consumption of cultural objects. The concept of high Culture relates to the belief that certain artistic and literary products in our society are better in scope and form than others. Classical music, for example, is viewed in higher cultural regard than 'popular music' producers such as David Bowie or the Arctic Monkeys.

Low Culture, then, refers to cultural items and hobbies that are produced for and consumed by "the people." Low cultural forms have included cinema, comic books, television, magazines like 'Heat,' and newspapers like 'The Sun' in various eras. In this regard, high cultural products and endeavors correspond to the wealthy and powerful's cultural interests. On the other hand, low cultural products and interests are linked with the generally poorer and less powerful.

CULTURE AND BEHAVIOR

Cultural elements are so pervasive in human society that no human behavior is free from their influence. In terms of our acting, thinking, and feeling, we are products of our Culture. It regulates our behavior by prescribing standards through values and norms.

Thus culture:
- Prescribes specific patterns of behavior.
- Prohibits certain other patterns of behavior.
- Sets standards of permissiveness or tolerance.

Men get potentialities through heredity, but these potentialities, in a real sense, grow only in an appropriate cultural milieu. Our biological needs are also regulated and served through the prescriptions provided by the Culture. The sheer biological explanation shall hardly serve any purpose in understanding human behavior. Human behavior can be explained only with the help of its cultural context. Culture has such a profound influence on human behavior that even societies and nations are characterized by the Culture (s) inherited from their predecessors.

CULTURAL MEANING OF SICKNESS

In every society, sickness is explained in the context of shared understanding. In primitive societies and even in modern complex industrial societies, disease, sickness, and other human sufferings are ultimately tried to be understood by supernatural power, evil spirits, etc. Thus, we find traditional healers in every society, including modern industrial and high-technology societies. Culturally, a sick person is unfit to carry out the assigned roles per cultural values and social norms. The recognition, in this sense, relieves him from normal expectations by others as long as he is sick. Moreover, the person is looked after by the social support system such as family, neighborhood, healthcare institutions, community, state, etc.

As birth and death are explained in a cultural context, so is the sickness in every society. With the advancement of science and technology, the concept of disease, sickness, and treatment measures is also fast-changing. The evolution of medicine and surgical treatment has passed through the phases of the growth of scientific knowledge. There is increasing awareness about the empirical causes of sickness rather than supernatural ones due to a change in the cultural perception of sickness.

CULTURE AND HEALTH DISORDERS

Health

The World Health Organization (WHO) defines health as "a state of complete physical, mental and social well-being and not merely an absence of disease or infirmity." Health is not an easy term to define. For some, physical and mental health is compartmentalized.

The patient's health or mental health concept is determined by medical and socio-cultural circumstances, including family and social networks and a diverse range of prospective providers. Such definitions may differ from one Culture to the next. A study of ethnic groups in the United States reveals the complexities of a non-clinical definition of health and illness (Maloof, 1991).

Physical appearance, emotional temperament, and behavioral qualities are three major areas for children and adults. For many individuals, the functional component is crucial in determining health or illness; there is no disease without symptoms. Many cultural groups' worldviews integrate physical, emotional, and spiritual well-being and believe all three are required for full health. Even within the biological approach, cultural values are represented in disease diagnosis and treatment (Helman, 1990).

Illness

The socio-cultural context in which disease is experienced is referred to as illness. The patient and their family identify, categorize, and explain the illness episode for it to be personally and socially relevant (Kleinman, 1978).

Sickness

Sickness can also be viewed as a notion that blends the biological model (disease) with the patient's socio-cultural milieu (illness) **(Fig. 8.1)**. Spirituality and religion can play a crucial role in defining, comprehending, and responding to diseases inside illnesses. Personal opinions of a health or mental healthcare professional must also be considered for the 'illness' aspect of the sickness, as they affect patient-provider communication.

The following are:
- The well-being of a member of any society is also culturally determined. Those members relegated to the lower rung of society often live under total subjugation and deprivation. Their health problems are hardly given the attention that they deserve. As a result, the poorer people are forced to live amidst suffering and health disorders.
- The belief in supernatural power and the evil spirit is a cultural impediment in motivating people to adopt healthy practices and lifestyles. Such a situation aggravates the problem of health disorders.
- Cultural practices relating to maternity and childcare often ignore the requirement of cleanliness, nutrition, standards of health, etc. As a consequence of such practices, the problem of infant mortality becomes acute due to the higher vulnerability of infants to an ailment such as diarrhea, malnutrition, etc. The mothers

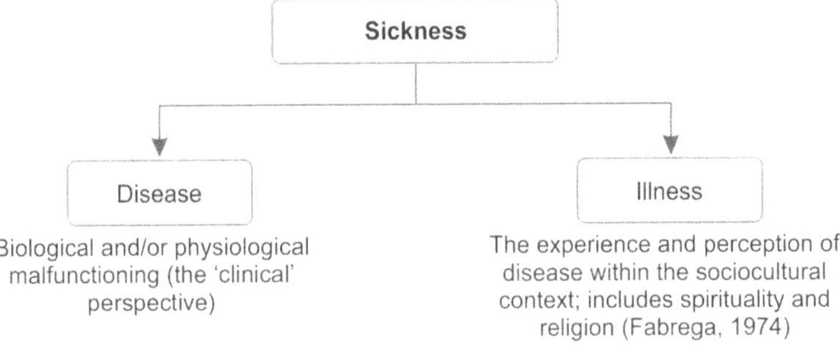

Fig. 8.1: Sickness.

are also subjected to several elements, especially among the socioeconomically poor classes.

- Rapid social change leads to maladjustment problems, causing mental stress and cardiac ailments. Highly urbanized societies also suffer from health disorders of these types.
- Environmental pollution due to heavy industrialization and technological advancements has led to the acute degradation of human conditions for a decent living. This has given birth to several health hazards that adversely affect the community and individuals' health. In a recent report by WHO, it has been pointed out that due to environmental degradation during the last 20 years, more than 30 new diseases have surfaced.
- Cultural stigma toward certain communicable diseases such as leprosy, sexually transmitted diseases such as acquired immunodeficiency syndrome (AIDS), tuberculosis, etc., perpetuates health disorders. This is true with mental illness as well. The fear of social rejection by one's people often results in a refusal to seek proper treatment and care.

The cultural environment works as a factor fostering health disorders under specific circumstances. These can be made ineffective only through effective education, community awareness, and adequate institutional arrangements involving people's participation and healthcare programs.

INFLUENCE OF CULTURE ON HEALTH AND ILLNESSES

The socio-cultural factors affect health as people are exposed to risk-taking behaviors, and some are vulnerable to disease. Analyzing actions and cultural activities that foster health and quality care are critical for the physiotherapist/nurse as socio-cultural influences play a vital role in influencing attitudes and reactions to health problems and their effects and well-being. So, every health professional should understand the factors that influence illness; and promote wellness.

Cultural Factors Affecting Health Care

Many factors in a particular culture affect people's health care. They are as follows:

- The decision was taken by the family members and their role in health care.
- The functional role of the community where the person lives.
- Influence of religion on diet, beliefs, illness, and treatment.
- People's view of their health and wellness.
- Cultural beliefs of death and dying process.
- Cultural views about Eastern, Western, or alternative medicine.

Beliefs in the Family

Citizens in India's rural communities have many misunderstandings about the size and structure of the family. Many believe children are born with the gift of God. The wealth of the family is determined by the birth of a child. Families are also fond of male children, leading to less childbirth gap. Lack of gap between childbirths leads to severe anemia for mothers, malnutrition, low birth weight, and a high infant mortality rate.

Sex and Marriage

Sexual customs and practices differ from one ethnic group to another. For example, Muslims have religious restrictions on performing oro-genital sex, especially during menstruation. Similarly, orthodox Jews are prohibited from having intercourse during menstruation, even seven days after the completion of menstruation. Such practices definitely influence oral health and family planning because they are stressed as they explain the maintenance of oral and sexual hygiene and the prevention of oral and genital infections.

Marriage practices such as polygamy, which is marrying one man to several women, and polyandry, which is marrying a woman to several men, are even practiced in Nilgiri hills, Nayars of Malabar coast in Kerala, and also among Jaunsar-Bawar in UP. Because of such practices, venereal diseases or sexually transmitted diseases occur if a person has sexual contact with more than one partner. Such diseases are prevalent since these marriage practices do not follow monogamy.

Maternal and Child Health

There are many customs and beliefs concerning mother and child health care; some are good, some are terrible, and some are unimportant. Some recommended practices include prolonged nursing, giving an oil bath, massaging the infant, and exposing the baby to sunlight after a morning bath.

Avoiding 'colostrum,' avoiding foods such as papaya, milk, fish, eggs, meat, and green leafy vegetables during pregnancy and nursing, and offering a light diet are some evil customs (this practice is seen in Tamil Nadu and Puducherry, where they believe that eating heavy foods will induce heat and cause problems to newborn).

Unimportant customs like applying turmeric, considered a holy spice, on the baby's head, piercing the ears and nose, balding the head, and applying kajal on eyelids are thought to ward off an evil eye on the head of the baby. In rural people, horrible practices include the application of cow dung in the umbilicus, which causes tetanus in newborns.

Religious Restrictions in Food Habits

Many religious beliefs and differences have significant health and disease consequences. Hindus, for example, do not consume beef since the cow is revered as 'Gaumata' and a holy animal known as 'Nandini.' Similarly, Muslims do not consume pork because they believe it is an unclean animal that eats dirt from sewers. However, these practices are beneficial in that they help to prevent cysticercosis, which is caused by tapeworms in undercooked beef and pig and results in severe anemia. This disease is mostly a foodborne disease that causes mouth ulcers and gingival bleeding and spreads through contaminated food and drink via the faecal-oral route.

Personal Habits

Purdah System

Muslims practice the Purdah system, where females are expected to cover their entire body, rendering them vulnerable to deficiency in vitamin D, teeth hypoplasia, and osteoporosis. Since skin is not exposed to sunlight, as most women wear black purdah that absorbs harmful ultraviolet rays, the risk of basal cell carcinoma is lower. However, droplet infections such as tuberculosis and diphtheria are high in prevalence.

Smoking and Alcoholism

Most religious traditions, especially among Muslims and Hindus, are against smoking and alcoholism. This promotes oral health. The younger generation of the present era is vulnerable as they consider smoking and alcohol consumption a symbol of machoism and status.

It forms acceptable behavior among peer groups and especially in tribal populations. For example, in the districts of Srikakulam and Vishakhapatnam in Andhra Pradesh, these habits were more prevalent among fishing communities earlier but now prevalent in nearly every part of India, more among young people and adolescents. Although the government has passed many laws and regulations to regulate this, tobacco consumption and alcoholism predominate. The high frequencies of oral and throat cancers reflect this.

Drug Addiction

Hindu sadhus have a habit of consuming *charas*, *bhang*, and *ganja* for pleasure and comfort. This habit has spread to youths in India, becoming addicted. Similarly, in western Culture, families have a habit of consuming alcohol as a common practice. This leads to addiction and subsequent illnesses.

Sedentary Lifestyle

The sedentary lifestyle followed by urban people is the leading cause of obesity-related illnesses. Sitting for a long time, watching television, and eating junk food lead to coronary artery diseases, hypertension, diabetes mellitus, etc. Carbonated beverages contain lots of phosphates and cause the demineralization of bones. It is dangerous to consume such drinks; it causes dry mouth and buccal keratosis. Lack of physical activity in sedentary life decreases the individual's lifespan.

Pan Chewing as a Custom

Offering pan with betel leaves, slaked lime, areca nut, and catechu is a way of welcoming guests in North India. However, continuous eating leads to oral diseases and oral submucosal fibrosis.

Social Change

LEARNING OBJECTIVES

☞ Describe meaning and nature of social change.
☞ What are the three basic sources of social change?
☞ Describe the factors affecting social change.
☞ What is social planning?

▦ MEANING AND NATURE OF SOCIAL CHANGE

Social change means the change in society's size, composition, and organization and the resultant change in the interrelationships between individuals and groups. In sociology, we see social change as alternations in social structure and relationships. Norms, values, cultural items, and social symbols can all alter. Other definitions of change suggest that change implies, above everything else, changes in the structure and function of a social system.

Social change is how human interactions and relationships transform cultural and social institutions over time, profoundly impacting society. Society is in a perpetual state of flux. The word "social change" describes the evolution of human society, and the changes in human interactions and interrelations indicate social change. Society is a network of social relationships. Hence, social change implies a change in the system of social relationships. As a result, any variation, modification, or transformation in the established pattern of human interaction and rules of behavior is considered a change. Child marriage has been abolished, inter-caste marriage has been legalized, and Indian women have a high social status.

Three Aspects of Social Change

Due to social change, institutions, patterns of interaction, work, leisure activities, roles, norms, and other aspects of society can be altered over time.

From various definitions of social change, we can see that:

1. Social change is essentially a process of alteration with no reference to change quality.

2. Because changes in society are linked to changes in culture, it is sometimes helpful to refer to 'socio-cultural change.' However, some sociologists distinguish between social and cultural change. Changes in the social structure (including changes in society's size), specific social institutions, or the connection between institutions are all examples of social change. They believe that social change primarily pertains to human behavior. On the other hand, cultural change refers to changes in cultural phenomena, including knowledge and ideas, art, religion, moral principles, values, beliefs, symbol systems, etc. This distinction is abstract because it is difficult or nearly impossible to decide which type of change occurs in many situations. For instance, the growth of modern technology as part of the culture has been closely associated with alterations in the economic structure—a critical part of society.

3. Social change can vary in scope and speed. We can talk of small-scale or large-scale changes. Change can take a cyclical pattern, e.g., when centralization and decentralization occur in administrative organizations. It can also be revolutionary. Revolutionary changes can be seen when there is an overthrow of the government in a particular nation. Change can also include short-term changes (e.g., in-migration rate) and long-term changes in economic structures. We can grow and decline the membership and size of social institutions in social change. Modification may consist of continuous processes such as specialization, bureaucratization, and discontinuous methods such as a particular technical or social invention, which appears at some point.

The change also varies in scope in that it may influence many aspects of society and disrupt the whole social system. The process of industrialization affected many aspects of culture. In contrast, substituting matchsticks (matches) for rubbing sticks to start a fire had a relatively limited scope.

Some changes happen quickly, while others take time. Many Western countries took decades to industrialize, but developing countries aim to do it faster. They achieve this by borrowing or adapting from countries that have already done so. Most sociologists believe change is an unavoidable, ever-present component of life in every culture. When we talk about social change, we're talking about changes in social structures, institutions, and social interactions, not individual experiences.

Some Allied Concepts

Social change is seen to be a neutral concept. 'Evolution' and 'progress' are two other terms that have frequently been associated with this concept:

1. Evolution expresses continuity and direction of change. It means more than growth. Growth suggests a change in direction, but mostly in size or quality. Evolution involves something more intrinsic, a change not only in size but also in structure.
2. Progress implies a change in direction toward some final desired goal. It involves a value judgment.

Not all changes are progressive or evolutionary. There is no need to make value judgments when discussing the direction of change. It is a historical fact that family sizes are shrinking while economic units grow in size. 'Social change' is a value-neutral term because sociologists do not study social changes in terms of 'good or bad,' 'desirable or undesirable.' However, one must accept that making a value-free critical analysis of changes in a society's structure is a difficult task.

▮ THREE BASIC SOURCES OF SOCIAL CHANGE

Some sociologists propose that social change occurs in one or more of three ways.

Discovery

It shares human perception of an aspect of reality that already exists, e.g., the discovery of blood circulation in biology. It is an addition to the world's store of verified knowledge. It is only when it is put to use, not when it is just known, that it becomes a factor in social change.

Inventions

A new combination or use of existing knowledge, e.g., assembling the automobile from an existing idea. The idea of combining them was unique. Inventions can be material (technology) and social (alphabet, trade union). Each invention may be unique in form (i.e., in shape or action), function (what it does) or in, meaning (its long-range consequences), or principle (the theory or law on which it is based).

Diffusion

The transmission of cultural traits from one group to another is diffusion. It works both within and between societies. It takes place whenever cultures come into contact. Diffusion is a two-way process. The British gave us their language and made tea a vital ritual. Diffusion is also a selective process. Most Indians may adopt the English language, but not their beef-eating habit. Diffusion typically involves some form, function, or meaning modification of the borrowed cultural elements.

■ FACTORS AFFECTING SOCIAL CHANGE

Robert Bierstadt has listed the following factors of social change:
- Geographical
- Biological
- Demographical
- Political and military
- Technological
- Economical
- Ideological
- Role of great men
- Education and learning
- Social legislations
- Social movements, psychological factors, and cultural factors also bring about social change
- Fear is also perhaps one of the crucial factors of social change.

Geographical Factors

Geographical or physical factors comprise all the inorganic (non-living) phenomena that influence human life. Natural events such as floods, drought, earthquakes, climate changes, exhaustion of natural resources, changes in the course of rivers, excessive soil erosion, etc., lead to demographic changes and trade routes.

Biological Factors

The plants and animals in an area constitute the biological factors that influence the lives of human beings. Man utilizes the available flora and fauna in ways determined by their culture and keeps off from poisonous plants, bacteria, insects, pests, and dangerous creatures. Biological processes determine the number, the compositions, the selection, and the hereditary qualities of succeeding generations. Social attitudes and interests may influence these processes as the latter control sex relations, interracial, inter-religious, and inter-caste marriages, the size of the family, etc. Social behavior of various kinds induces biological changes. Social conventions, such as taboos on inter-caste or religious marriages, child marriages, etc., affect offspring quality adversely. Race is an essential biological factor.

Demographical Factors

The size of a population is an essential factor. Tiny societies seldom rise to positions of historical imminence. Huge ones exert influences not only upon their neighbors but also on the course of history. An expanding population in any country brings many changes in the nation's economy, and a contracting population has contrary effects. In short, we can say that the demographical variables—fertility, mortality, and migration affect the social order, and the social order, in turn, affects the demographic variables. The effectiveness of medical care has improved throughout the world, which has impacted demography. Better surgical procedures and potent drugs have lowered mortality rates around the world.

Political and Military Factors

The emergence of democracy, communism, or socialism results in several societal changes; for example, democracy establishes political, economic, and social equality. Individuals can express their opinions, create associations, and engage in constitutionally allowed activities in a democracy. It shows a government "of the people, by the people, and for the people." Democracy seeks to provide equal opportunity for all citizens.

Technological Factors

The industrialization process alters society's structure and its members' behavior patterns. Specializations, mass production, and integrated organization govern both industry and business. Modern technology in instituting large-scale enterprises has accelerated the process of urbanization and has already changed and is also changing the whole socio-cultural life of human beings. Capitalism has brought about changes in the property system and the division of labor and has given rise to new social strata and classes. Technology has also brought about unemployment due to the displacement of work. Ogburn mentions that introducing a self-starter in the course has revolutionized the lives of many women.

Economical Factors

An economic interpretation of social changes is associated with the name Karl Marx. Karl Marx asserted that economic conditions and economically-oriented actions constituted the base of the social structure and profoundly influenced all other aspects of human society. The relations of production form society's financial system and the fundamental foundations for the legal and political superstructures. Marx stressed that economic conditions and production techniques significantly influence human activities and social institutions. The accumulation of capital by an organization of labor, labor relations, etc., have brought about socialistic measures to alleviate labor hardships and share the benefits of enterprise in various forms.

Ideological Factors

Ideologies are ideas that people in a given society value and respect. Thus, ideologies are powerful motivational forces in social change. What people think, what they do and want, etc., concerns prevailing ideologies. For example, the capitalist or communist ideology may initiate corresponding social changes among its adherents.

Role of Great Men

The great social reformers of India worked hard to bring about a new social order. Mahatma Gandhi, Raja Ram Mohan Roy, Ishwar

Chandra Vidyasagar, Swami Dayanand Saraswati, and a host of other social reformers have brought about changes in our society; the removal of untouchability, equal rights for women, removal of Sati custom, etc.

Education and Learning as Sources of Change

Education is perhaps one of the most critical factors in social change. Through education, knowledge is gained, and awareness is created. Studies on community development help change the community and realize the potential of community organizations with a technical understanding of how it may be brought about through childcare, nutrition, health education, etc. Food, health, population, family life, sex, and extension studies could bring about the desired social changes among people.

Social Legislation and Social Change

The law or social legislation brings about social change by creating norms and sanctions. Examples include the Sati Prohibitions Act, the Widow Remarriage Act, and the Untouchability Offences Act. Acts allowing inter-caste and inter-religious marriages, divorce, adoption, equal share for women in property, etc., were instrumental in bringing about social change.

Social Movements and Social Change

Social movements have occurred throughout history, but significant and far-reaching changes in the world's social order occurred during the 18th–19th century as products of social movements. The French, Russian, and American Revolutions transformed the prevailing social orders. Women's movements, student's movements, peasant and tribal movements, labor movements, nationalist movements, social reform movements, and a wide variety of resistance or counter-resistance movements are the order of the day. These movements have directly or indirectly affected the social order and the life of the people. Likewise, professional organizations have started functioning as pressure groups, changing many aspects of our lives. Medical and paramedical associations have also gained a lot due to their organized, professional movements.

Fear as a Cause of Change

Fear of a nuclear war caused leading world powers to unite and cooperate to control these weapons and use atomic energy for peaceful purposes. The danger arising from the uncontrolled use of drugs and narcotics has forced world powers to make concentrated efforts to control them. The fear of dire consequences of unprecedented population expansion has compelled many countries to adopt family planning as a state policy and take steps to prevent population growth.

■ OBSTACLES TO SOCIAL CHANGE

Anderson and Parker state that social change does not come in a society without resistance. Many forces tend to block acceptance. Those obstacles are inertia, habit, suspicion, tradition, vested interests, lack of knowledge, etc. These factors opposing social change are all closely interrelated. Inertia may grow out of habits, while practices are founded on habits, and lack of knowledge supports inertia. Vested interests also support these. In some cases, each of these forces may be the major obstacle to social change. In most cases, they combine to form a formidable opposition, which multiplies the effects of each separate force.

■ PLANNED SOCIAL CHANGE

Many Asian, African, and Latin American countries gained political independence in the second half of the twentieth century, particularly after World War II. These independent states' main concern was to accomplish their citizens' welfare. The government resorted to various types of planning for development. Planning is a conscious attempt to achieve a given goal. Planning implies that society is not satisfied with the status quo and desires to improve the quality of life for all. The government considers its resources at the national level, fixes its priorities, and allocates funds accordingly. Thus, planning means a consciously designed advancement toward a new social and economic order. Regional planning and planning at the grassroots and family levels are also encouraged through family welfare schemes, rural development, village and cottage industries schemes, etc., to supplement national planning.

■ SOCIAL CHANGE AND HUMAN ADAPTATION

Change is the law of nature; man must adjust, accommodate, and adapt to life's changing needs and demands. He molds his personality and leads his life as per societal norms. If he is unable to adjust or adapt himself to the changing scenario, then it causes stress, conflict, adjustment problems, and psychosomatic diseases, etc. Man adapts according to the situation and acquires new habits, customs, and values to lead a better, happy, and satisfactory life. Man has to quit the old roles/norms and get adjusted to new roles/norms by adapting to new situations to avoid stress. Changes in societal norms over time cause many adjustment problems for individuals. So, everyone has to accept reality and balance their thoughts to adjust to societal changes.

Social Change and Health Programs

Health programs are developed for the welfare of society at large. These programs were devised to reduce morbidity and mortality, protect the vulnerable population, and improve sanitation. Social change is a universal phenomenon observed throughout the world. The changes take place continuously. Without any change, society will stagnate. This will lead to multiple health-related and psychological problems. Social change and the developments or modifications in health programs are interrelated. New diseases or health-related issues also crop up as any advancement occurs in science, technology, agriculture, or industry. To protect the health of members of society, the government has implemented and amended many health programs to fulfill the requirement. For example:

- National Family Planning was launched in 1952 with the concept of 'small family norm' emphasizing three children. Then, it was amended to two children norm; now, it is amended to the 'one or none' formula. The Family Planning Program was renamed in 1977 as 'the Family Welfare Program' to improve the quality of living.
- In 1978, an expanded immunization program was launched, where pregnant women and 5-year-old children were protected against six killer diseases. In 1985, the government changed to the Universal Immunization Program (UIP), which beneficiaries are children under one year and pregnant women.
- To eradicate polio, in 1995 Pulse Polio Program was implemented.

Social Change and Stress

Social stress is defined as stressful social behaviors and situations. This includes stress from friends, work, academic clubs, or family. Social anxiety causes everyday anxiety, self-consciousness, and embarrassment because a person fears being judged negatively by others. Fear and anxiety can disrupt a person's life with social anxiety disorder.

Social anxiety can affect daily routines and activities, leading to isolation. Social stress and anxiety are emotional responses, but social stress is usually external. Social anxiety causes persistent, excessive worries even without a stressor. Social stress can threaten relationships, esteem, or belonging between two people, a group, or a larger social context. This feeling can stem from tumultuous marital or family relationships.

Social Stress at Work

Examples of social stressors in the workplace include:
- Verbal aggression in the workplace
- Co-worker conflict
- Negative group environments
- Organizational politics
- Unfair treatment

Social stress can manifest in performance situations, when co-workers or managers are judgmental or critical, or when one feels rejected, ostracized, or ignored. Workplace social stressors can harm positive organizational behaviors and consequences. This occurs due to social stressors depleting a person's coping resources or ability to cope with the strain. It has the potential to erode their fortitude. According to research, social stressors can result in the following:
- Lower job satisfaction
- Feelings of failure
- Increased turnover
- Decreased productivity
- Reduced altruism and teamwork

Social Stress Management

Want to reduce social stress and its adverse effects? Below are ways to minimize work and home social stress.

- Managers can help prevent co-worker aggression and conflict. Social conflict is generally negative and causes social stress.
- Focus debates on tasks, not people, to avoid social conflict. Forbes suggests that managers mediate disputes to resolve them positively. Ensure both parties are heard and valued. Help them align expectations.
- Forbes says divisive conversation topics can cause social stress. In today's hypersensitive political climate, political debate can cause anger, resentment, and stress. Avoid sensitive issues with co-workers to preserve relationships and a peaceful workplace.

SOCIAL PLANNING

Social planning is a concept of recent origin and is an instrument made by the government to achieve desired social and economic developments. It is part of national development planning. Man must plan based on facts, analyses, and scientific methods to deal with social problems. Man can control his destiny by remedying social issues, as social problems are artificial. Social planning is a process in which preventive, promotive, protective, and control measures have used to remedy social problems. It is done by adequately utilizing material, human resources, and social resources.

A social plan is 'an achievement to be realized within a fixed period.' It is based on a practical approach, a means of social progress.

Aims of Social Planning

- To check the recurrence of social problems
- To bring harmony in relationships between various social groups
- To maintain social order
- To adapt our culture to meet the present needs
- To hasten the social progress
- To develop gainful social habits and customs
- To compel social institutions to adapt to the present-day requirements of life.

Difficulties in Implementing Social Planning

- An accurate understanding of human society is a problem (emotional, raw material).

- Lack of scientific study to investigate thoroughly the social problems (planning without adequate scientific knowledge results in failure).
- Lack of human resources to carry out the work of social planning.
- Vested interests of society members, who exercise a powerful influence over the government machinery.
- Indifference and apathy of the ordinary people: The general public must learn to look at social issues objectively and participate in formulating and implementing social policy.

Social Planning in India

The government of India formulated the Planning Commission to promote social welfare activities and coordinate welfare services. Social welfare organizations were developed to strengthen, improve, and extend the existing social welfare activities, create new programs, and carry out new projects. Central Bureau of Correctional Services was developed as 'aftercare homes' to provide appropriate training and meet the needs of the especially needy population, such as rescued women, girls, economically deprived groups, and scheduled caste populations.

Role of Social Planning for the Improvement of Health and Rehabilitation: Preplanning

- **Government interest:** Any social welfare plan must be based on a strong 'political will' as manifested by clear directives, policies, or legislation given by the political authority. The social and health policies were formulated and translated into legislation to safeguard disabled individuals, e.g., the Disability and Workmen's Compensation Act.
- **Organization for planning:** The Central Planning Commission, Which consists of technical experts in the field of social and economic development. Central Ministry of Social Welfare Board coordinates and plans several social welfare programs.
- **Administrative capacity:** The state government and different voluntary agencies distribute funds for implementing the programs and looking after the welfare activities' execution. Welfare extension projects were carried out for the rehabilitation of disa-

bled delinquents. Establishment of craft centers and recreational homes, training centers, correctional institutions are focused on these people. Welfare officers have been appointed to rehabilitate individuals who are in need.

Steps in Planning Cycle

- **Analysis of social situation:** Collection, assessment, and interpretation of information related to a factual situation. For example:
    - The society and its characteristics and mortality/morbidity pattern of disabilities.
    - Social factors which promote the causation of social problems.
    - Social welfare facilities and resources (government and private).
    - Technical workforce of various categories.
    - Existence of training facilities and rehabilitation homes.
    - Attitudes and beliefs of society toward occurrence, preventive and curative measures of social problems.
- **Establish objectives and goals:** Short-term and long-term plans and general and specific purposes have to be formulated based on problem orientation to guide the activities and make a benchmark to measure the activities oriented towards achievement.
- **Assessment of resources:** Manpower, money and material, skills, knowledge and needed technique available, occupational/vocational training programs, and resources available and needed will be estimated.
- **Fixing priorities:** By the priority ranking method, the magnitude of the problem, social investment, community interest, social pressures, etc., can be fixed.
- **Alternate plans:** Formulate and suggest alternate methods to meet the needs of the disabled. It provides operational guidance to all those responsible for executing and allocating resources.
- **Programming and implementation:** Policy-making authorities approve the plan, and various procedures must be followed by a delegation of authority and fixation of responsibility to multiple categories of therapists (specialty-wise) to achieve the predetermined objectives and goals.
- **Monitoring:** Observing the day-to-day follow-up activities during the implementation, recording, and reporting objectives to the

concerned, to have a track throughout activities, identifying the deviation, and taking corrective actions for solving the problem and limitation of disabilities.

- **Evaluation:** To assess the achievement, adequacy, and efficiency of a rehabilitation program's objectives and quality assurance. Based on the result, a modified strategy can be implemented.

Social Problems

- ☞ Define social problem.
- ☞ Describe elements of social problems.
- ☞ What are the characteristics and causes of social problems?
- ☞ What are the sources and types of social problems?

▇ INTRODUCTION

A problem is a state of dissatisfaction felt by someone. However, when many people detest it, it becomes a social problem. A social problem must involve many people, often groups and institutions, who regard a specific condition as undesirable or unacceptable and wish to remedy it by collective action.

Thus, not all problems are social unless dissatisfied people gather together, vocalize their dissatisfaction, and band together to find a solution. When a problem is conveyed to others, it becomes social, and one person's involvement leads to comparable activity by other people. As a result, a social problem differs from an individual one.

A single person or a small group is affected by an individual problem. It has little effect on the general populace. Its answers are contained within the individual's or group's authority and immediate environment. On the other hand, a public issue necessitates a collaborative approach to its resolution. No one or a few people are to blame for the emergence of a socially harmful situation. This scenario is likewise beyond the control of a single or a small group of people.

"A social problem is a generic term that refers to a variety of conditions and abnormal behaviors that are indications of social disorder. It is a condition that the majority of people in a society consider unpleasant and wish to change through social engineering or social planning" (Oxford Dictionary of Sociology, 1994).

Reinhardt defined it as a situation that presents a group or a section of society with potentially harmful consequences that can only be addressed collectively.

Raab and Selznick think that the social problem is 'a problem of human relationship which gravely threatens society or impedes the critical goals of many individuals.'

'The social problem is a condition many people find undesirable and seek to improve,' write Horton and Leslie. It is a problem that affects many people negatively, and it is believed that something can be done by collective means.'

As a result, two things must be present in social problems:

1. The presence and magnitude of an objective state, such as crime, poverty, or communal tensions that can be witnessed, verified, and measured by objective social observers; and
2. The subjective definition of the objective condition as a "problem" that some members of society must solve. This is where values enter the picture. People begin to believe those specific ideas are under attack.

■ ELEMENTS OF SOCIAL PROBLEMS

The following are critical components of social problems:

- A condition or circumstance that many people find undesirable.
- It is seen as unfavorable due to its negative implications.
- All social problems require collective action to be addressed. They call for a change in circumstances through social engineering.
- Crime, juvenile delinquency, prostitution, rape, drug addiction, domestic violence, and ethnic or communal hostility are societal problems.
- Social problems are dynamic, changing with time and space. The idea of the social problem changes as laws and customs change.

Recognizing an undesirable situation and labelling it a social problem are not synonymous. There may be disagreement if some people believe a condition or situation is undesirable but also believe it is unavoidable because it is a part of the human condition or the price we pay for 'progress,' as in the case of environmental imbalance caused by tree cutting for road construction, dislodging people for dam and canal construction, air and noise pollution due to increased motor vehicles, and the rising rate of automobile-related accidental deaths.

The constantly rising rate of automotive-related fatalities has long been considered unavoidable, but automobile safety has become a social issue after widespread criticism. Slums and ghettos were seen as inescapable and not a societal concern during the early stages of industrialization.

People may not consider a situation a problem if it is desirable and natural and does not jeopardize their values. People who believed castes/genders were born unequal did not face caste/gender discrimination. They may argue that differential treatment is not discrimination (for them, integration threatens their values and, thus, a social problem).

In truth, defining discrimination as an issue necessitates a belief in equality. Some people continue to deny that poverty is a social issue. They see it as the inevitable fate of the people. Poor people are to blame for their predicament. Poverty, according to these people, is a personal failure of impoverished people, not a result of social structure.

Such archaic ideas, however, have transformed modern communities. People began to believe that something could be done about such conditions and that society (government) should take action.

CHARACTERISTICS OF SOCIAL PROBLEMS

Based on the above definitions, we can identify the following characteristics of social problems:

- All social problems are situations that have injurious consequences for society.
- All social problems are aberrations from the *'ideal'* condition.
- All social problems have some everyday basis of origin.
- All social problems are societal in origin.
- Pathological social conditions cause all social problems.
- All social problems are interrelated.
- All social problems are societal in their results; they affect all segments of society.
- The responsibility for social problems is societal; they require a collective approach for their solution.
- Social problems occur in all societies.

■ CAUSES OF SOCIAL PROBLEMS

Pathological social conditions give birth to social problems. They occur in all societies, both simple and complex (which are characterized by impersonal secondary relations, loneliness, anonymity, high mobility, and extreme specialization, and where change is faster), that is, wherever and whenever a relationship between a group of individuals is affected, leading to maladjustments and conflicts.

■ SOURCES OF SOCIAL PROBLEMS

There are no social problems in a properly integrated community. However, utopian hopes are unfounded because no society is, or can be, flawless. In an otherwise good society, social problems suggest certain undesirable and value-threatening characteristics.

The sources of social problems are numerous and can be categorized as follows:

- Social difficulties arise because modern society's internal organization is so complicated and intricate that an uncoordinated and loosely woven social structure cannot help but cause stress and social conflicts. Housing, poverty, unemployment, and inequality are complex and intertwined societal issues.
- Even though modern civilization is immensely productive and rewarding in terms of status and material things for many people, it nonetheless has a dark side. Every social system has costs and casualties. Progress, it is often said, comes at a cost.
  Many development initiatives have resulted in many challenges for the population, such as the eviction of many people from their villages due to the construction of dams on rivers. Similarly, road building has necessitated tree chopping, resulting in environmental damage. Many people have been relocated as a result of road building.
- As the social structure changes, established relationships between social groups (such as the relationship between Gujjars and Meenas in Rajasthan) are disrupted, social roles are redefined (such as between working husband and wife), and some beliefs and behavior patterns are rendered obsolete or dysfunctional.

TYPES OF SOCIAL PROBLEMS

There are two categories of societal problems, according to sociologists. To begin with, social organization issues are caused by how a community or society is formed. Some individuals in the community or society refuse to accept appropriate, necessary, or inevitable situations. For example, these examples are communalism, casteism, regionalism, poverty, gender inequality, population, and environmental imbalance (different kinds of pollution, health hazards, etc.).

Second, deviance-related issues relate to people's adaptation to traditional lifestyles. Delinquency, alcoholism, drug addiction, mental illness, various forms of sexual conduct (rape, incest, sodomy), bigamy, prostitution, vandalism, and a variety of other actions, the majority of which are illegal, are among them.

10.1 POPULATION EXPLOSION AND POPULATION CONTROL

LEARNING OBJECTIVES

- ☞ What is the population explosion?
- ☞ What are the causes of over population?
- ☞ Explain population growth characteristics.
- ☞ What is the impact of population growth on society and the economy?
- ☞ What measures can be adopted to control the population?

INTRODUCTION

A discrepancy in birth and mortality rates has resulted in the rapid rise of the world's population over the last century. The influence of global population expansion on the economy and the environment impacts everyone.

The current rate of population expansion is putting a strain on human well-being. Understanding the elements that influence population growth trends might aid in future planning.

POPULATION EXPLOSION

By population explosion, we mean a very rapid and unprecedented growth of population, which creates many problems in the country.

By population control, we mean controlling population growth through family planning or birth control. Today, the population explosion is a significant problem developing countries face globally. When we look at the figures of the Indian census from time to time, we observe an enormous growth in our population from 1931 onwards **(Table 10.1)**. Any population grows at an annual rate of 2% and can double in 35 years **(Fig. 10.1)**. It has happened in the Indian population.

As we've already mentioned, the time it takes for the global human population to double has decreased dramatically. The human population rose at a significantly quicker rate in the twentieth century. Between 1950 and 1990, the population surpassed 5 billion people in just 40 years, with an annual increase of nearly 92 million people, or roughly the equivalent of adding a New Mexico yearly. The world population was 6.3 billion in 2000, expected to expand fourfold in the next 100 years. This extraordinary increase in the human population is causing a population explosion at an alarming rate **(Fig. 10.1)**.

With almost 1 billion people, India is the world's second-most populous country. If present growth rates continue, it will surpass China as the most populous country in 2050, with 1.63 billion people.

Table 10.1: Growth rate of population in India.

Census year	Total population (Crores)	Annual growth rate (%)
1901	23.84	–
1910	25.21	0.56
1921	25.13	0.01
1931	27.9	1.01
1941	31.56	1.33
1951	36.11	1.25
1961	43.92	1.94
1971	54.64	2.22
1981	63.38	1.21
1991	84.93	2.01
2001	102.3	–

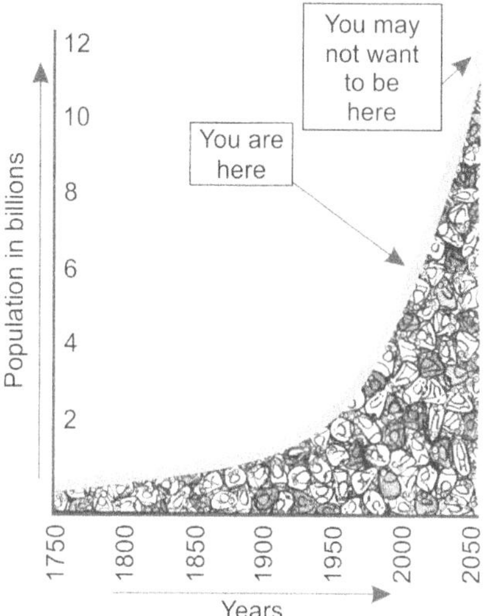

Fig. 10.1: Population growth in India.

As a result, we are on the threshold of severe consequences due to population growth.

If we look at our country's population figures, we can see that we have added another India in terms of people just 35 years after independence. We passed the one billion mark on May 11, 2000, and now every sixth person on the planet is an Indian.

By 2050, it is expected that we will be the most populous country in the world. The people of the Republic of China may be pushed to the second position because the rate of population in their country has come down with the enforcement of one child to a family. This sudden outburst in our population is mainly due to the sudden fall in our death rates. With antibiotics, more comprehensive immunization programs, and overall medical facilities, the death rate fell sharply, with no corresponding decrease in the birth rate. This led to a population explosion, and almost all other problems our country faces today are rooted in this. This will be very clear if we look at the fertility and mortality figures **(Table 10.1)**.

The rapid growth of the human population is depleting natural resources and degrading the environment. Land, water, fossil fuels, minerals, and other resources are limited, and they are depleting due to over-exploitation.

Many renewable resources, such as forests and grasslands, are under severe stress. Industrial and commercial development improves our living standards and introduces hazardous contaminants into the air, water, and soil. As a result, environmental life-support systems are compromised.

There is an intense debate about whether we should immediately reduce fertility rates through global birth control programs to stabilize or even shrink the population or develop new technologies for alternative resources so that the problem of exceeding the earth's carrying capacity never arises.

The ill-effect of such an explosion in the population is devastating to the national economy. All our planning and efforts become futile under these unfavorable demographic conditions. Our national leaders have correctly said that planning is like constructing a house on a flooded river in the present situation.

■ CAUSES OF OVERPOPULATION

- **A decline in the death rate:** One of the primary causes of overpopulation is decreased death and mortality rates. Man has discovered remedies for formerly fatal diseases due to medical advances. New medical discoveries have resulted in treatments for most of the world's most severe conditions. Individuals' life expectancy has grown as a result. The mortality rate has decreased, resulting in a rise in population.

  The death rate has dropped because of modern pharmaceuticals and improved treatments for many illnesses. On the plus side, we've been able to combat various diseases and prevent deaths. On the other side, the medical boon has brought the curse of overpopulation.

- **The rise in the birth rate:** We have been able to enhance human reproductive rates thanks to advances in medical science. Modern medicines can increase human reproduction rates. There are medications and treatments available to aid in conception. As a result, science has resulted in a rise in the birth rate. This is the apparent cause for celebration, yet medical breakthroughs have also contributed to overpopulation.

- **Migration:** In some places of the world, immigration is an issue. If people from different countries relocate to a specific section of the world and reside there, the area is bound to suffer from the negative impacts of overpopulation. Overpopulation occurs when the rates of departure from a particular country do not match the rates of immigration to that country. The country grows overcrowded. The overcrowding of immigrants in various places of the world causes an imbalance in population density.
- **Lack of education:** Another primary source of overpopulation is illiteracy. That lack of education fails to see the importance of limiting unsustainable population expansion. They are unable to comprehend the negative consequences of overpopulation.

They have no idea how to keep the population under control. The uneducated world is notorious for its lack of family planning. This is one of the primary causes of overpopulation. Due to ignorance, they do not use family planning methods, adding to population growth.

When looking at the issue of population growth positively, one may argue that overpopulation equals more human resources. As the population increases, so does the number of working hands and creative minds. However, we must overlook that an increase in the number of producers inevitably leads to an increase in the number of consumers. A growing number of people necessitates a larger amount of resources.

Not every country can provide enough resources to its citizens. With the world's population growing exponentially, no country can provide its citizens with the resources they require to survive. Overpopulation is a calamity when the ecosystem cannot handle the live beings occupying it.

POPULATION GROWTH CHARACTERISTICS

- **Exponential growth:** It is called linear growth when a quantity increases by a constant amount per unit of time, e.g., 1, 3, 5, 7, etc. However, it is known as exponential growth when it increases by a fixed percentage, e.g., 10, 102, 103, 104, or 2, 4, 8, 16, 32, etc. Population growth occurs exponentially, explaining the dramatic increase in the global population in the past 150 years.

- **Doubling time:** The amount of time it takes for a population to double at a constant annual rate is called doubling time. The formula is as follows:

  Td = 70/r

  Where,

  Td = Doubling time in years

  r = annual growth rate

  If a nation has a 2% annual growth rate, its population will double in 35 years.

- **Total fertility rates (TFR):** A country's population growth is one of the most important indicators. The average number of children born to a woman in her lifetime if age-specific birth rates remain constant is called TFR. TFR ranges from 1.9 in wealthy countries to 4.7 in impoverished countries. The TFR has been 6.1 since the 1950s. The TFR has decreased due to changes in society's cultural and technological setup and government legislation, which is a good shift.

- **Infant mortality rate:** It's a crucial factor in determining a population's future growth. It is the number of infants that died in a given year as a proportion of all those born in that year. Although this rate has decreased over the last 50 years, the pattern in industrialized and developing countries is somewhat different.

- **Zero population growth (ZPG):** When birth plus immigration in a population equals deaths plus emigration, it is said to be zero population growth.

- **Male-female ratio:** For society to thrive, the boy-to-girl ratio should be fairly balanced. The ratio has been thrown off in several nations, including India, due to female infanticide and gender-based abortions. In many parts of China, the boy-to-girl ratio reached 140:100, resulting in a shortage of brides.

- **Life expectancy:** It is the average age at which a newborn infant in a particular country is predicted to reach. Over the last century, the global average life expectancy has increased from 40 to 65.5 years. In 1900, males and females in India had life expectancies of only 22.6 and 23.3 years, respectively. Improved medical facilities and technical innovation have boosted the life expectancy of Indian males and females to 60.3 and 60.5 years, respectively, in the last 100 years. Japan and Sweden have a higher life expectancy, with ladies living 82.1–84.2 years and males living 77–77.4 years.

- **Demographic transition:** Economic development is frequently linked to population growth. A process known as the demographic transition happens when death and birth rates reduce due to improving living conditions, resulting in low population growth. It happens in four stages and is linked to urbanization and growth:
  i. The pre-industrial phase is characterized by high growth and death rates and low net population growth.
  ii. The transitional phase that occurs with the advent of industrialization provides better hygiene and medical facilities and adequate food, thereby reducing deaths. However, birth rates remain high, and the population shows a 2.5–3% growth rate.
  iii. Industrial phase, while there is a fall in birth rates, lowering the growth rate.
  iv. Post-industrial phase during which zero population growth is achieved.

  In most developing countries, demographic transition has already begun. The affluent countries are now increasing at around 0.5%, with a doubling period of 118 years due to demographic shifts. However, more than 90% of the world's population is concentrated in developing countries, with a growth rate of just over 2% and a doubling time of less than 35 years, which is cause for concern.

IMPACT OF POPULATION GROWTH

As a result of high fertility and fairly high mortality, developing countries like India have a huge young population. The total population of India is almost three times that of America. The number of people above 65 years in both countries is the same, but the 0–4 years age group is six times more in India than in America. Because of the vast young population, the dependency rate is very high. Any population with a large percentage of dependents and a small percentage of working people will be economically backward. The young population incurs huge national expenditures in many other ways. The rearing of children necessitates a considerable sum of money. The demand for primary and secondary schools, in turn, necessitates a significant financial investment. The medical and other needs of the growing population are pretty more extensive. Due to the high infant and child mortality rate, the rate of national waste is also high because expenses on the children go waste in the event of their death. The population will increase whenever this percentage of the young population is high because all these children will be growing into adults and producing more children **(Table 10.2)**.

Hence, despite the wide acceptance of family planning methods, population growth cannot decrease. Further, with a largely dependent population, the per capita income and the standard of life cannot improve. Even with a remarkable increase in the national income, the per capita income of Indians is still inferior. A large population is mainly responsible for this.

Such a large population also greatly hampered the country's capital formation. The lion's share of the national income is spent on unproductive items like food, shelter, clothing, education, health facilities, etc. These day-to-day needs are to be met before we can devote more capital to significant work. In the absence of capital, large-scale development projects cannot be implemented. The industrialization process becomes slow, affecting the country's economic growth and the people's standard of life. With good economic development and industrialization, new employment opportunities become limited.

On the other hand, many people enter the labor market as job seekers every year. This gives rise to acute unemployment, which our country is currently facing. Overpopulation results in food problems as well. The cultivable land of any country cannot increase to any remarkable extent. Therefore, food supply to the increased population may be a significant problem.

About 15% of the world's population lives in India, whereas we have only 2% of the cultivable land. McNamara has estimated that at least 100 million people worldwide are severely malnourished. Indian women and children suffer from malnutrition. Pregnant and lactating mothers also suffer from malnutrition and poor health. Deficiency diseases such as blindness, beriberi, rickets, and scurvy are prevalent.

With tremendous population growth, economic and several other problems have come up. Housing is a significant problem, especially in cities, and in the absence of cheap and hygienic facilities, the number of slum dwellers is shooting up. Inflation is increasing day by day due to limited resources and increased demands. Communalism,

Table 10.2: Growth rate of population in Ind a with birth and death rates.

Rate (%)	Years											
	2000	2001	2002	2003	2004	2005	2006	2007	2008	2009	2010	2011
Birth rate (births/1,000 population)	24.79	24.28	23.79	23.28	22.8	22.32	22.01	22.69	22.22	21.76	21.34	20.97
Death rate (births/1,000 population)	8.88	8.74	8.62	8.49	8.38	8.28	8.18	6.58	6.4	6.23	7.53	7.48
Growth rate = Birth rate– Death rate	15.91	15.54	15.17	14.79	14.42	14.04	13.83	16.11	15.82	15.53	13.81	13.49

Adapted from http://www.medindia.net/health_statistics/general/birthdeath.asp

regionalism, crime, and violence are rooted in poverty and economic discontentment. The pressure of the population on the land is increasing. Though additional land is being made available through land reclamation, the per capita land decreases due to population increase.

With a lack of additional employment facilities, more and more people are turning to cultivation. The availability of cheap labor inhibits the development of technology and labor-saving devices. In the long run, this will affect the cost of production. The scope for skill improvement and productivity is limited due to the slow industrial and technological development rate. All these factors result in a country's standing in the world market. We cannot compete and enter a highly competitive world market due to poor production technology standards. Thus, our international trade is greatly affected.

All the abovementioned factors will result in slow economic development and a poor standard of life. If we have to improve our standard of living, the first and foremost necessity is to control our population. The idea of a small family should be spread far and wide. Today, information technology is widely disseminated with improved communication techniques such as television. What remains is to study the rate of attitude change and the extent of adoption of family planning techniques.

An awareness regarding our population should be created in the young generation and the general public. We have already included population education as a part of the curriculum in schools. It should be effectively taught with the help of audio-visual aids, and children should be made aware of the extent of the problem and their responsibility to cope with the problem in the future.

Similarly, the general public should be aware of the problem, especially the less educated and privileged class. All measures should be taken to check infant mortality and birth rate. When the survival rate of children improves, the birth rate also gradually decreases. All village-level workers should be trained and motivated to contact eligible couples in their areas and persuade them to accept family planning techniques. These workers must have the proper knowledge of each technique. Primary health centers should also be adequately equipped.

It should be added that while family planning and birth control devices have been accepted and followed by educated urban people of India, it is not so in rural areas. Illiteracy and ignorance are a setback. So, special attention is paid to our villages for population control.

■ POPULATION CONTROL

The population is one of most developing countries' most serious development concerns. According to UN population data, the global population increased by 30% between 1990 and 2010, which is an alarmingly high rate. The excessive population has several negative consequences, including undue strain on natural resources. More people equal more consumption, which equals more exploitation of fixed and finite resources. Furthermore, the population is not a universal issue. It only applies to countries whose economies have not yet reached their full potential and growth. Along with China and India, Africa and certain Latin American countries are rapidly increasing populations. Instead, China, the world's most populous country, has accomplished a remarkable level of population control through highly dictatorial methods that cannot be imitated in other countries.

The following are the most successful methods for limiting population growth:

Consequences of Early Marriage

Child marriage is a significant problem in nations with large populations, such as India, Pakistan, and Bangladesh. Marriage at a young age results in an extended gestation period. Furthermore, young age marriage prevents people from receiving the necessary education and awareness to be sensitive to and grasp the effects of having too many children. According to a UN report, delaying marriage legalization for 20 years would significantly reduce the global population.

Medical Facilities

One of the significant disadvantages of developing countries is the scarcity of medical services. The availability of good hospitals and doctors is limited in developing nations due to the vast rural-urban divide, resulting in a high infant mortality rate in rural areas. Rural people give birth to more and more children to ensure that at least some of their children survive, leading to population expansion. The population rate will undoubtedly decrease if the best medical facilities are available.

Legislative Actions

If family planning and contraception remain optional rather than mandatory, little progress will be made. To reap significant benefits, strict legislative actions are required for child marriage, schooling, prohibiting child labor and beggary, and family planning. Child labor, slavery, and beggary laws that are adequately enforced will prevent parents from selling or sending their children to work, compelling them to raise fewer children.

Providing Incentives

Incentives are an effective policy tool for addressing most development challenges, including population. A highly effective population measure is to provide health, education, or even a financial incentive. There are specific incentive policies in most developing countries facing population-related challenges, such as paying a certain amount of money to people with no more than two children or providing free or discounted education to single children, etc., which have proven to be practical measures.

Spread Awareness

The implications of having too many children must be explained and clarified. Government and non-government organizations can run public awareness campaigns to tell people how having too many children mean they won't be able to provide sufficient nutrition, education, or medical care. Malnutrition and its negative repercussions must be presented to the general people to increase their reasoning and understanding.

Women Empowerment

In most developing countries, women are not considered equivalent to men in force and might. Such opinions are prevalent in Islamic countries and even India and Bangladesh. Gender discrimination is a primary reason for population growth. People keep giving birth to kids to have more sons than daughters. Empowering women with a say in childbirth and educating them to fight against discrimination will ensure a healthy and aware society.

Eradicate Poverty

Why are developing countries experiencing the fastest population growth rather than developed countries? Poverty and population increase are inextricably linked. Child labor, slave trade, and human trafficking are common in Asia and Africa's emerging nations. Slave selling is illegal everywhere globally, yet African countries, for example, continue to have the highest reporting levels. People give birth to children and then sell them to wealthy individuals who employ them in different arduous and unethical tasks. If not sold, these parents force their children to beg or work for a pittance to supplement the family's income. These individuals believe having more children means having more hands available for begging and work, hence more money. Other population control approaches may be ineffectual unless concrete measures for growth and poverty eradication are implemented.

Education

An individual's and the economy's backbones are formed by education. People who have been educated know the dangers of rapid population increase. Education, particularly women's education, can hugely impact population control. A well-educated man or woman can easily comprehend the advantages of a small household. Most efforts, such as awareness campaigns and women empowerment, will be ineffective and worthless if insufficient education exists.

Easy and Cheap Availability of Contraceptives

Providing people with accessible and affordable access to contraception can assist in preventing undesired pregnancies and births. Because impoverished individuals do not have the means or awareness to utilize contraception, every state-owned hospital should provide low-cost, effective birth control drugs or surgery.

Contraceptives and Condoms must be advertised and promoted, and they must be inexpensive and readily available. Contraceptives are a vital population control measure because they reduce the spread of sexually transmitted illnesses such as AIDS, resulting in small, healthy households.

Development

The most significant issues facing Africa and Asia's developing countries are their massive populations and growth rates. At the same time, countries such as America, Europe, and Japan face little or no threat. Lack of development is associated with high poverty, illiteracy, discrimination, a lack of awareness, and a lack of medical services, which contribute to higher population growth. Any modern economy has a population that is non-discriminatory and just. The difficulty of population increase could be eliminated by reducing gender and class inequality and ensuring the development of the entire population rather than a specific part of society.

10.2 POVERTY

LEARNING OBJECTIVES

- ☞ Explain the concept of poverty.
- ☞ What are the causes of poverty?
- ☞ Which factors are responsible for poverty?
- ☞ Suggest remedial measures for the eradication of poverty.

■ INTRODUCTION

Poverty is relative to richness. The sting of poverty is only felt when people resent their situation compared to others. They cannot achieve more than they have, and this failure produces animosity against poverty. People are impoverished not because of increased hardship but because of a resentful attitude toward what they lack and what others have. When people feel deprived of what others have and enjoy, they think of themselves as poor. Poverty becomes a social problem at this point.

Poverty is the most crucial problem for rural people in India. The vast majority of our villagers live below the poverty line. Rural sociologists like Sorokin and Zimmerman have held that about 30% of rural people worldwide are poverty-stricken. In India, it is much more.

CONCEPT OF POVERTY

- According to Gillin and Gillin, "Poverty is the condition in which a person, either because of inadequate income or unwise expenditure, does not maintain a scale of living high enough to provide his/her physical and mental efficiency and to enable him/her and his/her natural dependents to function usually according to the standards of the society of which he/she is a member."
- According to TG Goddard, "Poverty is an insufficient supply of those things, which are requisite for an individual to maintain himself/herself and those dependents upon him in health and vigor."

Somebody else has defined poverty as a condition of chronic insufficiency. Further, it is a condition in which a person cannot lead a life according to the desired standard of society.

There are two types of poverty, namely:
1. Abject poverty
2. Relative poverty

Abject poverty is when a person has nothing to eat or put on or have no proper housing. *Relative poverty* means that a person lacks certain things compared with others in a particular society.

For example, poverty in the United States (different from India) may mean that a person does not have as many cars or television sets as others in that society.

CAUSES OF POVERTY

Some of the important causes are mentioned here.

Landlessness: Land is the chief means of production for a rural man. Many ruralites in India do not possess any land; they are called landless agriculturalists. They work as agricultural laborers and are engaged in some other non-agricultural occupations. They are very poor. The wages they receive are also meager.

Sickness: Chronic ailments like malaria, tuberculosis (TB), and other diseases make the villagers weak and physically incapable of working. No proper medical treatment is available in most of the villages.

Illiteracy and ignorance: It makes rural people lead a life of superstitions and inefficiency. Others can easily exploit illiterate, uneducated people, including moneylenders, government officials, and traders.

Extravagancy: These are non-essential items of expenses. Much money is spent on shraddhas, festivals, marriages, and pilgrimages.

Unhealthy habits: Bad habits like drinking and smoking make the villagers poor.

Natural calamities: Famine, pestilences, floods, and earthquakes are the natural calamities that destroy the life and property of rural people. These make them destitute.

Unemployment and underemployment: Non-agricultural people in the villages face unemployment very often. Farmers are underemployed. Agriculture is a seasonal occupation and is wasted most of the year. There is no work between the time of sowing and harvesting.

Exploitation by the elite groups: The moneylenders, wealthy farmers, middlemen, or even government officials like 'patwaris' or 'tehsildars' often exploit poor villagers.

Overpopulation: Birth control methods are not yet fully used in our villages. While most educated urban people take to family planning, most rural people do not, with the result that the rural population is fast increasing. There is overcrowding in the villages. Subdivision and fragmenting of land make the holding of land uneconomical. Lack of supporting industries, lack of facilities for transportation, poor marketing system, and defective social organization cause poverty.

■ FACTORS RESPONSIBLE FOR POVERTY

Poverty is caused by three things, according to the Gillins:
1. The individual's incapacity may be due to faulty heredity or the environment.
2. Unfavorable physical conditions include insufficient natural resources, lousy climate and weather, and epidemics.

3. Inequitable wealth and income distribution, as well as the ineffectiveness of our economic institutions. The last two elements are primarily responsible for India's poverty. Our country is endowed with natural resources, but we have yet to exploit them fully.

 REMEDIAL MEASURES FOR ERADICATION OF POVERTY

Some of the remedial measures for poverty eradication in rural India are below.

Agricultural development: Better farming, redistribution of land, development of animal husbandry, poultry, and small cottage industries suiting the rural environment are needed.

Development of supporting occupations: Facilities for supplementary employment, such as handicrafts, weaving, and pottery, may be helpful.

Spread of education: Education should be made compulsory, at least up to high school standards. This will broaden rural people's outlook and help them adopt better lifestyles.

Family welfare programs should be intensified at the village level to avoid unwanted births and reduce the burden of overpopulation.

Fixing minimum wages: As in the factory, minimum wages should be set for agricultural labor and implemented.

Better marketing facilities: A farmer should get a reasonable price for his produce. Cooperative societies can be beneficial in this regard.

Redistribution of land: The unequal land distribution should be changed so that some justice is done concerning land ownership and use. The land already in people's ownership should be in their actual possession and use. All exploitation in this regard should be stopped.

Rural electrification: Even now, some villages are not electrified. Electricity is needed for irrigation and house lighting.

Other skills: Like social security schemes, implementation of all legislation and rules, and regulations concerning rural people. Social security schemes such as unemployment allowances, old-age pensions, and sickness assistance may be complex in a country like

India, where most people live in villages. However, some measures must be introduced, like compulsory insurance for human beings, animals, crops, and assistance in sickness and old age.

Many poor people cannot change their situation unless economic progress occurs. Drastic economic reforms are necessary. Our progress has fallen short of the goals we set for ourselves. There are numerous ailments. Bureaucratization, excessive industrial control, undue priority given to the public sector without assuring its profitability, and a lack of clear political leadership due to a fractured mandate have set the country back compared to many emerging nations.

10.3 UNEMPLOYMENT AND UNDEREMPLOYMENT

LEARNING OBJECTIVES

- ☞ What is the concept of unemployment?
- ☞ Describe the types and causes of unemployment.
- ☞ Describe the remedies for unemployment.
- ☞ Define underemployment and its types.
- ☞ What are the causes of underemployment and its effects on society?

▆ INTRODUCTION

Unemployment and underemployment are serious problems for the villagers in India. Millions of rural people in India are unemployed, as well as underemployed. These have several causes and effects. We must control and prevent much unemployment in our villages, though complete success may be a Utopia.

▆ CONCEPT OF UNEMPLOYMENT

- "Unemployment is a labor market condition in which labor supply exceeds the number of available openings."
- "Unemployment is a state of affairs in which a high number of able-bodied persons of working age are prepared to work but unable to find a job at present wage levels in a country."

Thus, we find that unemployment is a particular condition in a society where people are able and willing to work but cannot find jobs. It is a negative aspect of the economic process; it is enforced or involuntary separation from remunerative work.

Underemployment is a condition of not being fully employed, i.e., the time and capacities of the workers are not fully utilized. For instance, in Indian villages, the farmers worked only for 100–200 days; on the other days, they were idle. There is no supplementary employment. Similarly, educated men and women are employed in jobs much below their qualifications or ability in urban areas. For example, a graduate or postgraduate works as a menial worker or a small office assistant.

TYPES OF UNEMPLOYMENT

There are mainly three types of unemployment:
1. **Seasonal:** This is caused by seasonal changes in production, e.g., in the case of agriculture or work in a dockyard.
2. **Cyclical:** Caused by economic ups and downs. When there is economic depression, there is much unemployment.
3. **Normal:** This unemployment is the inevitable concomitant of any economic system based upon a free labor market, as we find in England, America, or India. Thus, the minimum amount of unemployment is inevitable.

CAUSES OF UNEMPLOYMENT

Some of the leading causes of unemployment in Indian villages are:
- **Population explosion:** The excessive increase in population is the leading factor in unemployment.
- Division and fragmentation of agricultural land: Due to –
  - population increase, the landholding size becomes too small.
  - Seasonal nature of agriculture.
  - Vagaries of climate.
  - Lack of literacy, education, and technical training.
  - Too many festivals, pilgrimages, and other traditional, religious,
  - And cultural activities. These hinder the villagers from working.
- **Chronic diseases:** Chronic ailments make the farmers unfit for work; inadequate medical facilities keep the villagers sick for extended periods.

REMEDIES OF UNEMPLOYMENT

Preventing unemployment or underemployment in Indian villages is difficult, looking at the magnitude of the problem, aggravated by population increase, poverty, and illiteracy. However, we may suggest the following remedies.

Land reclamation, conservation, and improvement: Though the country is overpopulated, much land remains unused, as they need reclamation and improvement. If all wasteland is used, more land will be cultivated, creating more employment.

Improvement in the agricultural system: Better seeds, manure, pesticides, and modern techniques can improve agriculture. This may create more employment avenues.

Other: Development of cottage industries, animal husbandry, poultry farming, food preservation, and fisheries.

Population control: Plays a significant role in India.

Assessment problem: Rural unemployment has not yet been studied scientifically. Therefore, there is a great need for a scientific assessment of rural unemployment, particularly the type of unemployment, the extent of the problem, the age group involved, and causes, and then suggest ways and means to control and prevent the problem of rural unemployment. Mere guesswork will not be sufficient. In this connection, starting employment exchanges in rural areas may also be explored.

Organization of rural labor: While there are several associations and unions to safeguard the interests of urban labor, there is not much in rural India. So, there should be rural labor organizations to promote the welfare of rural labor.

Development of rural areas as a whole: The development of our villages needs the construction of roads, irrigation canals and projects, dams, working of different types of cooperatives, and revival of cottage industries. When such developments occur, underemployment will also be solved to a great extent.

There are millions of people unemployed in India, both urban and rural. The urban unemployed is educated, while those of the rural are illiterate or semi-literate. At the end of the second Five-Year Plan, it was estimated that there were about 20 million unemployed in rural India. This may have doubled now. The evil consequences like poverty, frustration, and revolution result in crimes and social disorganization. Therefore, all efforts must be made to have maximum employment facilities. The Government of India has already announced that the question of payment of unemployment allowance cannot be considered in India.

▣ UNDEREMPLOYMENT

Introduction

Underemployment is the underuse of a worker because a job does not use the worker's skills, is part-time, or leaves the worker idle. Examples include holding a part-time job despite desiring full-time work and over-qualification. The employee has the education, experience, or skills beyond the job requirements.

Underemployment has been studied from various perspectives, including economics, management, psychology, and sociology. In economics, for example, underemployment has three different meanings and applications. All the meanings involve a situation where a person is working, unlike unemployment, where a person searching for work cannot find a job. All implications involve under-utilization of labor which is missed by most official (governmental agency) definitions and measurements of unemployment.

Definition

Underemployment is a measure of labor utilization and employment in the economy that looks at how well the workforce is being utilized in terms of skills, experience, and availability. Highly skilled workers who work in low-paying or low-skill positions are considered underemployed, as are part-time workers who prefer to work full-time. This differs from unemployment in that the individual is employed but not to their full potential.

Underemployed refers to "the condition in which people in a labor force are employed at less than full-time or regular jobs or jobs inadequate for their training or economic needs."

Types of Underemployment

Underemployment is calculated by dividing the number of unemployed people by the total number of workers in a labor force.

There are two types of underemployment:

1. **Visible underemployment** occurs when a person works fewer hours than is required for a full-time job in their chosen field. They work two or more part-time jobs to make ends meet due to the reduced hours.
2. **Invisible underemployment** is the second category of underemployment. It refers to a circumstance in which a person cannot obtain work in their desired field. As a result, they work in jobs that are not a good fit for their skills and, in most cases, pay well below industry standards.

The critical points of underemployment are:

- Underemployment is a measure of labor utilization and employment in the economy that looks at how well the workforce uses skills, experience, and availability.
- It refers to a situation where individuals must work in low-paying or low-skill jobs.
- Visible underemployment and invisible underemployment are forms of underemployment.
- Underemployment can be produced by various factors, from economic recessions to business cycles.

Causes of Underemployment

Several factors can contribute to underemployment. Underemployment occurs when businesses shrink and lay off qualified workers during and after a recession. Underemployment reached an all-time high during the recession that followed the financial crisis.

Another cause of underemployment is changing the job market due to technological shifts. Layoffs can be retrained or retired from the workforce as job descriptions change or are automated. Those who do not have the resources or means to retrain are more likely to be underemployed.

Business cycles can also result in underemployment. Seasonal staffing trends, especially in the hospitality industry, can result in more workers opting for the most straightforward available job and staying on. According to some estimates, nearly half of restaurant workers consider themselves underemployed.

For example, a person with an engineering degree who works as a pizza delivery man is considered underemployed as his primary source of income. In addition, someone who works part-time in an office but would prefer to work full-time is considered underemployed. In both situations, the economy underutilizes these people even if they can contribute more to the economy.

Effects of Underemployment

Underemployment has a tremendous impact on society. Here are three significant consequences of underemployment:

1. Unemployment leads to rising poverty levels because people pay for schools and training but do not acquire jobs that pay off their obligations, let alone pay what they should earn, given their backgrounds and credentials.
2. Unemployment can cause psychological issues in unemployed persons. They may feel stressed and anxious as a result of not being able to make ends meet. Furthermore, they may feel they have squandered their time and money when they cannot put their skills to use.
3. Unemployment can result from underemployment since underemployed workers cannot update their resumes with skills, on-the-job training, etc. This, of course, can make it difficult for them to apply for jobs in the future, and it may even prohibit them from finding another career.

10.4 BEGGARY

LEARNING OBJECTIVES

- ☞ What is beggary? Define beggary.
- ☞ Explain the meaning and concept of beggary.
- ☞ Describe types of beggars.
- ☞ What are the causes of beggary?
- ☞ How can beggary be managed?
- ☞ Suggest measures for eradication of beggary.

▨ INTRODUCTION

Of all social evils today, begging is perhaps the most demoralizing one. It constitutes a very complex socio-economic problem. Beggary is an age-old social evil, and so far as India is concerned, it has assumed a stunning proportion. However, the issue of Beggary does not have an economic dimension; it only has social and moral aspects.

A beggary is a form of personal disorganization because it indicates an individual's failure to adjust to his social milieu. It is a symptom of social disorganization because the beggar in the street immediately reminds us of an unorganized society that cannot adjust to him.

Beggary is a curse for any society, regardless of its condition or circumstances. It is, however, not the only curse for a developing country like India, but also a huge financial burden. India is a beggar's paradise. There are over 500,000 beggars in India, increasing to a few million if we include those who beg occasionally.

Even the foreign press and television have put India to shame by graphically showing pictures of beggars fighting like dogs for a few coins, swarming like bees for food leftover in hotels and restaurants, naked women sleeping on the floor, and children sucking. These scenes show India in very lurid colors.

Beggars contribute to the impoverishment of society. The beggars are the source of disease spreading. The beggar represents a section of society that was rotted and is further petrifying. They spoil the beauty and cleanliness of the environment because they use the streets and pavements as lavatories, resulting in sanitation problems. The beggars are chronically diseased and, physically weak, morally corrupt as a rule.

The beggars of today have adopted Beggary as a profession, it has changed its form in the modern period, and the problem has become colossal. Considering Beggary's social and moral aspects, we cannot help concluding that Beggary must be uprooted from a society that wants to progress. The beggars perform no proper social function; their existence is parasitical. In most cases, the beggars are found to be professionals who otherwise could have earned a decent living. They do nothing except begging and lead a life of horrible moral corruption. Many superstitions and orthodox Indians consider it a moral duty to give charity. However, any intelligent man can readily appreciate that giving charity amounts to society's social and moral cancer perpetuation.

Beggary means 'the state or condition of a habitual beggar.' A beggar begs one who lives by asking for alms. Beggars were found in ancient times. Beggary was a profession or way of life that has come into being in modern times. India is a country where a considerable number of beggars are found. According to one estimate, at least 15 million beggars are in India. These beggars roam around the country and are located at railway stations, bus stands, places of pilgrimage, temples, and mosques. Beggary has become a big nuisance in Indian cities.

Begging is the practice of pleading with others to grant favor with little or no expectation of reciprocation, often a gift of money. A person who does so is called a beggar. Beggars may be found in public places like transit routes, urban parks, and markets. They may also ask for food, drink, cigarettes, or other small items and money.

Internet or online begging is the modern method of asking people to give beggars money, maintaining their anonymity. Internet begging is generally targeted at people who know the beggar, but it may be advertised to strangers.

Internet begging may include requests to help meet basic needs such as medical care and shelter and demands for people to pay for holidays, school trips, and other things the beggar wants but cannot afford comfortably.

There are several causes of Beggary in India. Beggary has serious ill effects too. Further, the incidence of Beggary is steadily on the increase. Therefore all steps ought to be taken to control and remedy the situation.

DEFINITION OF BEGGAR

The Bombay Prevention of Beggars Act defines a beggar as "A person without subsistence wandering about or found in public places, or allowing him to be used as an exhibit to beg."

Beggary is also defined as—soliciting or receiving alms in a public place, whether or not under any pretense such as singing, dancing, fortune-telling, performing or offering any article for sale, entering on any private premises to solicit or receive alms, exposing or exhibiting with the object for obtaining or extorting alms, by showing any sore, wound, injury, deformity or disease; whether of a human being or animal or having no visible means of subsistence and wandering, about or remaining in any public place in such condition or manner.

■ MEANING AND CONCEPT

Beggars have existed in society since the inception of human civilization. Begging is witnessed in almost all cultures around the world. In India, beggars may be begging in crowded places like bus stands, railway stations, marketplaces, and near worship sites. Many religions have prescribed begging as an acceptable means of support for certain classes of adherents, including Hinduism, Islam, Buddhism, Jainism, etc. The religious beliefs provide that the disciples should focus exclusively on spiritual development without the possibility of becoming caught up in worldly affairs.

■ TYPES OF BEGGARS

There are various types of beggars, some of which are described below:

- **Child beggars:** There are vagrant children engaged in begging. They may be poor at home or have stopped school education as dropouts, run away from home, do odd jobs and then beg. Most of these children are between the ages of 10 and 16.
- **Physically handicapped:** They are blind, lame, deaf, and people who have lost their arms or feet owing to accidents or diseases.
- **Mentally sick beggars:** They are lunatics and mentally deficient people, men, and women, who seldom live in their homes.
- **Able-bodied beggars:** They are physically and mentally fit to work but have taken begging as a profession. They do not want to get rid of their habit.
- **Tribal beggars:** This category includes those who have migrated from rural and tribal areas.
- **Religious mendicants:** Religions like Buddhism and Hinduism have encouraged beggaries.
- **Small trade beggars:** Some people are engaged in small trades but occasionally resort to begging.
- **Temporarily unemployed beggars:** Unemployment paves the way to poverty. So when people are rendered jobless, they take to begging.
- **Permanently unemployed:** These fail to secure employment for their livelihood. Although physically and mentally all right, they find it difficult to have proper jobs.

- **Orphans and destitute:** In a country like India, thousands of orphans and destitute. They are helpless. The state does not provide social security facilities to them. Therefore, they take to begging.

CAUSES OF BEGGARY

Every social problem we encounter demands a solution, but a practical solution can be arrived at only by understanding the problem's nature, extent, and root cause. The Beggary is no exception to this rule. While the Beggary in India has always been an object of charitable attention, the beggar issue has seldom been a subject of rigorous scientific inquiry. The practice of asking for alms has become a tremendous socio-economic problem. As with a criminal, it is impossible to attribute a particular cause or set of causes to the institution of beggary.

There is a relationship between the types of beggars and the causes of beggary. Some essential reasons for beggary, especially in India, are the following.

Poverty: Millions of people live in chronic poverty in India. They are found in tribal, rural, and urban centers. There is no exaggeration in saying that at least 50% of our population is poor or has a poor standard of living. Many are in abject poverty, i.e., there is nothing to eat, wear, or live on. Some of them take to begging.

Loss of agricultural employment in villages: Due to overpopulation and fragmentation of land, the ruralities have serious economic problems. There are millions of landless agriculturists in our villages.

Physical defects and diseases: Physical deformities like blindness, deformed legs and hands, hunchback, deafness, and several other conditions make a person unable to work. Similarly, people afflicted with chronic debilitating diseases like TB and malaria also lose their ability to work regularly.

Mental disorders: In a developing country like ours, family members cannot support abnormal persons at home.

Leprosy: This deserves a special mention as a cause of Beggary because many beggars are formed of lepers. Severe stigma is attached to leprosy, and anyone afflicted with it is thrown out on the streets to beg. In India, it is estimated that there are not less than four million leprosy patients.

Children uncared for: Marriage is a universal phenomenon in India. Everybody ought to marry. However, nobody worries about the number of children and the means to bring them up nicely. So, poor children go out of their homes and take to beggary.

Desertion or death: The death of the family is also a cause of beggary.

Natural calamities: Famines, floods, pestilences, and earthquakes turn many orphans and destitute. There are institutions run by the government and non-governmental agencies to take care of them to some extent, but then all cannot be looked after.

Laziness and indifference: Some people do not want to work. They are indifferent to work. They start begging, and then it becomes a habit. Thus, they become habitual beggars.

Cruelty: The unimaginable cruelty of some guardians and other ruthless persons who disfigure, maim, and blind the children, force them to beg and live on their earnings, the destitution of the deserted wife, the helplessness of the widows, the willingness of many parents to use their infirm and disabled children as means of earning more income.

Desire to give alms: Human nature worldwide is to donate to the poor and beggars. Often, it is not realized that we encourage Beggary by providing donations. There are religious, moral, and humanitarian motives behind this. All religions impart their followers to be kind, loving, hospitable, and help the needy. According to Dr Clifford, there are six reasons why people give alms, religious, custom, personal, fear, pity, and carelessness.

■ MANAGEMENT OF THE PROBLEM

Most civilized countries have long ago prohibited begging and declared it an offense. In India also, various states have made legislation against Beggary. Even before independence, Maharashtra, West Bengal, Tamil Nadu, Karnataka, and Kerala have passed acts against Beggary. Legislations are also given in Madhya Pradesh, Punjab, Uttar Pradesh, etc. Police Acts of Bombay, Calcutta, and Madras cities also provide measures against Beggary.

These laws follow a more or less uniform pattern, as shown below:

1. They prohibit and penalize begging in public places.
2. Some classification is made based on the age, and physical condition of the beggar juveniles are taken care of under the provisions of the children act.
3. Most of them are operative in areas notified by the government.
4. All the legislations penalize escape or violation of discipline with imprisonment, fine, or both.

There are state institutions for custody, care, assistance to beggars, and rehabilitation. The inmates of these institutions are provided with food, clothing, sanitation, education, and vocational training. These homes also try to provide religious and moral instructions and facilities for the physical well-being of beggars. Employment facilities are provided so that all non-disabled beggars may learn to work and support themselves.

 SUGGESTIONS FOR THE ERADICATION OF BEGGARY

Legal measures are often inadequate to solve a social problem. Though several acts have been passed against Beggary, we still find hordes of beggars in streets, bus stands, railway stations, religious places, or any other public place where the public is likely to gather. Hence, society has to look for additional measures to prevent the problem. In this connection, some suggestions are given below:

- The law concerning Beggary should be made more stringent and uniform for India. Any beggar found in public should be arrested immediately. The beggars should not be allowed to move from place to place.
- More orphanages, shelter homes, and beggar homes should be established so that orphans, the destitute, and the disabled can receive proper care and protection. Old age homes should be set up so that the citizens may be looked after well. This is especially so in cases where the children do not care for their old parents.
- Any non-disabled persons found begging should be severely dealt with. The names of such persons should be registered and listed. Further, they must be made to work.
- Any person found begging should be fined heavily. He should be sent to a beggar home and made to work.

- Try to educate beggars and develop a sense of self-respect and the dignity of labor.
- The public should be educated not to give alms indiscriminately. By giving alms, we are not helping the person but are encouraging him to become a parasite. If people are interested in donating to the beggars' welfare, they should do so to establish and manage beggars' homes.
- More organized community efforts should be made to eradicate the problem.
- All efforts should be made to create social awareness in public about the problem of Beggary so that a collective effort is made to solve it. The existing legislation against Beggary also should be made known to the public.
- Different states have passed anti-beggary legislation, and the Union Government also contemplates having all-India legislation. However, whatever legislation or rules and regulations are there must be enforced. For example, the Indian railways have prohibited beggars on their premises. However, the maximum number of beggars is found at railway stations and even inside railway compartments. It sometimes makes railway travel very inconvenient.

10.5 JUVENILE DELINQUENCY

LEARNING OBJECTIVES

☞ Describe the concept of juvenile delinquency.
☞ Who is a juvenile?
☞ What are the causes of juvenile delinquency?
☞ Describe the classification for juvenile delinquency.
☞ Which preventive programs can be adopted to eliminate juvenile delinquency?

■ INTRODUCTION

Juvenile delinquency is a criminal activity done by a person under 18 years. These illegal activities have increased rapidly in recent years for many reasons. In most places, juveniles are charged with serious crimes, such as robbery or murder, transferred to criminal courts, and tried as adults. Sometimes prosecutors make this decision or allow transfers requiring a hearing to consider the age and record of the juvenile, the type of crime, and the likelihood that the juvenile court can help the youth. As a result of a strict attitude towards juvenile crime, many countries have revised their juvenile codes to make it easier to transfer juvenile offenders to adult courts.

In short words, juvenile delinquency is participating in illegal activities by minors. A juvenile delinquent is a person under 18 who commits an act that would typically result in an adult being charged and tried. So it is clear that juvenile delinquency is also a part of all those behavioral changes that occur in a person's life while passing the stormy phase of adolescence. However, it is not found in every adolescent. The degree of delinquency varies from one to another, and it remains unnoticed unless and until the particular act becomes society's concern.

Since adolescence is the transitional period of life, one passes through rapid evolutionary changes in one's physical, mental, moral, spiritual, sexual, and social outlook during this phase. They become emotionally unstable, and frequent mood change is observed. It is a period of anxieties, conflicts, worries, and complexities. Therefore, during this period, they do certain things to satisfy their needs, often leading them to become delinquent.

Delinquent children are exceptional children who exhibit significant deviation in their social adjustment and are thus labeled as socially deviant. They display criminal behavior and are punishable under legal procedures. Violation of social norms and values threatens the peace of society and is therefore considered a criminal act. The nature and kind of crime may range from very mild to severe. However, they are all antisocial and are subjected to legal criminal acts.

In this regard, they resemble criminals and antisocial elements. However, legal terminology refers to them as delinquents, not criminals. Juvenile delinquency is a legal term that denotes the act of varying social consequences, from mere naughtiness to major assault punishable by law.

WHO IS A JUVENILE?

A juvenile is someone under the age of 18. A juvenile is a child who has not reached the age at which he, like an adult, can be held legally responsible for his illegal conduct. The juvenile is a child accused of committing a crime through some act or omission on their part.

Juvenile and minor in legal—terms are used in different contexts. The term juvenile refers to young criminal offenders, whereas the term minor refers to legal capacity or majority. The idea of a juvenile differs from one state to another.

CONCEPT OF JUVENILE DELINQUENCY

Sethna states, "Juvenile delinquency (JD) involves wrong doing by a child or young person under an age specified by the law of the place concerned."

According to Robinson, JD is *"Any behavior, which a given community at a given time considers in conflict with its best interest, whether or not the offender has been brought to court."* Thus, JD is an act of a child that is against the norms and values of society and violates the state's law.

Juvenile delinquency is the involvement of a juvenile between the ages of 10 and 17 in illegal activities. When a person deviates from the normal course of social life, his behavior is called 'delinquent.' When a youngster under the age stipulated by a statute demonstrates behavior that may be dangerous to society or himself, he is referred to as a juvenile delinquent. Offenders who are under the age of 18 are classified as juvenile delinquents. A juvenile delinquent is a young individual who is persistently disobedient.

All children, somehow, do something that violates society's norms or the provisions of the law. This may be due to their ignorance. It is not with any intent. However, sometimes the acts of some children become so grave that some action is to be taken against them by the state. For example, some children steal, fight, and indulge in violent activities.

Acts of delinquency may include:
1. Running away from home without the permission of parents.
2. Habitual behavior beyond the control of parents.
3. Spending time idly beyond limits.
4. Use of vulgar language.
5. Committing sexual crime.
6. Visiting gambling centers, etc.

■ CAUSES OF JUVENILE DELINQUENCY

Understanding the causes of juvenile delinquency is critical for preventing young people from engaging in inappropriate, harmful, and illegal behavior. Individual, family, mental health, and substance abuse are four primary risk factors that identify young people as prone to delinquent behavior. A juvenile is frequently exposed to more than one risk factor.

■ INDIVIDUAL FACTORS

Several risk factors are identified with juvenile delinquency. A minor with lower intelligence and who does not receive a proper education is more prone to become involved in delinquent conduct. Other risk factors include impulsive behavior, uncontrolled aggression, and an inability to delay gratification. In many instances, multiple individual risk factors can contribute to a juvenile's involvement in harmful, destructive, and illegal activities.

■ FAMILY FACTORS

Young individuals' development of delinquent behavior is linked to a consistent pattern of family risk factors. A lack of sufficient parental supervision, continuing parental conflict, neglect, and abuse are examples of family risk factors (emotional, psychological, or physical). Parents who disrespect the law and societal conventions are likelier to have children who do the same. Finally, the children that have the least relation to their parents and families are the same ones who participate in unsuitable activities, including delinquent behavior.

■ MENTAL HEALTH FACTORS

Several mental health factors are also seen as contributing to juvenile delinquency. However, it is crucial to remember that a diagnosis of certain types of mental health conditions- primarily personality disorders—cannot be made regarding a child. However, there are precursors to these conditions that can be seen in children and usually manifest as delinquent behavior. A common one is conduct disorder. Conduct disorder is a lack of empathy and disregard for societal norms.

■ SUBSTANCE ABUSE FACTORS

The majority of cases of juvenile delinquency involve substance misuse. There are two patterns in substance abuse and minors. Juveniles today utilize more potent narcotics than they were ten years ago. Second, some youths start using drugs at an earlier age. It has been discovered that primary school children abuse dangerous illegal narcotics. The unlawful use of these illicit or legal substances pushes young people to conduct crimes to earn money for drugs. Furthermore, when using drugs and alcohol, juveniles are significantly more prone to engage in destructive, hazardous, and unlawful actions.

■ CLASSIFICATION OF JUVENILE DELINQUENCY

Hirsch classified them into six groups based on the types of offenses committed:
1. Incorrigibility (for example, disobedience and keeping late hours),
2. Truancy (staying away from school),
3. Larceny (ranging from petty thefts to armed robbery),
4. Destruction of property (both public and private),
5. Violence against individuals or communities, and
6. Sexual offenses range from homosexuality to rape.

■ PREVENTIVE PROGRAMS FOR JUVENILE DELINQUENCY

First, we should identify such juveniles and, after that, give them treatment. They will become a habitual offender if they are not timely approached for therapy and counseling. The most effective way to prevent juvenile delinquency is to assist children and their families as early as possible. Numerous state programs attempt early intervention, and federal funding for community initiatives has allowed independent groups to tackle the problem innovatively.

Delinquency prevention is the broad term used to prevent youth from becoming involved in criminal or other antisocial activities.

Increasingly, governments recognize the importance of allocating resources to avoid delinquency. Preventive services include substance abuse education and treatment, family counseling, youth mentoring, parenting education, educational support, and youth sheltering.

There are two types of programs for preventing juvenile delinquency:

1. **Individual program:** Individual program involves the prevention of delinquency through counseling, psychotherapy, and proper education.

2. **Environmental program:** Environmental program involves employing techniques to change the socio-economic context likely to promote delinquency.

Crime prevention programs use the following two preventive approaches.

1. **Individual program**

   - *Clinical program:* This clinic aims to provide aid through Psychiatrists, Clinical Psychologists, and Psychiatric Social workers to help Juveniles and delinquents understand their personality problems. Taft and England have listed the function of clinics as follows:

     - To participate in the discovery of pre-delinquents.
     - To investigate cases selected for study and treatment.
     - To treat patients by themselves or refer cases to other agencies for treatment.
     - To interest others against psychiatrically oriented types of treatment of behavioral disorders in children.
     - To reveal the community's unmet needs of children.
     - To cooperate in the training of students intending to specialize in the treatment of behavioral problems.

   - *Educational program:* In countries where every child attends school, educational institutions have a huge impact, and preventive programs can be efficiently introduced through schools. Teachers should not discriminate against pupils; they should be treated equally and supplied with moral education, which is extremely beneficial to students' future lives. Moral education is an important aspect for kids who make life decisions. They must comprehend the distinction between right and improper thoughts that benefit them and those that are not.

- *Mental hygiene:* The value of psychotherapy in addressing a mental disturbance cannot be over emphasized to prevent mental conflict and bring about a proper mental adjustment in childhood. Life's mission must be determined, and energies must be directed toward fulfilling the high mission. The development of high sentiments and values in a child also prevents juvenile delinquency.
- *Parent education:* Every community should ensure opportunities for parental education, which will help make good homes, improve the family relationship, and educate and care for children. Some educational programs inform parents on how to raise healthy children.
- *Recreational programs:* Recreational programs curb delinquency. Youth can make friends through recreation programs. Positive companies may help children later. Youth programs may include sports, dancing, music, rock climbing, drama, karate, bowling, and art. Youth energy can be channeled into sports, games, and other healthy activities, reducing delinquency.
  Establishing recreational facilities like sports playgrounds, community centers, concerts, drama, and puppet shows is essential for preventing delinquency and developing social group work and youth groups. Recreational agencies should provide open-air meeting halls and playgrounds for sports and cultural activities in rural areas. Youth organizations and groups/agencies should be responsible for organizing these programs so that juveniles may be kept away from delinquency.
- *Removal of inferiority complex:* Inferiority complex, dread, and apprehension may occasionally cause a child to commit a crime under the mistaken and erroneous belief/impression that he is proving himself. Children deserve to be encouraged to grow into self-assured, positive individuals. Discouragement drags people down in life. They should be prepared to go through numerous ups and downs in life, and their failures should not be condemned. Praise, applause, sympathy, and love should be poured on the child to eliminate the inferiority complex.

2. **Environmental program**
   - *Community programs:* The primary goal of the community program is to reach out to those in need of assistance rather than having them approach employees and agencies. Another

relevance of this program is that the engagement of the local community is regarded as crucial, and the role of professional leadership is tried to be maintained to a minimum.

Clinard has outlined the critical points of these programs as follows:

- Local people will participate in efforts to change neighborhood conditions.
- Moreover, they do not accept an adverse social and physical environment as natural and enviable.
- Because self-imposed modifications in the immediate surroundings will have a significant impact on the resident and, as a result, will last longer.

- *Publicity:* This method can also be very useful in preventing juvenile delinquency. The newspapers, magazines, radio, television, motion pictures, etc., should honestly show juvenile delinquency from a proper perspective. They should also present reports about the juveniles' various wrongs, analyze their true causes, and protect the juvenile against false and misleading reporting. The exact position should be presented and produced before society about their delinquent behavior so that they may be appropriately assessed.

- *Parental love and affection:* The child requires his mother and father's unconditional, instant, and real love, care, and protection. Because of the lack of such affection and care, the child may develop discontent and unhappiness, leading to criminal behavior. As a result, parental love, care, and protection are required to keep the child from committing the crime.

- *Family environment:* Family factors that may influence offenders include parental supervision, the way parents discipline a child, parental conflict or separation, criminal parents or siblings, and the parent-child relationship quality. Many studies have found a strong correlation between a lack of supervision and offenders, which appears to be the most critical family influence on offenders.

CONCLUSION

The question that emerges is, "What should be done?" In the best interests of the delinquent, they should be rehabilitated and integrated back into society as soon as feasible. Furthermore, the state must defend these children's rights and devise reformative methods to instill in their ideals that can socially uplift them and give them renewed confidence to play a productive part in society.

10.6 PROSTITUTION

LEARNING OBJECTIVES

- ☞ Define prostitution.
- ☞ What are the causes of prostitution?
- ☞ What are the types of prostitution?
- ☞ How to prevent and control prostitution?

▣ INTRODUCTION

Prostitution is considered one of the oldest professions. It has existed in all communities in some form or the other. There is mention of prostitution in ancient texts like the Vedas, though it probably developed in the post-Vedic period as an institution. The institution has grown with civilization; it can be said to be a necessary accompaniment to civilized life.

▣ DEFINITION

A prostitute may be defined as "An individual (male or female) who for some kind of reward (monetary or otherwise) or some other forms of personal satisfaction and as a part, or full-time profession, engages in normal or abnormal sexual intercourse with various persons who may be of the same sex or the opposite sex to the prostitute".

From this definition, a prostitute need not be a woman as commonly understood. Anyone who indulges in sexual relations for monetary benefits may be a prostitute. Thus, three essential constituents of prostitution are:

1. Promiscuous sexual relationship.
2. Mercenary basis, whether in cash or kind.
3. Lack of affection or personal interest.

▣ CAUSES OF PROSTITUTION

Many causes are responsible for the occurrence and perpetuation of the problem of prostitution, which is as follows:

Poverty: 'The foundation of prostitution is hunger.' Several studies have shown that 80% of prostitutes enter this profession out of sheer economic necessity. It is the tragedy of women who are illiterate, unfortunate, and poor.

Religious factor: In several places in India, young girls are dedicated to temples as 'devadasis.' They sing and dance during the daytime but are used as prostitutes and concubines by the influential class of the people.

Child widows: In our country, widow remarriage is strictly prohibited. Child marriage was widely practiced in states like West Bengal, Bihar, and Odisha, and child widows were abundant. Once widowed, they were neglected, ill-treated, or even abandoned. Most of these young widows often become prostitutes.

Broken homes and neglected girls: The father or mother abandons the children in many broken homes. Without proper care and guidance, many of them turn to prostitution.

A desire for luxury: Many young women are turned toward prostitution today to lead a life of affluence. Their parent's or husbands' meager salaries or income cannot buy the luxuries they desire, and they often take up prostitution as a part-time activity. Call girls associated with modern hotels are an excellent example of this.

Excessive sexual drive: Some women are hypersexual and crave to fulfill their sexual desire by indulging in prostitution.

Laziness: Prostitution is taken as an easy way to earn money. Lazy women may think of this as an excellent opportunity to make money.

Growth of modern cities: Modern industrial and urban centers facilitate prostitution in many ways. All the cities have a large number of unattached men. Even married men are forced to leave behind their wives because of the housing problem in cities. This bulk of single men is the customers who patronize prostitutes. The anonymity existing in cities facilitates the prostitutes to operate unobtrusively.

Unsatisfactory home and marital life: The poor conditions in the home often drive women to prostitution. Dissatisfaction with sex life may be one-factor pushing women into prostitution.

Mental deficiency: Certain studies have shown that many sex offenders and prostitutes have poor intelligence. Women of poor intelligence may be easily exploited and misled.

Enticement by antisocial elements: Since prostitution is a lucrative trade, many intermediaries may lure young women into prostitution. In several cities, brothels employ pimps who bring customers and more women into the profession.

Demand for prostitution: Probably the most crucial reason for prostitution is its demand. Various types of men patronize prostitutes. The unmarried men, old bachelors, widowers dissatisfied with their marital relations, those who desire variety, and men with excessive and perverted sex urge all go to prostitutes. If there is no demand for prostitution from men, this profession cannot continue. In other words, men and their needs are mainly responsible for perpetuating this trade.

TYPES OF PROSTITUTE

Prostitutes can be classified into two major groups: The overt group and the clandestine group. The overt group includes those who live in brothels. The clandestine (secret) prostitutes have a wide variety of women who enter into sexual relationships for mercenary considerations. They may be women employed in several occupations, students, or married women, who use sex to procure monetary benefits. They usually have a restricted clientele. Modern facilities like posh hotels and telephone network help their operations.

PREVENTION AND CONTROL OF PROSTITUTION

The measures to be adopted to fight this vice may be grouped into four:
1. Preventive
2. Prohibitory
3. Prophylaxis
4. Legislation

Preventive Measures

- Facilities for vocational and moral training for women of lower economic stratum should be provided

- As far as possible, women workers should not be retrenched from jobs
- Rescue homes, shelter homes, and other facilities should be provided for the destitute women; girls who are in danger should be put in reformatories or institutions where they can be kept safe from the clutches of antisocial elements; in these institutions, facilities for vocational training should be provided, so that girls will be economically independent
- Males should be taught to respect women folk and not to exploit them sexually
- Unhealthy social customs such as 'devadasis' should be abolished completely
- There should be sex education at school and college levels; girls should be taught in their curriculum the danger of sex exploitation by males
- Social education and propaganda also are essential measures to fight this evil; a healthy public opinion should be created against illicit sex relations
- Pornographic literature and obscene films should be banned entirely
- The existing legislation against prostitution should be adequately and realistically implemented.

Prohibitory Measures

Medical examinations of all prostitutes should be conducted frequently. Any woman, who is found to be infected, should be segregated immediately and should not be allowed to receive customers till she is cured. The Licensing system for prostitutes will be helpful if the law permits it. This licensing will facilitate help constantly check over them. Medical personnel dealing with prostitutes should be specially trained. Compassionate, efficient, and accessible care should be provided to prostitutes because many are very poor and helpless. Many of the brothels are situated near marketplaces or industrial areas. No prostitution should be allowed in or near the workingmen's residences or educational institutions. Employment of women in hotels and similar institutions should be under close supervision.

Prophylactic Measures

The prophylactic measures include the prevention of communicable diseases and improving hygienic conditions. Many of the brothels are dirty and overcrowded. The prostitutes and the customers should be instructed to use protective measures. Males may use condoms, and females can use chemical disincentives after exposure. These will prevent the communication of venereal diseases. Young men should be educated to practice celibacy and develop healthy recreation habits.

Legislative Measures

There is a good deal of opinion about the efficacy of legislation in combating vice-like prostitution. Legislation alone may not be effective. Industrialization, the growth of unhealthy slums, the excess of the male population in urban centers, employment of female labor in the factories and workshops in unhealthy social environments, poverty, and alcoholism all demand proper attention to prevent the problem of prostitution. The development of a single standard of ethics for men and women, education and economic freedom of movement, widow remarriage, and the establishment of rescue and destitute homes are all measures to be considered for preventing moral danger to women.

According to the law, prostitution is not an offense where both parties to the act are adults and no fraud or force has been used. It is regarded as a personal affair beyond law cognizance. The Indian law concerns prostitution when it offends public decency or its practice amounts to public nuisance.

▮ REHABILITATION OF PROSTITUTES

Rehabilitation of those prostitutes who want to quit their profession is crucial. We cannot expect these unfortunate women to leave their ways unless and until society welcomes them back and offers them shelter, protection, and assurance. Adequate arrangements should be in place to train them in other jobs and educate them, particularly younger women.

Older women should be assisted through social security schemes and free medical assistance. If prostitutes have children, the state should take care of them. Especially girls should be protected because they should not follow in their fallen mothers' footsteps.

CONCLUSION

Prostitution is a case of sexual gratification where the commodification of female sexuality leads to the devaluation and objectification of women. Prostitution today results from the disappointment and unsatisfied desires of young men and women who find it convenient to enter this relationship for money. Studies in various parts of the country show a very high percentage of sexually transmitted diseases among prostitutes.

10.7 ALCOHOLISM

LEARNING OBJECTIVES

- ☞ What is alcoholism?
- ☞ What are the characteristics of alcoholism?
- ☞ How does one become an alcoholic?
- ☞ Describe the symptoms of alcoholism.
- ☞ List the causes of alcoholism.
- ☞ How to control and eradicate the problem of alcoholism?

INTRODUCTION

Alcoholism is not only a moral issue or a form of deviant behavior. It is also a deadly and costly disease. The victim of alcoholism needs systematic treatment from specialists such as psychiatrists, doctors, social workers, and family members. These are the people who will help the victim to reconstruct his personality. A physiotherapist/ nurse should consider an alcoholic person as a patient who needs treatment and rehabilitation.

WHAT IS ALCOHOLISM?

Alcoholism is a condition in which the individual has lost control over their intake of alcohol, and they cannot refrain from drinking once they begin **(Fig. 10.2)**. Drinkers may be broadly classified into two groups:

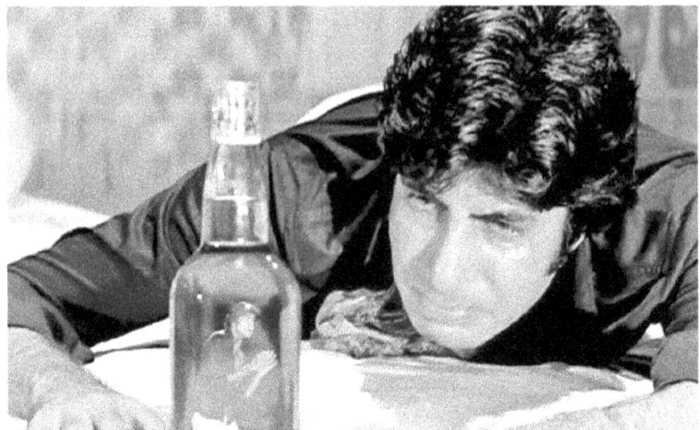

Fig. 10.2: Dramatic presentation of an alcoholic.

1. Moderate drinkers who consume alcohol moderately and their drinking habit does not cause much problem.
2. Problem drinkers: According to Durfee, A problem drinker is one if, as a result, of drinking, his health is endangered, his peace of mind affected, his home life made unhappy, his business jeopardized, and his reputation clouded, and drinking has become his routine.

Richard Waskim says, *"An alcoholic is a compulsive drinker."* Further, *"an alcoholic is an excessive drinker whose dependence upon alcohol has reached such a degree that it results in a noticeable mental disturbance or interference with his bodily and mental health, his interpersonal relations and his smooth social, and economic or one who shows the early signs of such developments."* Thus, an alcoholic is different from an *'occasional'* or *'social'* drinker.

Also, alcoholism is defined as an illness in which the sufferer experiences a strong need for alcohol, a loss of control during limiting alcohol intake, developing tolerance, and needing more alcohol to get the same effect. If he tries to withdraw from drinking, he sees withdrawal symptoms.

■ CHARACTERISTICS OF ALCOHOLISM

The following four characteristics are identified:
1. Excessive intake of alcoholic beverages.
2. Individuals increasingly worry over his drinking.

3. Loss of drinker's control over his drinking.
4. The disturbance in his functioning in his social world.

▪ PROCESS OF BECOMING ALCOHOLIC

A drinker or an alcoholic person is not born. It is one's socio-cultural milieu that leads one to initiate the act of drinking. It is a process that has the following stages.

Prealcoholic symptomatic phase: In this phase, an individual starts drinking to reduce tension and solve his problem.

Prodigal phase: In this phase, along with the increase in the frequency of drinking, there is an increase in the quantity of drinks. However, there is a 'guilt feeling.'

Crucial phase: In this phase drinker's habit of drinking becomes conspicuous. However, he develops rationalization to face social pressure and assure himself that he has not lost control over himself. Nevertheless, his physical and social deterioration becomes evident to everyone.

Chronic phase: The alcoholic starts drinking even in the morning during this phase. He is experiencing prolonged intoxication, impaired thinking, indefinable anxieties, tremors, and skill loss. He is constantly thinking about drinking and feels restless when he is not drinking.

▪ ALCOHOLISM SYMPTOMS

Alcoholism can be mild, moderate, or excessive. The three conditions will exhibit symptoms accordingly. The more severe the symptoms, the more critical the condition of alcoholism is signs and symptoms of this condition include:

- Inability to control alcohol intake
- Inability to cut down on intake despite several attempts
- Wanting to cut down on how much one drinks or attempting to do so
- Despite physical and social harms, continuing to drink alcohol
- Spending a considerable time drinking
- Failing to fulfill work or home responsibilities
- Reducing social activities

- Consuming alcohol in unsafe situations, such as when driving
- Needing more quantity of alcohol to reproduce a similar effect
- Experiencing nausea, sweating, and shaking (withdrawal symptoms) when you avoid drinking, delay or stop it
- Excessive alcohol intake can affect one's speech, muscle coordination, and brain. It may also prove life-threatening to the patient.

Drinking excess alcohol can lead to the following health problems:
- **Liver disease:** Drinking excess alcohol can lead to fat in the liver (hepatic steatosis), inflammation of the liver (alcoholic hepatitis), or irreversible destruction and scarring of liver tissue (cirrhosis).
- **Heart problems:** Alcoholism may cause high blood pressure and increase the risk of an enlarged heart, heart failure, or stroke.
- **Digestive problems:** Alcoholism can cause inflammation of the stomach lining (gastritis) and stomach and esophageal ulcers. It can also hinder the absorption of nutrients and lead to inflammation of the pancreas.
- **Diabetic complications:** Alcoholism can increase the risk of low blood sugar (hypoglycemia).
- **Congenital disabilities:** Alcoholism may lead to miscarriage or physical and developmental problems in the child.
- **Increased risk of cancer:** The risk of cancer in the mouth, throat, liver, colon, and breast increases with excessive alcohol consumption.
- **Weakens immunity:** Alcoholism can weaken the immune system, making the person more prone to various illnesses, especially pneumonia.
- **Neurological complications:** Alcoholism can affect the nervous system, causing numbness, disordered thinking, dementia, and short-term memory loss.

CAUSES OF ALCOHOLISM

One thing should be clear about those who drink, 90% are not alcoholics. Some become alcoholics because of anyone or a cluster of the following reasons:
- Environmental pressures – social, cultural, etc.
- Peer pressure
- Authoritarianism

- A dominant subculture
- Over rejection–emotional pressure
- Success worship.

The current approach to handling the problem of alcoholism is to understand the problem in terms of character and motivation. An alcoholic is seen as a sick person. Their personality is a victim of self-destruction. Hence, they need proper treatment rather than condemnation and blame.

Suggestions for Controlling and Eradicating the Problem

- Alcoholism is found among industrial workers, agricultural laborers, and those in strenuous manual occupations. This alcoholism is more so in India. The working conditions are to be improved if the problem is eradicated.
- Mass education should be provided through various means of communication about the evils of drinking. Public lectures, film shows, songs, radio, and television should be adopted to convince the people.
- Recreational facilities should be provided. Healthy recreation will divert people's minds and keep them away from the habit of drinking.
- Brothels should be away from the residence of industrial workers. It is said that wine and women usually go together.
- Workers are given housing by management or the government to bring their families to the cities where men work. Family living might help keep people away from evil habits.
- High officials in the administration should not indulge in drinking. If found drunk, anyone in a responsible position should be seriously dealt with because the senior responsible people should set an example before others. Here, it may be mentioned that a study abroad showed that "the higher the education one has, the stronger the possibility of one's being a habitual drinker or consumer of more alcoholic beverages than the one with lower education."
- The practice of serving drinks at parties should be banned.
- Women should undertake anti-drinking movements, for women are the worst sufferers if men drink and behave irresponsibly.

- Early detection and treatment of addicts: In several cities, now de-addiction services are available. Parents, spouses, or other close relatives should take the addict to such places and help them get treatment. It is their responsibility to rehabilitate the addict and help them get readjusted in life. Without family support, this cannot be achieved.
- The Central and State governments, local self-government, and private agencies should see that stopping the production, sale, and consumption of alcohol imposes complete prohibition. The economic loss caused by this due to the loss of revenue should be gained through other means. It will be a vicious circle if we say that we cannot impose prohibition, as we will lose revenue through excise duty or license fees. The constitutional provision of implementing a ban throughout India should be put into actual effect.

10.8 PROBLEMS OF EMPLOYMENT AND HEALTH OF WOMEN

LEARNING OBJECTIVES

- ☞ How are biological, social, and cultural factors influence women's health?
- ☞ Describe the social factors affecting women's health.
- ☞ How sexual health affects women's health?
- ☞ How do life stages affect women's health?
- ☞ What are the issues of working women in third-world nations?
- ☞ How sex ratio and life expectancy is affecting women's health?
- ☞ What are the effects of work or employment on women's health, and what can be done about this?

▦ INTRODUCTION

The health of Indian women is intrinsically linked to their status in society. Women's health concern is influenced by interrelated biological, social, and cultural factors. *Understanding the multifaceted character of women's health has led to increased acceptance of the impact of social, cultural, and economic variables on women's health. There is mounting evidence that women are more vulnerable to these issues. Furthermore, some health concerns impact women disproportionately or are unique to women.*

Women's changing roles have also had an impact on their health. Despite contributing significantly to household income, many women continue to bear primary responsibility for the care of the family, particularly its health.

Most poor people are women, emphasizing their economic vulnerability and the health hazards of inadequate diet and housing. Indeed, the link between women's health and concerns like poverty, powerlessness, discrimination, and fertility is well established.

Major life transitions such as pregnancy, motherhood, and menopause can create physical and emotional stress for women. Negative life experiences—infertility and perinatal loss, poverty, discrimination, violence, unemployment, and isolation—also impact women's mental health and well-being. Unequal economic and social conditions also contribute to women's higher risk of depression.

Women's roles in the workforce vary by society's structure, needs, customs, and attitudes. Women and men hunted and gathered food in prehistoric times. Agricultural communities shifted women's work to the home. They cooked, sewed, and cared for children while plowing, harvesting, and tending animals. Women sold or traded goods as cities grew.

In industrial nations, the proportion of women in the labor force is rising, family responsibilities are decreasing (due to smaller families and technological innovation in the home), and more middle- and upper-income women are working for pay.

SOCIAL FACTORS AFFECTING WOMEN'S HEALTH

The social factors impacting women's health vary according to society and economic growth. Factors such as various roles, discrimination, and sexual health influence women's health in India, as in other modern cultures. The research being conducted on the impact of women's many roles emphasizes the complexities of the results on their health (**Fig. 10.3**).

Some studies demonstrate that women who are employed and are married parents have the healthiest profile. However, women's physical symptoms and diseases are unaffected by their role status.

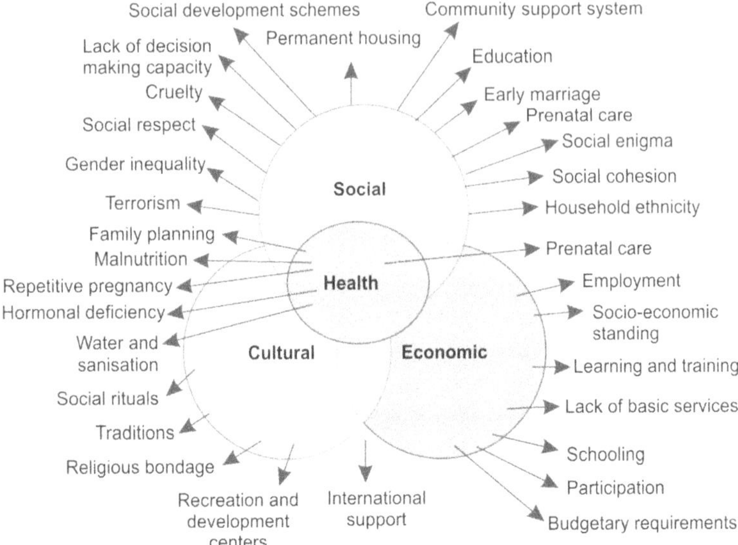

Fig. 10.3: Major issues related to women's health, social, cultural, and economic development.

Discrimination is an example of a more unfavorable societal factor impacting women's health. In terms of working conditions and salary, women face discrimination in the workplace. Employment policies can also harm health. Maternity leave is an example of such a policy, which, while intended to shield women from wrongful dismissal, typically leads to lower breastfeeding rates. This practice may have special repercussions for women in India, where, despite the known benefits of nursing for both women and infants, maternity leave is only ten weeks long. This is in contrast to countries such as the United Kingdom, where women enjoy around 19 weeks of paid leave. Changing family patterns due to rising divorce rates and increased single-parent households have contributed to women facing discrimination in acquiring housing and jobs, negatively impacting their psychological health.

Some causes of anxiety and depression in women are:

- **Caring for or supporting others:** Two-thirds of primary caregivers are women who care for partners, parents, and children. Managing paid and unpaid work can affect health, financial security, and independence.

- **Relationship breakdown:** When a relationship fails, it can result in losses in all areas of life, including financial security, social ties, housing, and relationships with children. As a result, separated, divorced, or widowed women are more prone to suffer from mental health problems such as despair and anxiety. It is normal to feel disturbed or depressed once a relationship ends – or to lose interest in your specific interests. When these feelings linger and begin interfering with your everyday life, you must talk to someone about how you feel and seek help.

- **Violence or abuse:** To maintain good mental health and well-being, women must feel safe and respected in their relationships. Violence and assault, as well as emotional, physical, and sexual abuse, have severe repercussions on the health and well-being of women. Depression and anxiety, drug and alcohol abuse, suicidal thoughts or attempts, and post-traumatic stress disorder are examples. Women frequently stay in relationships that bring them great grief and misery out of fear and a conviction that there are no other options.

- **Discrimination based on sexuality or gender identity:** Lesbian, bisexual, and other sexual women had greater rates of depression and anxiety than heterosexual women. If these women face prejudice, marginalization, bullying, and abuse, they are more likely to commit suicide or self-harm. If they do not have family or community support, they are more likely to develop mental health problems. Transgender women and other gender-varied persons have been demonstrated to have higher rates of anxiety, despair, and suicidal ideation due to hurdles to assistance, discrimination, and isolation.

SEXUAL HEALTH

Sexual health issues have major implications for women's health status **(Fig. 10.4)**. Contraception—a fundamental right of all women—has transformed the health of many women who now have control over their fertility. However, their choice of delaying pregnancies has led to infertility and associated psychological morbidity among some women.

Sexual health includes sexually transmitted infections (STIs), such as human immunodeficiency virus infection (HIV). The

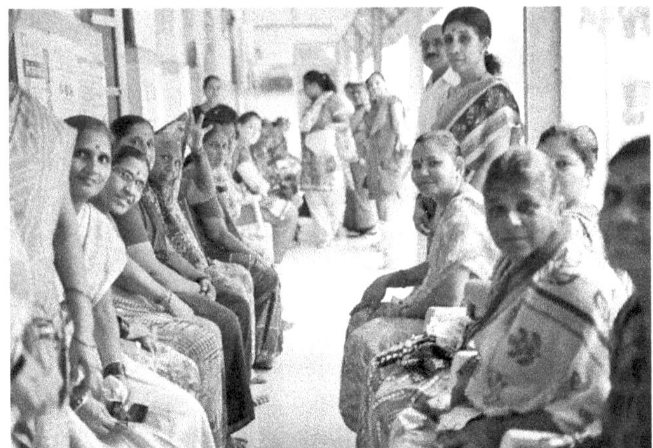

Fig. 10.4: Women seeking healthcare outside a hospital in India.

similarities between STIs and HIV infection in terms of behavior, transmission, and control measures highlight the importance of HIV infection to women's health, particularly given the steady increase in the number of newly reported infections among women and the fact that heterosexual relationships are the most common mode of transmission.

Cervical cancer, which claims thousands of lives in India each year, is another factor to consider in the context of sexual health. Cervical cancer is an example of the implications of poor sexual health for women, and it may be of special interest to healthcare practitioners because many have the opportunity to discuss these issues with women during screening programs or opportunistically.

The main issue is that women are unaware of the significance of cervical screening to their sexual health. Women who are sexually active but do not have children usually indicate that they are too busy to have a cervical smear. However, as women became parents of small children, their acknowledged responsibility for their children indicated that they were more likely to attend the screening.

Women want more information about the screening method and are unhappy with what's offered. Their lack of knowledge was due to information provided at the clinic and in the media, which did not sufficiently emphasize the importance of cervical screening. The absence of information also affected women's attendance habits, making them unaware of the importance of regular cervical smears and relying on practitioners' advice to return for more smears. Some women's views on the disease and screening method are revealing. Because of a lack of knowledge, the disease has been associated with promiscuity. Although having multiple sexual partners is a risk factor, many women are unaware that being sexually active raises their risk. Embarrassment over the screening procedure and fear of discomfort and agony affect women's attendance. Indeed, a practitioner's technical ability to reduce pain and interpersonal and communicative skills to reduce anxiety and shame are important.

The third point to consider is age and the unique needs of older women. Although younger women have identified rising age as a risk factor, many older women are unaware of any increased danger with age. Furthermore, many women may believe they are no longer in danger after menopause.

Another important issue relates to older women's lack of knowledge about their cervical smear status. Although many of these women have children and have undergone gynecological examinations, they have little knowledge about what is involved in the investigation or whether they have undergone cervical smear screening. These women are, however, keen to receive information about screening so they can make an informed decision about their attendance pattern.

Some of these factors also affect women's health and well-being:

- **Infertility and perinatal loss:** Infertility and miscarriage are everyday experiences for women. Some people's desire to be parents is unfulfilled. One in every six couples has infertility, one in every four recognized pregnancies ends in miscarriage, and one in every 100 births results in stillbirth or newborn mortality. These losses can devastate the emotional and mental health of women who want to be mothers. Grief over these losses is generally secret and rarely acknowledged. Without acknowledgment or assistance, a woman may feel lost and alone, thus impacting her mental health. Speaking with someone a woman can trust is essential for preserving mental health during the difficulties and anguish of infertility and perinatal bereavement.

- **Pregnancy, having a baby, and becoming a mother (perinatal):** Depression and anxiety are common in pregnancy and after childbirth. 1 in 10 pregnant women and 1 in 6 postpartum women experience depression. Many women experience both conditions simultaneously. Adjusting to this major life change and coping with early motherhood's daily challenges can make some women more prone to depression or anxiety, especially if they've experienced it before.

- **Menopause:** Menopause increases mental health issues. Perimenopause hormone fluctuations cause mood swings, irritability, sadness, and anxiety. Hormonal changes can cause hot flushes, night sweats, disrupted sleep patterns, and weight gain, affecting mental health.

  Menopause can occur when duties and relationships change. Some raise children, help adults and children live independently, or care for the elderly. Many people have more job opportunities and responsibilities now.

  Surgical or early menopause increases depression risk. A doctor should check mental and physical health. Help is available. Healthy eating, staying active, and doing what one enjoys is essential for menopause wellness.

■ EFFECTS OF LIFE STAGES ON WOMEN'S HEALTH

The health needs of women differ through the stages of their lifecycles. Physical and social circumstances, starting before birth and continuing through childhood, influence physical health and the ability to maintain health. Key transition points in women's lives are important in developing good or poor health. These include pregnancy and childbirth, school entry, puberty, workforce entry, partnering, menopause, leaving the paid workforce, and widowhood.

Health issues may be more relevant to women's lives at varying stages. For example, young women and risky behavior; mid-age women and sexual and reproductive health; and older women and recognition of how social isolation, caring role, and financial insecurity can impact health.

This makes age-appropriate health information and health promotion material particularly important. Transition points are opportunities to target health promotion material.

- **For young women**, pressures to achieve academically and socially and conform to stereotypes about appearance can push them into risky behavior, including high-risk drinking, unprotected sex, and unhealthy body image. Young women are experiencing high rates of smoking and violence, as well as obesity and overweight, which are increasing amongst young women at a higher rate than in past generations. The increasing rates of sexually transmitted infections, such as chlamydia, amongst young women, have the potential to impact fertility later in life. Mental health issues are a particular concern for young women.

- **Pregnancy, managing fertility, and having children are prominent issues for women in their reproductive years.** The age of first birth is getting older in India. There is a need for education about fertility and the reproductive system to help Indian women understand the factors that may impact their fertility and their baby's health during pregnancy (such as obesity, smoking, alcohol, STIs, and maternal nutrition).

  Women going through the transition to becoming a mother can experience mental health issues. Support services are vital at this life stage, especially concerning antenatal support, to address issues such as postnatal depression.

  Balancing work and family commitments can substantially influence women's physical and emotional health, especially because women continue to bear more caring responsibilities.

- **For women in mid-life**, symptoms of menopause and other life-stage factors can affect women's mental and physical health. It is a time of transition physically and can be in different ways, with children reaching adulthood and gaining independence and aging parents requiring care.

  Several health issues are particularly important to mid-age women, including mental disorders, musculoskeletal diseases, and breast cancer. Anxiety and depression are leading burdens of illness for adult women. Intimate partner violence is a leading burden for females up to 44 years of age.

- **Older women** are more likely than men to be widowed, live alone or in residential care, experience financial insecurity, more chronic illness, multiple disabilities, and greater health service use. Furthermore, older women are often marginalized or regarded as 'socially invisible.' Violence against older women has been increasing but is still underreported.

Older women experience much higher rates of disability, partially due to the high rates of dementia and musculoskeletal diseases in older women.

■ WORKING WOMEN IN THIRD WORLD NATIONS

Even though women make up more than one-third of the global labor market, they are concentrated in a small number of low-paying conventional jobs. According to ILO data, as countries industrialize, more women gain jobs in various fields.

Africa, Asia, the Middle East, and Latin America have poor agricultural economies. Most women work in fields and markets, but their economic contributions are unrecognized. As men migrate to cities for cash incomes, many rural women support families alone.

Higher female illiteracy than male. High unemployment affects women even in countries with some equality. In India, women's employment is expanding. These women still lack equal access to education and training, especially in nation-building skills.

■ WOMEN AND HEALTH

In India, within the given socio-cultural matrix, women get less access to medical care. Women belonging to lower strata of the socio-economic hierarchy and the rural areas are the victim of this. Women's health is affected by a series of interrelated economic and socio-cultural factors, viz. levels of earnings and educational background, and "the attitudes to marriage, age of marriage, the value attached to fertility and sex of the child, the pattern of family organizations and the ideal role demanded of women by social conventions."

Here we discuss Indian women's health:

Sex Ratio and Life Expectancy

The sex ratio (females per 1,000 males) indicates women's social status. The female population increased from 117 million in 1901 to 321 million in 1981, but the number of females per thousand males is declining. By 1971, there were 930 females per 1,000 males, compared to 972 in 1901. The female-to-male ratio in 1981 was 933 to 1,000.

Despite increased life expectancy for both sexes, the gap is widening. The low female sex ratio and life expectancy are partly due to the differential sex ratio of newborns and the high female mortality rate. Neglect in early childhood, childbirth deaths, and infant mortality contribute to female mortality.

- **Neglect during early childhood:** Girl child neglect begins very early in life. The degree of negligence varies from family to family, depending on their financial situation. However, in most socioeconomic strata, a female youngster is neglected compared to her male equivalent. It has been discovered throughout the country that when a girl child relies on breastfeeding, her chances of survival are substantially higher. Data from many sources reveal that the mortality rate of a female child significantly outweighs that of a male child from infancy to age 15. This can be attributed to several factors.

  Female children are breastfed for significantly less time than their male counterparts. Second, during illness, parents are more concerned about their male offspring. Poor economic conditions frequently exacerbate this carelessness. Finally, female youngster is subjected to heavier task early in life without adequate and healthy food intake. In lower-income homes, the girl kid is often found doing household chores and caring for her younger brothers and sisters.

- **Death during childbirth:** Early marriages expose women to longer childbearing periods. This means more significant health hazards to women and children. Several studies show that teenage mothers are at risk of poor health for themselves and their children. This risk is further enhanced by poor nutrition. Various surveys indicate that women's caloric content is about 1000 calories (per woman per day) which is far less than they expend, whereas men show an 800 calories surplus intake. Women spend much energy working inside and outside the house, and they often get insufficient food. They usually eat after the men and other family members have eaten. This is especially true in joint families in both urban and rural areas. Besides these, lack of knowledge, improper care during the postnatal period, and frequent pregnancies lead to fetal wastage, the birth of a more significant number of low-weight babies, and the death of young pregnant women.

- **Female infanticide and fetal killing:** This refers to killing the infant soon after birth or at the fetus stage. The former is common amongst certain tribes and caste groups, such as the ***Kallars*** of Tamil Nadu. The ***Kallars*** live in abject poverty. They work in illicit liquor distilleries and coconut groves for livelihood, which requires more male hands. The birth of a daughter is a burden for them because not only is there an insufficient occupation for her, but also dowry has to be given for her wedding and other gifts to be given to her husband's family on various occasions after the solemnization of the marriage.

  Fetal killing has been a crucial problem in some urban areas. In a medical diagnostic procedure called Amniocentesis or ultrasound, parents use these two to find out the sex of the fetus, and consequently female fetus is aborted with the help of unethical medical practitioners or quacks.

Early Marriage and Women's Health

Early marriage harms women's health. A large number of adolescent girls marry. It leads to adolescent pregnancy and a variety of physiological issues. In India, 50 percent of teenage girls are introduced to sexual life and reproduction procedures. These pregnant females endanger their lives due to starvation, overburdening of work, illiteracy, and ignorance of sex behavior. These adolescent women account for approximately 10–15% of all births annually. However, most of their newborns are malnourished, have low birth weight, and have a high mortality rate.

Pregnancy and Women's Health

In India, women have 6–7 pregnancies on average, spending around 80% of their reproductive years in pregnancy and lactation. Study shows that pregnant women have a deficiency of 1,100 calories in the low-income groups of people and lactating women 1,000 calories. Women of the lower socio-economic groups gain only around 3–5 Kg during pregnancy, which is far less than the required weight. Anemia in pregnant women accounts for 15-20% of all maternal deaths in India.

Again, the mortality rate is increased because of untrained personnel; who carry out deliveries in rural and urban areas. In most rural areas, medical termination of pregnancy (MTP) services are unavailable. Besides, women are unaware of the MTP Act of 1971, which has made abortion legal. Hence abortions by incompetent persons continue, resulting in abortion-related mortality and morbidity as serious problems.

Effects of Work on Women's Health

Very little information is available about the effects of work on women's health and safety standards. Even though women make up almost half of the workforce in India. There are several industries where women outnumber males. Women are more likely to work part-time or casually, often performing many jobs simultaneously. Women face uncertain work, which has ramifications for reporting accidents and injuries and claiming, let alone receiving, compensation.

It is essential to look at the question of women's health for several reasons:

- Much less is known about the risks that women face;
- Women are concentrated in certain occupations and industries, and therefore certain specific risks apply;
- The legislation makes no distinction between women's and men's jobs, and men have developed many norms and standards for men;
- There are physical differences between men and women that have an impact on the workplace; and
- It is still the case that most women have the major responsibility for unpaid work at home and the paid shift in the workplace.

Women in traditionally male-dominated high-risk occupations faced far greater risks of impairment than their male counterparts. Musculoskeletal problems affect many women. They are most likely the most common work-related problem among female employees. These illnesses commonly involve heavy lifting, difficult postures, boring or repeated occupations, and insufficient work systems. Health care and home care workers, cleaners, catering, other hospitality professionals, and many office workers, primarily women, frequently work in similar environments. However, gender is not a factor that is frequently included during risk assessments.

Women are exposed to hazardous substances, such as solvents, in several industries, including cleaning. These drugs can interfere with fertility and pregnancy, resulting in miscarriages or premature births. It is uncertain what effect it has on menopausal women. Other disorders, such as dermatitis, allergies, and even cancer, may be exacerbated by such drugs.

Older women work longer hours than younger women, have lower-status professions, and are more likely to suffer from back pain and broken bones.

Aside from a few examples, women who encounter gynecological or reproductive difficulties or other potential work-related concerns are rarely linked to their job. Women's doctors do not inquire about their jobs or work schedules.

What Should be Done?

Urgent action is required to improve the jobs and health of women:
- **Employers:** There are numerous health and safety issues for women that employers fail to address effectively. Employers must consider their female employees when developing health and safety initiatives such as risk assessments, new work systems, work equipment, or personal protective equipment.
- **Standards:** The general view that women workers' health and safety problems and needs are identical to those of men is inaccurate, yet the same standards apply to women in the workplace. Government agencies must ensure that legal standards fully account for working women's occupational health and safety issues.
- **Compliance:** Employers who refuse to comply with their obligations under the Occupational Health and Safety Act and regulations must face legal action. Government agencies and non-governmental organizations (NGOs) must continue to campaign to prevent worker illness and ensure that women's health and safety are effectively addressed in the workplace.

◼ CONCLUSION

The evidence identifies social factors on women's health status, and the multidimensional nature of health highlights the complexity of these implications. There is a need for women to share concerns about their health with practitioners sensitive to their particular needs.

10.9 CHILD ABUSE

LEARNING OBJECTIVES

- ☞ What is child abuse?
- ☞ Describe signs of child abuse.
- ☞ Explain the causes of child abuse.
- ☞ List the risk factors for child abuse.
- ☞ Forms of child abuse.
- ☞ What are the effects of child abuse?
- ☞ Protective factors to lower the incidence of child abuse.
- ☞ What is the connection between child abuse and health problems?
- ☞ What types of prevention programs are available to address the issue of child abuse?

INTRODUCTION

Child abuse is the term that refers to children who have received a severe physical injury that was caused wilfully. This definition has not considered the neglect and maltreatment of children and mental and sexual harassment.

The broader meaning of child abuse includes three types of abuse—physical, sexual, and emotional. An adult or another child may cause the abuse. It causes serious injury to the child and even results in their death.

SIGNS OF CHILD ABUSE

If a child has been abused, their behavior shows apparent signs. Such signs have been discussed in **Table 10.3**.

Table 10.3: Signs of child abuse.

Child abuse	Characteristics
Physical abuse	• Unexplained or repeated injuries such as bruises or burns • Injuries that are in the shape of an object (belt buckle, electric rod, and so on) • Injuries are not likely to happen, given the age or ability of the child, e.g., broken bones in a child that is too young to walk or climb

Contd...

Contd...

Child abuse	Characteristics
	<ul><li>The disagreement between the child's and the parent's explanation of the injury</li><li>Unreasonable explanation of the injury</li><li>Blatant neglect of the child (dirty, undernourished, clothes inappropriate for the weather, lack of medical or dental care, etc.</li></ul>
Emotional abuse	<ul><li>Aggressive or withdrawn behavior</li><li>Shying away from physical contact with parents or adults</li><li>Afraid to go home</li></ul>
Sexual abuse	<ul><li>The child says that he or she was sexually mistreated.</li><li>The child has physical signs such as:<ul><li>Difficulty in walking or sitting</li><li>Stained or bloody underwear</li><li>Genital or rectal pain, itching, swelling, redness, or discharge</li><li>Bruises or other injuries in the genital or rectal area</li></ul></li><li>The child has behavioral and emotional signs such as:<ul><li>Difficulty in eating or sleeping</li><li>Soiling or wetting pants or bed after being potty-trained</li><li>Acting like a much younger child</li><li>Excessive crying or sadness</li><li>Withdrawing from activities</li><li>Talking about or acting out sexual acts beyond usual for his or her age</li></ul></li></ul>
Family characteristics	<ul><li>Families who are isolated and have no friends, relatives, or other support systems</li><li>Parents telling that they were abused as children</li><li>Families who are often in crisis (having money problems more often)</li><li>Parents who abuse drugs or alcohol</li><li>Parents who are very rigid with their child</li><li>Parents who are very rigid in disciplining their child</li><li>Parents who show too much or too little concern for their child</li><li>Parents who feel they have a different child</li><li>Parents who are under much stress</li></ul>

■ CAUSES OF CHILD ABUSE

Generally, the causes of child abuse are poverty, illiteracy, adaptation failure, family disorganization, parents' death, disobedience, lack of adequate control, and defective socialization. The irritable nature and rigidness of authorities, low income, lack of effective school education, and other factors also lead to child abuse.

■ RISK FACTORS OF CHILD ABUSE

Research has linked specific characteristics of the child and caregiver and features of the family environment to child abuse and neglect.

Child abuse, whether physical, sexual or neglect, is influenced partly by the child's age and gender. Young children are most vulnerable to physical abuse, whereas children who have reached puberty or adolescence have the highest rates of sexual abuse.

Boys are more frequently the victims of beatings and physical punishment than girls in most places. On the other hand, girls are more likely to be victims of infanticide, sexual abuse, forced prostitution, and educational and nutritional neglect. More than 130 million children between the ages of 6 and 11 are not in school worldwide, with 60 percent being girls.

Other factors that increase a child's vulnerability to abuse include being raised by a single parent or very young parents without the support of an extended family, household overcrowding, a lack of income to meet the family's needs, and other violent relationships in the home.

Parents more likely to abuse their children tend to have low self-esteem, poor control over their impulses, mental health problems, and antisocial behavior. They also tend to be uninformed and have unrealistic expectations about child development.

Research also shows that child maltreatment is more likely in communities with high poverty rates and with lesser social networks and neighborhood support systems, which have been shown to protect children.

■ EFFECTS OF CHILD ABUSE

a. Child abuse produces a negative attitude called social devaluation. It is called a loss of social esteem. It leads to deviant behavior.

b. Many victimized children indulge in violations of social norms. To their dependency, they try to escape from such a situation. Some common deviant behaviors among abused children are absent from school, running away, stealing money, drug addiction, etc.

c. Child abuse also leads to social and interpersonal problems like isolation, withdrawal from interactional settings, and antagonistic relations with parents or caretakers.

d. There are more chances of the children being re-victimized, which hinders the development of their personality. Hence, a majority of them are forced to become child laborers. They are exposed to work for long hours in hazardous work conditions. They miss education, and many of them become bonded laborers.

e. Most children work in fireworks, tea gardens, hotels, household work, mining, etc. Working under inhuman conditions and unhygienic surroundings, the children suffer from various diseases such as lung diseases, tuberculosis, eye diseases, asthma, bronchitis, etc.

■ MEASURES TO IMPROVE THE PROBLEM

- The first Factory Act to regulate the employment of children and their work hours was introduced in 1881. Later, the Child Labour Act of 1933 and the Factory Act of 1948 provided some safeguards for child laborers.

- The Juvenile Justice Act 1986 was introduced in different stages. Advisory boards and state children funds for preventing the abuse of children and providing protection and care, educational facilities, and training and rehabilitation facilities were provided.

- The government has tried to improve their working conditions, reduce working hours, and ensure minimum wages and health education. However, legislative measures have proved to be ineffective.

- The Union Government set up a National Advisory Board in 1993 to eliminate child labor in hazardous industries by 2000. The Government provided ₹ 850 crores to rehabilitate the child workers and educate them. However, the government was not serious about implementing the plan.

- The Supreme Court in 1996 banned child labor and ordered to set up of a child labor rehabilitation fund to safeguard the social and humanitarian rights of the children.

- UNICEF has taken up various ameliorative measures for child welfare.
- The present need is to enforce laws to curb this menace. People must change their attitude towards children, who must be provided opportunities to develop their potential in a healthy and free social environment and be protected against exploitation.

■ FORMS OF CHILD ABUSE

Child abuse falls into four categories: physical abuse, emotional abuse, sexual abuse, and neglect.

a. **Physical abuse:** Physical abuse may involve hitting, shaking, throwing, poisoning, burning or scalding, drowning, suffocating, or causing physical harm to a child. It may also be caused when a parent or caretaker fabricates symptoms of or induces illness in a child.

b. **Emotional abuse:** Emotional abuse is the persistent emotional ill-treatment of a child, causing severe and persistent effects on the child's emotional development. Emotional abuse is involved in most types of ill-treatment of children, although emotional abuse may occur alone. It may involve the following:
   - Conveying to a child that they are worthless, unloved, inadequate, or valued only in so far as they meet the needs of another person
   - Imposing developmentally inappropriate expectations, for example, interactions beyond the child's developmental capability, overprotection, limitation of exploration and learning, and preventing the child from participating in regular social interaction
   - Causing a child to feel frightened or in danger, for example, witnessing domestic violence and seeing or hearing the ill-treatment of another
   - Exploitation or corruption of a child

c. **Sexual abuse:** Sexual abuse involves forcing or enticing a child to participate in sexual activities, such as prostitution, whether they are aware of what is happening. Activities may involve physical contact, including penetrative and non-penetrative acts. 'Penetrative acts' include 'rape' (forced penetration of the vagina, anus, or mouth with a penis) and 'assault by penetration' (sexual penetration of the vagina or anus of a child with a part of the body or an object). Sexual activities may include non-contact activities such as involving a child in looking at abusive images, watching sexual activities, or encouraging them to behave in sexually inappropriate ways. It may include photos, pictures, cartoons, literature, or sound recordings via the internet, books, magazines, audio cassettes, tapes, or CDs. Children under 16 years of age cannot lawfully consent to sexual intercourse, although they may be involved in sexual contact to which, as individuals, they have agreed. According to law, a child under 13 years cannot provide consent.

d. **Neglect**: It involves the persistent failure to meet a child's basic physical and/or psychological needs, which is likely to result in the severe impairment of the child's health and development. Neglect may occur during pregnancy because of maternal substance misuse. Once the child is born, neglect may involve failure to:
   - Provide adequate food, clothing, or shelter (including exclusion from home or abandonment)
   - Protect from physical and emotional harm or danger
   - Meet or respond to basic emotional needs
   - Ensure adequate supervision, including the use of adequate caretakers
   - Ensure access to appropriate medical care or treatment
   - Ensure that their educational needs are met
   - Ensure their opportunities for intellectual stimulation are met.

CHILD ABUSE AND HEALTH PROBLEMS

There are four main types of abuse:
1. **Physical:** Parents or other adults intentionally injure their children or do nothing to prevent it. This includes not only physical violence but also giving children alcohol or drugs. The most severe cases can result in brain damage and death.
2. **Emotional:** It occurs when parents cannot show their child love and affection consistently. Sarcasm, threats, criticism, yelling, and taunting are all examples. The consequences are severe and long-term.
3. **Neglect:** It happens when parents fail to meet a child's basic needs for food, warmth, clothing, or medical attention. Neglected

children may be very withdrawn or aggressive, develop health problems, or have difficulty coping at school.

4. **Sexual:** It occurs when an adult, or occasionally a younger person, uses a child for sexual gratification. Forcing a child to commit sexual acts, showing child-adult pornographic videos or magazines, and filming or sexually photographing children are all examples of this. Sexual abuse occurs in both boys and girls, and it can occur in young children—even babies—and older children. Sexual abuse has long-term and severe consequences. Some children who are abused this way may grow up to be abusers.

PREVENTION PROGRAM FOR CHILD ABUSE

Statistics can be frightening. In 2006, approximately 9,05,000 children were victims of child abuse and neglect in the United States. Child abuse and neglect, on the other hand, are preventable. Every day, state and municipal governments, community organizations, and individual citizens work to keep children safe. According to studies, parents and caregivers who receive help from their families, friends, neighbors, and communities are more likely to provide safe and healthy environments for their children. When parents lack this support or feel alienated, they are more likely to make poor decisions, leading to child neglect or abuse.

Many states, local and tribal governments, and community and faith-based organizations, engage in preventive activities. The services they offer vary greatly. Some preventive services are intended for everyone, such as public service announcements (PSAs) to raise public awareness about child abuse. Others are aimed specifically at individuals and families who may be more vulnerable to child abuse or neglect. A parenting class for single teen mothers is one example. Some services are designed specifically for families who have experienced abuse or neglect to mitigate the abuse's effects and prevent it from happening again.

Typical activities of prevention programs include:

- Public awareness, such as PSAs, posters, and brochures, promote healthy parenting, child safety, and how to report suspected abuse.
- Skills-based curricula teach children safety and protection skills. Many of these programs focus on preventing sexual abuse.

- Parent education helps parents develop positive parenting skills and decrease child abuse and neglect behaviors.
- Parent support groups, where parents work together, help to strengthen their families, and build social networks.
- Home visitation focuses on enhancing child safety by helping pregnant mothers and families with new babies or young children learn more about positive parenting and child development.
- Respite and crisis care programs offer temporary relief to caregivers in stressful situations by providing short-term care for their children.
- Family resource centers work with community members to develop various services to meet the specific needs of the people who live in surrounding neighborhoods.

Two factors have increased the effectiveness of prevention programs, independent of the type of service or intended recipients. Involving parents in all stages of program planning, implementation, and assessment helps ensure that care providers collaborate with families. When parents are given the ability to discover viable options, they are more likely to implement long-term adjustments.

PROTECTIVE FACTORS TO LOWER THE INCIDENCE OF CHILD ABUSE

Prevention services increasingly recognize the importance of promoting protective factors and conditions in families and communities, which research has shown to improve children's and families' health and well-being. These factors assist parents who would otherwise be at risk of abusing or neglecting their children in locating resources, supports, or coping strategies that will allow them to parent effectively, even under stress.

The following protective factors have been linked to a lower incidence of child abuse and neglect:

- **Attachment and nurturing:** When parents and children have strong, warm feelings for one another, children develop trust that their parents will provide them with everything they need to thrive.
- **Parenting and child and youth development knowledge:** Parents who understand how children grow and develop can provide an environment where children can reach their full potential.

- **Parental resilience:** Emotionally strong parents have a positive attitude, solve problems creatively, address challenges effectively, and are less likely to direct their anger and frustration at their children.
- **Social connections:** Trusted and caring family friends offer emotional support to parents by encouraging and assisting them in dealing with the daily challenges of raising a family.
- **Concrete supports for parents:** Parents need essential resources such as food, clothing, housing, transportation, and access to critical services that address family-specific needs (such as child care, health care, and mental health services) to ensure the health and well-being of their children.

■ CONCLUSION

Child abuse and child labor are severe problems in India. Many Indian children are neglected by their parents, exploited by employers, harassed, and abused. They remain in distress and turmoil. Millions of children from low-income families are compelled to join the labor force. In India, 15% of the children are child laborers. Sexual abuse among children refers to the involvement of immature children in sexual activities, rape, prostitution, etc. Emotional abuse is the maltreatment of children. Children's social abuse includes kidnapping and forcing them to beg on the streets or using them for sexual gratification.

10.10 HIV/AIDS

LEARNING OBJECTIVES

- ☞ Describe the clinical features of HIV/AIDS.
- ☞ What are the effects of HIV/AIDS? How to manage?
- ☞ Discuss the nursing/physiotherapy concerns related to HIV/AIDS.
- ☞ Describe the National AIDS Control Programme in India.
- ☞ Discuss the attributable factors to the spread of HIV.
- ☞ Understand and describe the National AIDS Prevention and Control Policy (NAPCP) 2002.
- ☞ What are stigma and discrimination?
- ☞ What are the psychological and social impacts of HIV on individuals and families?

■ INTRODUCTION

Acquired immunodeficiency syndrome (AIDS) is a virus-borne communicable disease. This fatal disease is caused by the human immunodeficiency virus (HIV), transmitted through sexual intercourse, injection of drugs, and blood transfusion. HIV destroys specific antibody-producing white blood cells (WBCs), called T-cells, thus crippling the immune system. The first case of AIDS was discovered at the Centre of Disease Control in Atlanta, USA in 1981. The causative organism was found in 1983.

■ CLINICAL FEATURES OF HIV

Significant symptoms are weight loss, diarrhea for more than a month, fever for more than a month, and extrapulmonary TB at over one site.

Minor symptoms are persistent cough for over a month, swollen glands, itching skin diseases, chronic generalized herpes simplex (a viral illness), and thrush in the mouth and throat.

How HIV Spreads?

- The most important reason for the spread of AIDS is sexual contact. This includes homosexuality, group sex, sexual intercourse by persons infected with AIDS with persons of the opposite sex, and anal sex.
- The use of infected syringes, needles, or instruments transmits HIV. AIDS also spreads through blood transfusion.
- Injections of intoxicant drugs also spread HIV infection.
- A pregnant HIV-infected mother can transmit the infection to the fetus.
- Using an ordinary razor at the barber's shop or tonsuring at religious places is also a source of transmission of HIV.

How HIV Does Not Spread?

- Living with or caring for people with HIV or AIDS
- Using the same toilets used by the infected persons
- Swimming in pools used by the infected persons
- Shaking hands, hugging, or kissing the infected persons
- Drinking water from the same glass used by an infected person
- By bites of mosquitoes that have already bitten an infected person.

HIV Tests

The following tests are related to HIV:

- An enzyme-linked immunosorbent assay (ELISA) blood test is conducted to diagnose HIV.
- Western blot: The Western blot test must confirm the ELISA diagnosis. Generally, it takes 3 to 24 weeks for persons to test positive after being infected.
- Virus isolation.
- Murex SUD HIV-l test.
- T-4 cells and T-8 cells to find out the status of T-lymphocytes.

EFFECTS OF AIDS

People with AIDS may die of:
- Chronic pneumonia
- Chronic diarrhea
- Infections that block the throat, intestines, and lungs
- Cancer of the skin and bone
- Swelling in the brain
- Destruction of brain tissues, causing loss of memory and personality changes.

MANAGEMENT OF AIDS

Aims of the project made for AIDS control:
- Achieving a zero level of infection
- Blood protection and improvement in its rational use
- Encouraging public awareness and community support
- Developing capacity for observation and management
- Controlling over sexually transmitted diseases
- Strengthening program management capacity.

Control Over Blood-borne Transmission

- Test all blood products and blood for HIV/AIDS before transmission.
- Ensure proper sterilization process; take precautions in organ transplantation.

- Avoid using syringe, needles, or other skin-puncturing instruments, or use them with utmost caution.
- Use disposable syringes.
- Take precautions in ear piercing, tattooing, acupuncture, tooth extraction, etc.

Safe Sexual Relations

- Have a sexual relationship only within marriage. Have a sexual relationship with one husband or wife only.
- Use condoms for safe sex.
- Sexual relations should be moral. Sexual partners should be faithful to each other.
- Avoid unnatural sexual activities like anal sex, oral sex, homosexuality, and group sex.
- Avoid sex when there are injuries or lesions on reproductive organs.

Health Education

- Health education should include sex education in the general education curriculum to encourage healthy sexual relations.
- It should emphasize the restoration of moral values and characters.
- It is necessary to remove all erroneous ideas about AIDS. It should be made clear that AIDS does not spread through mosquitoes or other insects.
- AIDS does not spread due to sitting or having contact with the patient or through clothes.
- The staff who works with AIDS patients also does not get the disease, but the preventive measures should not be overlooked.

Other Measures

- Carrying out surveillance and research
- Reduction of impact
- Providing healthcare to people with HIV infection
- Providing antiviral treatment. Encourage research regarding AIDS control and eradication.
- Saving HIV/AIDS-infected people and providing them with psychological support

- Treating complications occurring due to AIDS immediately
- Conducting effective implementation and evaluation of the AIDS Control Programme.

AIDS AND NURSING/PHYSIOTHERAPIST'S CONCERNS

World AIDS Day is observed every year on the first of December to spread awareness of its prevention and control. The following approaches are described here to enable physiotherapists in the fight against stigma and discrimination:
- **Information-based approaches:** Giving factual information about HIV/AIDS.
- **Counseling:** Providing positive reinforcement and support to family members.
- **Coping skill acquisition:** Generating a positive attitude towards people living with HIV/AIDS through information and skill acquisition.
- **Contact with infected or affected people:** Reducing stigma and discrimination by interacting with the stigmatized group.
- Creating HIV/AIDS patient-friendly hospitals.
- Supporting general and specialist professional associations in AIDS care.
- Providing adequate supplies and equipment for AIDS prevention and control.

NATIONAL AIDS CONTROL PROGRAMME IN INDIA

HIV is a virus that belongs to the retrovirus family and is responsible for HIV infection and AIDS. Since the first case was reported in 1986, AIDS has emerged as one of the most serious public health issues. The first HIV/AIDS cases were discovered among commercial sex workers in Mumbai and Chennai and injecting drug users in the northeastern state of Manipur. The disease quickly spread in the areas surrounding these epicenters, and by 1996, Maharashtra, Tamil Nadu, and Manipur accounted for 77% of all AIDS cases. Tamil Nadu accounted for nearly half of these cases.

Burden of Disease

World

During 1998, 11 men, women, and children were infected per minute, according to UNAIDS/WHO estimates. More than 95 percent of HIV-infected people live in developing countries.

India

The trends of HIV infection in India are alarming. The following characteristics of the AIDS epidemic have been observed:

- In recent years, it has spread from urban to rural areas and individuals practicing risk behavior to the general population.
- More and more women attending antenatal clinics are being found to test HIV-positive, increasing the risk of perinatal transmission. One in every four cases of HIV-positive reported is a woman.
- About 84% of the infections occur through the sexual route (both heterosexual and homosexual).
- Another 4% through injecting drug use.
- Other transmission roots are blood transmission, injectable drug use, and perinatal transmission.
- About 80% of the reported cases occur in the sexually active and economically productive age group of 15–44 years.
- HIV positive in antenatal clinics varied from zero % in Assam to 1.71% in Maharashtra. The average prevalence was as low as 0.7%, with more than 500 million adults. NACO calculates that about 4.8 million people are infected.

Attributable Factors of the Spread of HIV

- Labor migration and mobility in search of employment from economically backward to more advanced regions.
- Low literacy levels lead to low awareness among the potential high-risk groups.
- Gender disparity.
- High prevalence of sexually transmitted and reproductive tract infections among men and women.
- The social stigma attached to sexually transmitted infections also holds good for HIV/AIDS, even much more seriously. This,

coupled with a lack of awareness, results in reporting of full-blown AIDS cases in cities like Mumbai and Chennai.

- There have been cases of refusal of AIDS patients in hospitals and nursing homes in the government and private sectors. This has compounded the misery of AIDS patients.
- Isolation of AIDS cases in the wards scares the general patients.
- On some occasions, discrimination in the workplace leads to loss of employment.
- The treatment options are still in trial and too expensive, and no effective vaccine is available.
- Multi-drug protease inhibitor therapy, popularly known as 'cocktail therapy,' helps only prolong the patient's life. There are fears of patients developing drug resistance and side effects if the therapy is not administered under proper medical supervision.
- There were instances of quacks taking advantage of the situation and promising cures through so-called herbal treatment providing only false assurances.
- Many unlicensed small and medium blood banks in the private sector have also compounded the problem.
- The twin problem of drug addiction and HIV transmission raises serious ethical and moral issues in needle exchange programs and condom distribution, as legally, no person should take the drug or go to prostitutes.
- Although transmission of HIV through the use of needles, razors, and other cutting instruments in the thousands of beauty parlors and hair-cutting saloons is insignificant, the lack of hygiene practices in the majority of these establishments also poses a health risk to the unsuspecting general population who visit these places every often.
- HIV–TB infection is another twin challenge. 60% of AIDS cases are TB opportunists. National TB Control Programme faces a new challenges with HIV-positive TB patients. Thiacetazone, an anti-tubercular drug, can cause skin eruptions in HIV-positive patients. There is no risk of HIV from any TB patient unless they practice high-risk behavior or get infected from a transfusion of HIV-infected blood.
- Inadequate understanding of the severe implications of the disease among the legislators, political and social leaders,

bureaucracy, media, trade and industry leaders, and even medical and paramedical personnel engaged in healthcare provision.

- Difficulty identifying, reaching, and reaching out to risk groups for interventions.
- Low NGO participation due to borrowers' and recipients' unfamiliarity with the guidelines and project processing requirements.
- Vacant positions, frequent transfers, holding dual charges, and changes in staffing patterns are major impediments to implementing preventive program strategies.
- Inconsistency in the processes of disbursement of funds across states.
- A large segment of civil society did not acknowledge HIV as a priority in the early 1990s. It was critical of the Central Government and the World Bank to draw attention to HIV/AIDS.

National AIDS Prevention and Control Policy (NAPCP) 2002

The NAPCP 2002 was announced to bring AIDS transmission to zero levels by 2007.

- Preventing the disease's spread by educating the public, especially high-risk groups, and providing them with tools to avoid infection. Controlling STDs among sexually active and economically productive groups and promoting condom use will be key to preventing HIV infection.
- Provide an enabling socio-economic environment so individuals and families affected with HIV/AIDS can manage their problems.
- Improve services for the care of People Living with AIDS (PLWA) in times of sickness, both in hospitals and at home, through community healthcare.

For these purposes, the policy addresses the following components of the National AIDS Control Programme for bringing in a paradigm shift in response to HIV/AIDS at all levels, both within and outside the government:

- Program management
  - National AIDS Committee
  - State Level Strengthening

- Empowered Committee
- State AIDS Control Societies
- Advocacy and social mobilization
  - Participation in NGOs or community-based organizations
  - Organizational counseling
  - Surveillance, monitoring, and research
  - HIV testing
- Research and development
- Target intervention
- People Living With AIDS (PLWA)
- Sexually Transmitted Disease Control Program
- Condom Program
- Policy for blood safety.

■ PSYCHOSOCIAL EFFECTS OF HIV-AIDS

Infection with HIV usually has a considerable physical, mental, social, and economic impact on infected individuals, their families, and the community in which they live. Stigmatization by other community members hinders HIV prevention, management, social support, and disclosure.

Another impact of HIV is depicted in the inequality and discrimination individuals living with HIV experience in matters such as securing or sustaining employment and vital services like life assurance. Children have born with the most significant effects of HIV, especially those orphaned and infected with HIV. The number of orphans has been steadily rising due to the AIDS-related deaths of guardians.

Psychological and Social Impact of HIV on Individuals and Families

Infection with HIV/AIDS causes many medical, mental, and social problems for individuals, their families, and communities. Currently, families must deal with HIV infection as a chronic disease that must be managed for the duration of the infected person's life.

The requirement to take a complex regimen of many drugs is the most significant burden for the HIV-infected individual; many patients experience anxiety, frustration, depression, and hopelessness, particularly when the drugs fail to achieve or maintain the perceived benefits expected from the treatment regime. This could be related to virus mutation and individual medication resistance.

Other issues, such as concerns about jobs, sexuality, relationship possibilities, and the social reactions of other community members, exacerbate the burden of HIV therapy.

Another effect of HIV is stigma and discrimination against HIV/AIDS patients. They must continually deal with rejection and social discrimination and suffer treatment with serious side effects. People living with HIV/AIDS must deal with being categorized as "victims," a term that suggests defeat, helplessness, and reliance on others.

Stigma from employers and coworkers encompasses social isolation and derision, as well as discriminatory behaviors such as dismissal or refusal of employment.

Stigma and prejudice linked with HIV/AIDS stymie efforts to combat the HIV/AIDS pandemic successfully. This fear of discrimination frequently inhibits people from seeking AIDS medication and management or reporting their HIV status publicly. In multiple situations, the stigma associated with HIV/AIDS can extend to the sick individual's relatives and siblings, creating an emotional burden on those left behind. HIV/AIDS stigma evolves as infection rates, disease understanding, and treatment availability change.

Economic Impact of HIV

HIV/AIDS has had the most significant adverse effect on the economies of many countries worldwide. The pandemic has been devastating for many nations, and it has caused deep poverty to the individual, families, and communities. The magnitude of HIV/AIDS infection's economic and demographic impact in third-world countries is pronounced because it affects persons at the most economically able and productive age. Besides, it also weighs down on the economic and health gains made in the last few decades. People with HIV/AIDS profoundly burden public finances, especially in the health sector.

The individuals and their families intensely feel the economic impact of HIV. HIV/AIDS, in many cases, results in the loss of income for the breadwinners and an increase in expenditures as a result of caring for the infected. Families affected by HIV deplete their savings and assets to cope with increased costs and income shocks. Firm profits, savings, and investments may reduce due to increased AIDS-related expenditure and lower labor productivity.

Impact of HIV on Parenthood and Children

HIV/AIDS affects parenting. Improved treatment regimens allow HIV-infected children to reach adolescence. This means more teens are infected. HIV/AIDS children are at risk for opportunistic diseases. The virus affects children psychologically and causes neurological impairment, resulting in cognitive insufficiency, behavioral issues, and low quality of life. Due to medication and reporting issues, HIV-positive children may have trouble leading normal life. Other effects of HIV on motherhood include ethical concerns about transmitting the virus to the newborn, the socioeconomic burden, anxiety, and the stigma of raising a child with a potentially fatal condition.

HIV/AIDS has caused a global rise in orphans. Older teens must assume parental responsibilities, while the majority are cared for by relatives or foster parents. Long-term care strains financial resources. Without parental care, guidance, and protection, social problems arise. Children must quit school. Many of these children drop out of school due to a lack of resources, stigma, and discrimination or to become early parents after their parent's deaths. Having both parents dead exacerbates these effects. Long-term HIV/AIDS causes crime, poverty, drug abuse, illiteracy, decreased production, and social collapse.

STIGMA AND DISCRIMINATION

Over the past two decades, HIV has emerged from an unknown virus to a pandemic of astronomical proportions.

The virus is relatively difficult to contract compared to others, such as Influenza. However, diverse social issues have allowed the virus to gain a significant foothold worldwide. The immense nature of this epidemic has led to mass fear, hysteria, and many misconceptions about the virus. This has led to the stigma and discrimination of those infected worldwide as people seek to explain what they do not understand.

Unfortunately, this hinders the fight against the global pandemic and makes populations vulnerable to infection. Stigma and discrimination must be adequately addressed to combat HIV/AIDS worldwide effectively.

What are stigma and discrimination?

- Stigma marks disgrace associated with a circumstance, quality, or person.
- People living with HIV are often believed (and led to believe) they deserve their status. By alienating and blaming others, people can avoid risk and not face the problem.
- A lack of understanding of HIV causes stigma, discrimination, lack of access to treatment, irresponsible media coverage of the epidemic, and prejudices related to sexuality, disease, drug use, and death.
- Discrimination results when stigmatization is acted upon and can take many forms, such as:
  - Lack of access to equal healthcare
  - Denial of equal opportunities for employment
  - Deprivation of education for HIV-positive children
  - Detention of HIV-infected persons

How do stigma and discrimination fuel the epidemic?

Preventing people from coming forward and getting tested

- "Internalized Stigma"
  - People with HIV can self-stigmatize themselves because of their views on infected individuals as they seek to adjust to their new status.
  - This can mainly occur in already stigmatized groups such as men who have sex with men (MSM), sex workers, injecting drug users, and migrants.
- People who do not know they are HIV positive can in no way use this knowledge to plan for their future.
  - Do not seek treatment until they begin showing symptoms of AIDS-related illnesses; it may be too late to start anti-retroviral treatment.

- Use knowledge of their HIV infection to protect their family members from infection or plan for their family's economic future after passing.
  - Leaving AIDS orphans
- Low perception of individual risk: Individuals do not see themselves at risk of contracting HIV because they do not belong to one of the stereotypically stigmatized groups.
- Preventing people from disclosing their status: Infected people may not want to disclose their status for fear of stigma and discrimination. This happens not only to them but also to family members.
- Denial goes hand in hand with discrimination. If one does not see themselves at risk or the potential for the epidemic to affect their community, they are at greater risk. Denial can even take the extreme form of not seeing the pandemic as a serious problem. Either way, denial silences open conversation about the epidemic, hindering preventative measures.

What can be done?

Society at all levels must be involved to counteract stigma and discrimination. The legal process must be applied at international and national levels to defend the rights of HIV-infected people. Measures must be put in place to ensure that this is enforced on a local level. Finally, education is the key.

Myths about HIV and its transmission contribute significantly to stigma and discrimination. Education initiatives around the world about HIV transmission techniques (particularly how it is NOT spread), measures to protect oneself from infection, and treatment alternatives will go a long way toward combating stigma and discrimination and, therefore, the global epidemic.

■ CONCLUSION

HIV/AIDS is different from most other fatal diseases because it affects both physical and social health. AIDS was first linked to gang members, drug addicts, sex workers, and other stigmatized groups. Because of fear, misunderstanding, and discrimination, HIV awareness can create enormous psychological pressures and anxieties that can delay constructive change or worsen the illness.

10.11 ELDERLY: A VULNERABLE GROUP

LEARNING OBJECTIVES

☞ Understand and describe the problems of the elderly.
☞ Classify old age and describe the types of age.
☞ Describe the services available for the aged.
☞ What type of services can be provided to the elderly?
☞ What are elderly abuse and its types?
☞ Recognize the health problems found in the elderly.
☞ Describe the role of HelpAge India.

■ INTRODUCTION

Because of education, urbanization, westernization, and industrialization, senior citizens' position and prestige have been seriously affected by causes such as shifting ideals, increased individualism, and rising expectations for consumer goods.

Also, people opt for few children because of acceptance of small family norms and hence greater vulnerability for elders.

When younger family members migrate to cities in search of a new source of income, the severe scarcity of housing and excessive rents are powerful deterrents to bringing elderly parents to live with them.

The participation of women in employment in cities in white-collar jobs has left the old unattended during the daytime, creating stressful situations. This situation prompts the younger generation to press for separate residences so that they will not be burdened with the complexities of modern living. Which discounts the value of the traditional systems and places a lateral transmission of knowledge in contrast to vertical information from the older generation, devaluing the expertise and experience of the old.

The fast pace of social change stresses the intergenerational differences in values and lifestyles. The increased expenses in children's education than in the past and the costly upbringing of children, together with the inflationary pressure, cause significant hardships to the old as less money is left for maintenance.

Life is the progression from youth to old. Aging is a complex process that significantly influences a person's biological, psychological, and sociological functioning. It is a normative process and not a fixed life cycle dimension. Like all life stages, aging comprises a series of status passages. A central concept in any discussion of aging is the meaning of age itself.

The aging cycle occurs from birth to death. The aging phenomenon has profound implications for individuals and society alike. Various countries devise specific laws for the elderly based on their need. There are many variations in defining aging. Some find aging relative, arguing that chronological age is not a reasonable indicator of anything due to the observed variations in the aging population.

◼ AGED AND SOCIETY

The elderly usually enjoyed a high status in older, civilized societies. The status was assumed due to the aged's experience and knowledge, which benefited the family and community.

Old age has been divided into the following categories:
a. Young old: 65 to 75 years
b. Old: 75 to 85 years
c. Old-old: 85 to 100 years
d. Elite old: over 100 years

Types of Age

- **Chronological age:** Chronological age markers may be associated with specific events. In most cultures, they have broad social and personal importance at all life-cycle stages. They also provide social regulation of the aging process. Chronological age is a weak aging measure because it does not consider the continuum of individual variations between people.
- **Biological age:** An individual's biological age can be described as a lifespan estimate. The biological age assessment will require measures of the functional capacities of the essential life-limiting organs.
- **Psychological age:** Psychological age is attained through an individual's adaptive capacity to change environmental demands —the ability to adjust with time and situation. Psychological age study involves researching memory, thinking, knowledge, competencies, feeling, motivation, and emotions.
- **Social age:** Changes in the individuals' social age are linked to the changing conditions or situations as members of the family, culture, and society. These could be termed sociological changes.

- **Functional age:** Functional age may be grouped within a given human society by the individual capacity level relative to others of the same age or functioning. The term functional is a double indication, on the one hand, of observable characteristics in the person and, on the other, of its functioning in the physical, social, or otherwise defined environment.

SERVICES FOR THE AGED

The family, community, and administration must contribute to providing essential services to the elderly. **Table 10.4** lists the services that elderly people require.

Table 10.4: Services needed for the elderly.

Types	Services
Social services	<ul><li>Medical services in hospitals or nursing homes</li><li>In the home for the aged</li><li>In families: a. Services for the incapacitated, such as home visits, home services, and escorting b. Recreational activities, consumer education, and legal aid for persons with physical capacity and social contacts c. Housing d. Adult education</li></ul>
Social welfare services	<ul><li>Daycare services</li><li>Institutional services</li><li>Infirmaries</li><li>Poor homes</li><li>Information and referral services</li><li>Services for old persons with special needs, such as the physically or mentally challenged who are unable to look after their interests</li></ul>
Socio-psychological services	<ul><li>Community education and awareness</li><li>Family support and care</li><li>Leisure activities</li><li>Religious activities</li><li>Preparation for retirement</li><li>Counseling services</li></ul>

Contd...

Contd...

Types	Services
Economic services	• If he belongs to a family below the poverty line • If he is ailing or infirm, requiring prolonged hospitalization • If he has some family responsibility such as education or marriage of his sons or daughters • Social employment

SERVICES PROVIDED TO THE ELDERLY

- Access to health centers is established for the elderly, and medical care is provided for the chronically ill elderly through mobile dispensaries.
- Providing aids such as spectacles, crutches, sticks, transportation, etc.
- Organizing social and religious functions in temples, mosques, churches, and spiritual gatherings
- Providing leisure activities such as low-cost movies, libraries, reading rooms, holiday centers, daycare centers
- Providing better living conditions in a healthy environment
- Helping the elderly in managing investments, tax exemptions, and legal aids
- Counseling service to overcome isolation
- Providing opportunities for community services.

ELDERLY ABUSE

The key to preventing elderly abuse is recognizing the warning signs. Signs of elderly abuse differ according to the type of abuse the victim is suffering. Each type of abuse has its distinct characteristics.

- Physical abuse can be identified by looking for bruises, scars, sprains, or broken bones on the elder's body. More subtle physical abuse indications include restraint signs such as rope marks on the elder's wrist or broken eyeglasses.
- Emotional abuse frequently occurs alongside other forms of abuse and is usually discovered by changes in the elder's personality or behavior. The elder may also display behavior that mimics dementia, such as rocking or mumbling.

- Compared with other types, financial exploitation is a more subtle form of abuse and, perhaps, more difficult to notice. Signs of financial exploitation include frequent withdrawals from the elderly's accounts, belongings or money missing from the elderly's home, many unpaid bills, and many unnecessary goods or services purchased from the elderly's account.
- Sexual abuse, such as physical abuse, may be detected through visible signs on the elder's body, particularly around the breasts or genital area. Inexplicable infections, bleeding, and torn underclothing are other signs.
- Neglect is a peculiar type of abuse. It can be inflicted either by the elder's caregiver or by himself. Signs of neglect include malnutrition and dehydration, poor hygiene, failure to take prescription medication, and unsafe living conditions.

Elderly abuse can also be detected by monitoring changes in the caregiver's behavior and observing certain signs in the elderly individual. The caretaker may, for example, refuse to allow the older to talk to or receive visitors, show apathy or lack of affection toward the elder, or refer to the elder as a "burden." Caregivers with a history of substance misuse or mental illness are more prone than others to commit elder abuse. Elder abuse can sometimes be subtle and hence, difficult to detect. So, any suspicion must be taken critically, and concerns must be immediately addressed.

HEALTH PROBLEMS IN THE ELDERLY

According to the World Health Organization, heart disease, cancer, and cerebrovascular disease are responsible for 75% of deaths in industrialized nations. Osteoporosis and postmenopausal bone loss cause osteoporosis and fractures in many women.

Governments and society are not aware of the problem, so millions of seniors do not get the proper care. By 2025, the UN estimates there will be 1200 million over-65s. Today's neglect of oral health could cost tomorrow. 7% of India's 1.1 billion people are 60+. They want better healthcare and a fun, healthy, dignified, financially independent, peaceful death. Sickness is too expensive.

Gray hair, wrinkles, and forgetting where you parked the car can be daunting. Age-related health issues are no joke. With seniors accounting for 12 percent of the world's population (and rising to 22 percent by 2050), it's important to understand the challenges they face and recognize that there are preventive measures that can lead to healthy aging.

Chronic Health Conditions

Generally, about 92% of seniors have at least one chronic disease, and 77% have at least two. The most frequent and costly chronic health problems are heart disease, stroke, cancer, and diabetes, which account for two-thirds of yearly fatalities. To assist in managing or avoiding chronic diseases, the National Center for Chronic Disease Prevention and Health Promotion recommends seeing a doctor for an annual checkup, eating a balanced diet, and exercising regularly. Obesity is rising among the elderly, and adopting certain lifestyle habits can help prevent obesity and its related chronic diseases.

Cognitive Health

Cognitive health focuses on a person's ability to think, learn, and remember. Dementia, or the loss of cognitive functioning, is the most common mental health problem among the elderly. Dementia affects around 47.5 million people globally, expected to nearly quadruple by 2050. Alzheimer's disease is the most common form of dementia, affecting up to five million people over 65 in the USA. According to the National Institute on Aging, other chronic health disorders and diseases, such as substance misuse, diabetes, hypertension, depression, HIV, and smoking, enhance the likelihood of acquiring dementia. While there are no cures for dementia, doctors can prescribe treatment and drugs to help patients manage their symptoms.

Mental Health

According to the WHO, over 15% of adults over 60 have a mental disorder. A common mental illness among seniors is depression, occurring in seven percent of the elderly. Unfortunately, this mental disorder is frequently underdiagnosed and mismanaged. In the United States, older individuals account for nearly 18% of suicide deaths. Because sadness can be a side effect of chronic illnesses, treating those illnesses can help. Furthermore, promoting a healthy lifestyle, such as improved living conditions and social support from family, friends, or support groups, can aid in treating depression.

Physical Injury

An older adult is admitted to the emergency room for a fall every 15 seconds. Every 29 minutes, a senior dies from a fall, making it the leading cause of injury among the elderly. Seniors are more prone to losing their balance, bruising, and breaking a bone as their bones weaken, and muscles lose strength and flexibility as they age. Osteoporosis and osteoarthritis are two disorders that lead to frailty. Falls, however, are not unavoidable. Education, more significant physical activity, and appropriate house adaptations can often be avoided.

HIV/AIDS and other Sexually Transmitted Diseases

While sexual needs and abilities may change as people age, sexual desire does not disappear completely. Seniors are unlikely to use condoms, making the elderly more susceptible to contracting HIV when combined with a weakened immune system. Late diagnosis of HIV is common among older adults because symptoms of HIV are very similar to those of normal aging, making it more challenging to treat and prevent damage to the immune system.

Malnutrition

Malnutrition in elders over 65 is frequently underdiagnosed, leading to additional health problems in the aged, such as a reduced immune system and muscle weakness. Other health issues (for example, the elderly with dementia may forget to eat), depression, alcoholism, dietary restrictions, poor social contact, and low income contribute to malnutrition. Minor dietary modifications, such as boosting fruit and vegetable consumption while decreasing saturated fat and salt consumption, can help with nutrition difficulties in the elderly. Food services are given to older persons who cannot afford or prepare meals.

Sensory Impairments

Sensory impairments, such as vision and hearing, are prevalent for older Indians over 70. Luckily, these issues are easily treatable by aids such as glasses or hearing aids. New technologies enhance hearing loss assessment and the wearability of hearing aids.

Oral Health

Oral health is one of the most critical issues for the elderly, although it is often disregarded. Approximately 25% of persons over 65 no longer have their natural teeth. Cavities and dental decay can make it challenging to eat a nutritious diet and cause low self-esteem and other issues. Dry mouth, gum disease, and mouth cancer are all oral health issues that affect older persons. Regular dental exams could help control or avoid specific problems. On the other hand, dental care can be complex for seniors due to the loss of dental insurance after retirement or financial constraints.

Substance Abuse

Substance abuse, typically alcohol or drug-related, is more prevalent among seniors than realized. Because many do not associate substance abuse with the elderly, it is often overlooked and missed in medical checkups. Furthermore, elderly persons are frequently prescribed many medicines for long-term use. Abuse is often the outcome of mental illness or taking another patient's prescription because they can't afford their own.

Bladder Control and Constipation

Incontinence and constipation are frequent in older persons and can negatively influence their quality of life. These may be a side effect of the difficulties stated above, such as not eating a well-balanced diet and suffering from chronic health disorders and age-related changes. To avoid these elderly health difficulties, the Mayo Clinic recommends keeping a healthy weight, eating a balanced diet, and exercising regularly. Medical therapies are frequently effective, and older persons should not be embarrassed to discuss them with their doctors.

ORGANIZATIONS ACTIVE IN ELDERLY CARE

HelpAge India

HelpAge integrates its programs and services and consciously moves from welfare to development and long-term sustainability for senior citizens. HelpAge works closely with Senior Citizen Associations and encourages seniors to speak up for their rights.

HelpAge has made considerable progress in a continuing fight against poverty, isolation, and neglect of elders in our society. The aim is to help elders rebuild their lives and take charge of their future, restoring a sense of self-worth and confidence. Advocacy is one of the most potent tools for impact and change; it is gaining impetus with the sensitization of school principals, urging them to include Value Education on Aged Care in school curriculums. HelpAge is also pushing for Reverse mortgages for seniors to create a secure financial net for elders. An awareness campaign was launched to deal with the rising crime against elders, sensitizing the decision-makers to take action.

HelpAge reaches out to the needy elderly through various financial, health, and emotional security services. HelpAge is slowly moving from welfare to integrated age care services for the elderly in urban and rural areas. New services have been started in the recent past, such as Elder Helplines and physio-care, and existing services are experimenting in new places. One example is the Mobile Medicare Unit (MMU) program. The MMU program delivers essential services in some areas and incorporates new programs such as disability assistance, housing assistance, yoga, personalized home visits, and psychological counseling.

HelpAge India manages and implements the following programs aimed at enhancing the quality of life for the elderly:

- **Mobile Medicare Units:** These are medical vans that take healthcare facilities to the doorsteps of needy older people. They dispense free medicines and health checks for the elderly. They are manned by a trained doctor, a pharmacist, and a social worker who counsels older people and the community within which they live. In complicated cases, the MMUs often allow references to nearby hospitals to which they have ties **(Fig. 10.5)**.

- **Restoring sight:** Every year, cataract destroys the vision of millions of the elderly across the nation. Due to a lack of access to this simple operation, many cannot see it. Nearly more than 12 million elders in India are blind due to cataracts. Every year, HelpAge India conducts thousands of free cataract operations **(Fig. 10.6)**.
- **Residential care:** These residential care facilities provide a safe haven for those who have been ejected from their families. Old age homes, according to HelpAge, are not the answer to the problem, and that the best care for an elderly person is provided by their

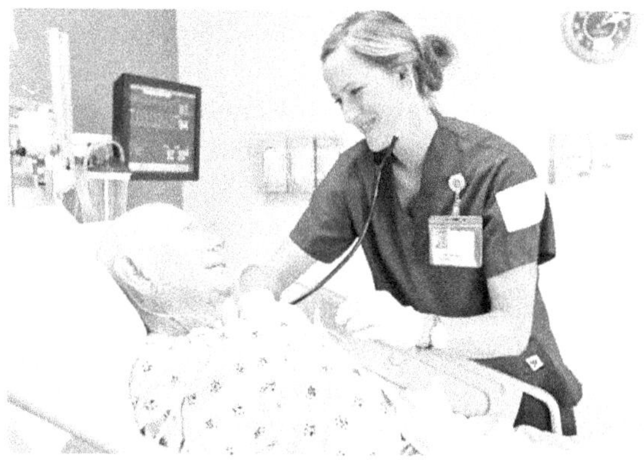

Fig. 10.5: Health problems of the elderly.

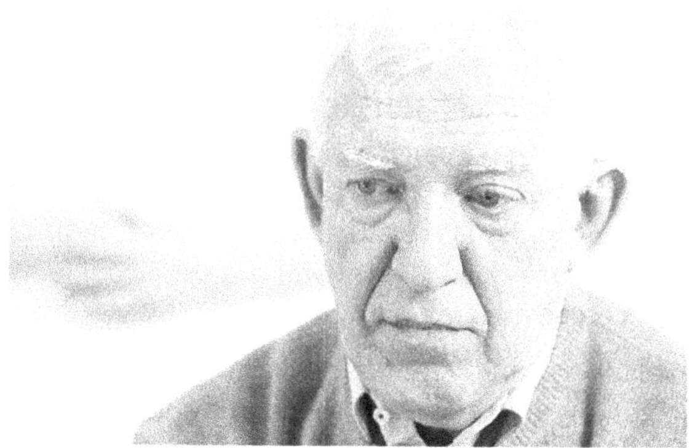

Fig. 10.6: Cognitive issues of elderly.

own family. Loneliness and depression are common among the elderly. HelpAge India's daycare centers serve as a gathering place for them to share their concerns. They spend their days interacting with one another and catching up on their lives; some even engage in recreational and income-generating activities like basket weaving and candle making.

- **Support a grandma or grandpa:** For those older people with no family and no financial or social support, HelpAge India links them to individuals and organizations who can care for their essential needs.
- **Income generation:** HelpAge has started income generation schemes to restore pride and dignity to thousands of elderly and make them financially self-reliant.
- **Advocacy:** HelpAge expresses the concerns of the elderly and has been fighting for their rights. It has also contributed to the government's National Policy on Older Persons. It has successfully pushed ahead with travel, tax concessions, and other benefits for the elderly.
- **Relief and rehabilitation:** Elder people are especially susceptible to disasters and often get sidelined when aid is distributed. HelpAge runs large rehabilitation programs in Gujarat, coastal India, and Jammu and Kashmir to help them regain their lives.

SOCIAL ISOLATION IN THE ELDERLY

Old age is a time for peace and relaxation. Old age is supposed to be the second childhood. However, with aging comes health problems and the inability to perform once-cherished activities. In addition, losing touch with near and dear ones leads to a recipe for emotional issues like depression. People's social age is determined by their habits or roles concerning social expectations. Growing older causes a steady decline in modern life's essential mental and physical qualities. Physical, psychological, and behavioral changes occur in the elderly. As people get older, their mental and physical abilities deteriorate.

There are many reasons for social isolation in the elderly:
- Loneliness due to the death of a spouse or friends
- Feeling of social isolation as children become busy with their own lives or move to a different city or country

- Dependence on caregivers to perform activities of daily living
- Stress due to financial issues from loss of regular income
- Struggling to cope with and difficulty accepting physical changes due to aging
- Advancing age severely limits mobility and the persuasion of hobbies
- Feeling of dissatisfaction due to retirement and lack of routine activities
- Depression due to ongoing or chronic medical problems and medication

For older people with dementia, relocation also causes social isolation. Moving away from their known surroundings confuses them, and their increasing dependence on others may lead to frustration. This may lead them to avoid social interactions.

Losing control or being unable to make independent judgments can sometimes aggravate depression. Loneliness can be caused by a lack of ability to articulate one's feelings or a lack of a confidante or companion.

REMEDIES FOR SOCIAL ISOLATION

- Take a brief journey with your partner now and again. Even a half-hour walk to a nearby park or hideaway can help them feel refreshed and relieve depression and loneliness. Giving children a ride keeps them connected to their social environment and gives them a sense of independence.
- Encourage them to pursue their hobbies and interests. Making volunteer activities available will give them a feeling of purpose and value.
- Those who are religiously inclined should be encouraged to visit their places of worship—praying regularly or meditation help to develop a mind that is fresh and free of unwanted thoughts.
- Caring for a pet or gardening might keep them occupied and satisfy their desire to nurture and care for others. These have also been shown to be effective in the treatment of depression.
- With old age come difficulties in hearing and vision. Older people who have such issues that are undiagnosed and left untreated hesitate to face social situations. Embarrassment due

to problems in communication with others slowly makes them avoid socializing. This leads to social isolation.

- Incontinence in the elderly causes them to stay at home and avoid social interactions for fear of embarrassment. To feel more confident and increase social connections, caregivers and family members of these elders should be more cautious and prompt in giving incontinence solutions. This will help them avoid feelings of loneliness.

A counseling session can help the elderly facing social isolation to adjust to lifestyle changes. This will better prepare them emotionally. Eldercare in Kolkata is a nascent field, but it is here to stay.

CONCLUSION

The elderly have different economic, social, and psychological needs in different societies. Social work must consider the interplay of physical, health, financial, and social factors. The elderly expect their children and grandchildren to live peacefully and with affection. Aging makes people more self-absorbed. They may become so self-centered that they don't care about others' interests or wishes.

10.12 DRUG ABUSE AND DRUG ADDICTION

LEARNING OBJECTIVES

- ☞ What is aberrant behavior?
- ☞ Describe basic concepts of drugs, drug abuse, drug dependence, and drug addiction.
- ☞ Explain the social effects of drug abuse.
- ☞ Describe the nature and impact of various abusable drugs.
- ☞ What is the extent and nature of drug abuse?
- ☞ What are the measures to combat drug trafficking?
- ☞ How do we treat addicts and prevent drug abuse?

INTRODUCTION

Drug abuse and addiction are significant social and public health problems worldwide, negatively impacting individual and social levels.

June 26th is celebrated annually as International Day against Drug Abuse and Illicit Trafficking. It is an effort by the international community to raise awareness about the dangers of drugs among the general public and youth in particular. The picture is bleak when global data on the drug situation is reviewed. It is the world's third-largest company, behind petroleum and the arms trade, with a market capitalization of over $500 billion. Around 190 million people use one or more drugs around the world.

Drug addiction is extremely distressing for people, and the illicit production and distribution of narcotics have resulted in crime and violence worldwide. No corner of the world today is free of the curse of drug trafficking and addiction. Hundreds of millions of drug addicts worldwide live on death's edge.

■ SOCIAL EFFECTS OF DRUG ABUSE

Addiction can cause permanent brain damage and severely affect the mind and body. People are experiencing substance abuse disorder often experience changes in their behavior, perceptions, judgment, and decision-making. People can begin taking drugs for a variety of different reasons, including:

Peer Pressure

Because everyone around them uses drugs and does not emphasize the dangers, an addict may consider drugs an accepted activity. Peer pressure, on the other hand, can lead to drug usage. This occurs when someone or a group repeatedly attempts to persuade someone to do something unpleasant.

Improve Performance

Someone may start using drugs to improve their performance in sports or academics. Aspiring college athletes may begin taking drugs to help perform better during their track meet. Unfortunately, this can have dangerous consequences.

Relieve Stress

An addict may have started using a drug to relieve pent-up stress because they heard that drugs produce an intense high feeling. Drugs release a very intense feeling of pleasure, but it continuously causes the brain to seek that same high.

To Feel Better

Someone who develops a drug addiction may have begun using them to self-medicate. They could be dealing with another underlying mental disease and are attempting to treat the symptoms. However, this will only add to the confusion.

PERMANENT EFFECTS OF ADDICTION ON THE BRAIN

Short- and long-term drug and alcohol use can damage the brain. The inability to resist drug-like highs causes brain changes. Nothing can compare to the high. Rewired reward pathways caused this. Still, there's hope. The De-Addiction Center helps patients manage symptoms and live full life.

Alcohol and drugs both have harmful effects. While taking medications, the brain will adapt to its feelings. The addict may also lose the ability to feel pleasure. This can lead to severe mental disorders.

SOCIAL IMPACTS OF DRUG ABUSE

Nobody's immune to addiction. Substance abuse has social costs. Substance abuse affects every aspect of an addict's life. A user may lose friends. Substance abuse often disrupts friendships and family ties. Emotions may run high, causing some to cut ties with the addict.

The addict may be denied higher education. Drugs and alcohol are banned on school grounds and can lead to legal action. College and high school students have been known to self-medicate to prepare for tests or other academic activities. Addiction paraphernalia can also be brought to class. Expulsion from school and criminal charges are possible.

The addict could be cut from the team or club. Drugs can boost academic or athletic performance and be used at special events. Breathing, heart rate, senses, and coordination can be affected by drugs. Using random variables in sports is risky. If someone gets sick, they'll be kicked off the team and face legal action.

An addict may lose their job for many reasons. A drug addict's overwhelming desire for a drug may lead to drug abuse rather than work. These missed days may result in dismissal. Under the influence, a drug addict may not work. Addicts may feel compelled to bring drug paraphernalia to work to experience the drug's effects, which can lead to job loss.

■ TEENAGERS AND DRUG OR ALCOHOL ABUSE

Teens are more inclined to notice the perceived good social benefits of drug and alcohol use than the potential negative consequences. Teenagers are more likely than adults to want to take risks.

As a result, drug and alcohol experimentation peaks throughout these years. Massive physical and mental growth spurts occur during the teenage years of development. The frontal cortex is mainly in charge of making good decisions. However, it usually does not fully mature until well into adolescence. The brain and body are both affected by drug and alcohol misuse.

Drugs and alcohol can force the brain to rewire itself, mistaking the high for what it needs to strive for. The adolescent brain can also be affected by short-term or long-term memory impairment during this critical developmental stage. The following is a list of what can happen to the teenage brain during substance abuse.

- Damaged synapses
- Memory problems
- Habits that are unhealthy for both the body and mind
- Limiting learning potential

If someone is addicted, the best action is to seek help as soon as possible. Addiction can harm the mind and the body, leaving addicts with long-term consequences. This addiction can break all elements of a person's life.

"Your brain alters by being unable to resist the temptation to experience the same high that you had when on drugs," states an insightful essay about the social impacts of drug misuse. All addicts deserve treatment for their addiction.

Aberrant Behavior

Drug abuse may be perceived as aberrant behavior and a social problem. In the former sense, it is regarded as evidence of an individual's social maladjustment; in the latter sense, it is viewed

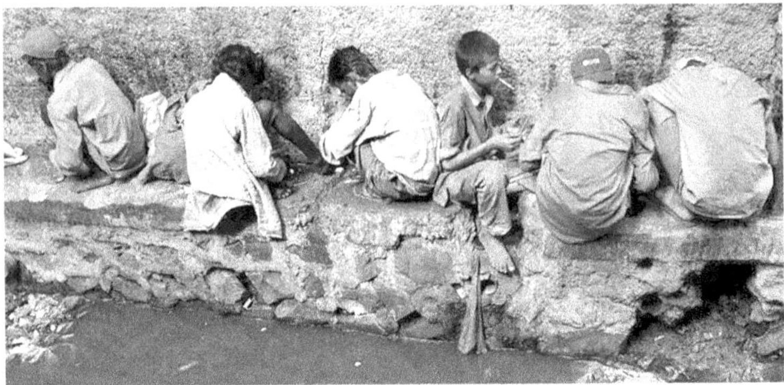

Fig. 10.7: Drug addicts in India.

as a widespread condition with harmful consequences for society. Several Western countries have regarded drug abuse as an actual social problem. However, it has become a crucial social problem in India only in the last two and half decades. It is said that India has become an important transit center for drugs, and the prevalence of drug abuse is also alarmingly increasing. Today's illicit drugs are not confined to the street urchins and the lower classes; more and more middle and upper-class youth succumb to drugs.

Despite this increase, drug abuse in India is still considered more aberrant than antisocial or non-conforming behavior. By this, one means that the aberrant person conceals their transgression from the social norms of the society, violates norms without questioning their legitimacy, and attempts to escape the penalties for violating norms without proposing changes to them. The aberrant person is believed to be out to satisfy their private interests **(Fig. 10.7)**.

■ BASIC CONCEPTS OF DRUG ABUSE

The concepts of drug abuse, dependence, addiction, and abstinence syndrome need clarification.

Drug

"Drug" is a chemical with physical and/or psychological effects. It affects body functions. Too broad a drug is a substance prescribed by a doctor or manufactured to treat and prevent disease by affecting a living organism's structure and functions. Drug refers to a habit-forming substance that affects the brain or nervous system.

It refers to "any chemical substance that affects bodily function, mood, perception, or consciousness and has misuse potential" According to this definition, frequent drug use is so dangerous, immoral, and antisocial that it causes public outrage and hostility.

Some drugs are not addictive or have harmful physiological effects. Using such drugs contrasts with illegal drugs like heroin, cocaine, and LSD or legal drugs like alcohol, tobacco, barbiturates, and amphetamines, which have harmful physical effects on the user.

Drug Abuse

'Drug abuse' is illicit drugs or misuse of the legitimate drug resulting in physical or psychological harm. It includes smoking ganja/hashish, taking heroin/cocaine or LSD, injecting morphine, drinking alcohol, etc. These are sometimes referred to as 'high on speed' or 'trip' or 'getting kicks.'

Drug Dependence

Drug dependence denotes habitual or frequent use of a drug. The dependence can either be physical or psychological. Physical dependence occurs with repeated drug use when the body has adjusted to a drug and will suffer pain, discomfort, or illness if the drug is discontinued. Psychological dependence arises when a person becomes dependent on a drug for the sense of well-being it provides.

Drug Addiction

Addiction is commonly used to describe physical dependence. Thus, 'addiction' or 'physical dependence' is a state whereby the body requires continued drug administration. Addiction to a drug occurs when the body gets so dependent on its toxic effects that it cannot function without it.

The characteristics of drug addiction are:
- An overpowering desire or need (compulsion) to continue taking the drug and to obtain it by any means
- A tendency to increase the dose
- A psychological and physical dependence on the effects of the drugs
- An effect detrimental to the individual and society.

Abstinence Syndrome

Body functioning is interfered with if the drug is withdrawn and withdrawal symptoms appear in a pattern specific to the drug. The total reaction to deprivation is known as 'abstinence syndrome.'

Tolerance

The chronic drug user feels he must constantly increase the dose to produce the same effect as the initial dose. This phenomenon is called tolerance. It represents the body's ability to adapt itself to the presence of a foreign substance.

However, tolerance does not develop for all drugs or individuals; though, with certain drugs (e.g., morphine), addicts have been known to build up greater tolerance quickly. Cross tolerance refers to tolerance development for one drug that may also result in tolerance for similar drugs.

■ NATURE AND IMPACT OF ABUSABLE DRUGS

The abusable drugs may be divided into six categories such as alcohol, sedatives, stimulants, narcotics, hallucinogens, and nicotine. Stimulants, depressants, narcotics, and hallucinogens are also called psychoactive drugs.

Alcohol

Some people use alcohol as a regular, pleasurable, and social activity, while others use it as a stimulant that allows them to work. It can also be used as a sedative to calm nerves or as an anesthetic to alleviate pain from daily living. Alcohol reduces aggressive inhibitions and relaxes tension. It also causes disorientation and hampers judgment.

Sedatives or Depressants

Sedatives or depressants relax the central nervous system (CNS), induce sleep, and provide a calming effect. Tranquilizers and barbiturates fall into this category. Medically, these are used for high blood pressure, insomnia, and epilepsy, and to relax patients before and during surgery. Like depressants, they depress the actions of nerves and muscles. They slow down breathing and heartbeats in small quantities and relax the user. However, the user becomes sluggish, gloomy, sometimes irritable, and quarrelsome in higher doses. Their ability to think, concentrate, and work is impaired, weakening emotional control.

Stimulants

Stimulants activate the CNS and relieve tensions, treat mild depression, induce insomnia (keep a person awake), increase alertness, contract fatigue, and expressive drowsiness, and lessen aggressive inhibitions. The most widely known stimulants and amphetamines (popularly called pep pills) are caffeine and cocaine.

Moderate doses of amphetamine, when popularly prescribed by a doctor, can check fatigue and produce feelings of alertness, self-confidence, and well-being. Heavier doses cause extreme nervousness, headache, irritability, sweating, diarrhea, and unclear speech.

Most stimulant medicines are taken orally. However, some (such as methedrine) are administered intravenously. These medications do not produce physical dependence, but they are psychologically addictive. Long-term heavy use of amphetamines causes varying intellectual, social, emotional, and economic deterioration. Withdrawing the drug abruptly can cause mental illness and severe suicidal depression.

Narcotics

Narcotics and sedatives produce a depressant effect on the CNS. They cause sensations of joy, strength, and superiority, a reduction in hunger, a reduction in inhibitions, and an increase in suggestibility. This category includes opium, marijuana, heroin, morphine, Pethidine, cocaine, and cannabis (charas, ganja, and bhang).

Heroin is morphine powder, cocaine is coca bush leaves, and cannabis is hemp. Marijuana is cannabis. Heroin, morphine, Pethidine, and cocaine are inhaled or injected. Smoke, sniff, or ingest opium and marijuana.

Physical dependence affects withdrawal symptoms. Shaking, sweating, chills, diarrhea, nausea, mental anguish, and abdominal and leg cramps occur 8–12 hours after the last dose. After that, symptoms worsen over the next 5–10 days, peaking between 36–72 hours. Muscle pain, weakness, insomnia, and nervousness may last weeks.

Hallucinogens

Hallucinogens produce distorted perception (seeing or hearing things differently than they are) and dream images. Medical practitioners do not advise their use. The well-known drug in this group is LSD, a synthetic chemical. An amount smaller than a grain of salt of hallucinogens can produce gross psychotic reactions in humans. Usually, LSD is taken orally, but it may also be injected. The effect of an average dose of LSD usually lasts 8–10 hours. Panic, depression, and permanent severe mental derangement can result from an attempt to withdraw from its use.

Nicotine

Nicotine includes cigarettes, bidi, cigars, snuffs, and tobacco. Nicotine has no medical use. The risk of physical dependence is always there. It leads to relaxation, stimulates CNS, increases wakefulness, and removes boredom. However, frequent or heavy nicotine use may cause heart attack, lung cancer, stroke, and bronchitis. This is not a controlled substance under the law.

■ EXTENT AND NATURE OF DRUG ABUSE

Drug addiction is a vicious chain in which one addict spreads the habit to others. So, for each known addict, there are at least ten unknown addicts.

It may be said that sandwiched between the Golden Crescent (Pakistan, Afghanistan, and Iran) and the Golden Triangle (Myanmar, Thailand, and Laos) countries, India was once only a conduit of drugs to the West but has become a ravenous consumer as well. After the urban centers, the menace is now spreading to the rural areas.

PREDISPOSING FACTORS OF DRUG USAGE

It may be pointed out that those persons who are predisposed to drug usage who:
- Have difficulties in assuming a masculine role
- Are frequently overcome by a sense of futility, apprehension of failure, and general depression
- Are easily frustrated and made anxious
- Find frustrations and anxieties unbearable.

MOTIVATIONS IN DRUG USAGE

Causes of Drug Abuse

The causes may be classified under four heads:
a. **Psychological causes:** Relieving tension, easing depression, removing inhibitions, satisfying curiosity, removing boredom, getting kicks, feeling high and confident, and intensifying perceptions.
b. **Social causes:** Facilitating social experiences, being accepted by friends, and challenging social values.
c. **Physiological causes:** Staying awake, heightening sexual experiences, removing pain, and getting sleep.
d. **Miscellaneous causes:** Improving study, sharpening religious insight, deepening self-understanding, solving personal problems, etc.

Role of Family and Peer Group in Drug Abuse

Family and peer group associations are the primary potent influences on the direction an individual takes and maintains in his/her life. Among college or university students, drug usage is influenced by the quality of affectionate family relationships. This term (affectionate family relationships) is operationalized on the following bases:

- Parents are interested in their children's careers and are conscious of their parental obligations.
- Relations between parents of drug users and between users and their siblings are based on harmony and solidarity.
- Parental control is neither very harsh nor lenient in allowing the child to self-express.
- The family size is so manageable in terms of family income that no child in the family suffers from a deficit in the necessities of life.
- Parents broadly conform to social and moral norms setting examples for their children to follow.
- The child exhibits trust and security in the parents by taking them into confidence and seeking their advice and help in facing perplexing problems.

Drug users' families were often not 'normal' or 'affectionate.' When the link between drug use and living away from parents was tested, parents' residence was more important than hostel living. Genealogy affects drug use. The nature of family control, the discipline imposed by parents on their children, the parents' interest in their friends, leisure activities, future career prospects, and parents' obligations toward their children are important factors determining children's drug use. Family drinking/smoking and drug use affected drug use. The family environment, therefore, influences drug use.

Peer pressure influenced drug use like family. Based on the analysis, the leading causes of drug abuse are family environment, mental condition, oppressive social system and power structure, subcultures (slum areas, college/hostel subcultures, etc.), peer pressures, personality factors (dependent personality), and pursuit of pleasure and fun **(Fig. 10.8)**.

■ MEASURES TO COMBAT DRUG TRAFFICKING

Over the last three to four decades, India has been facing the problem of increasing trafficking in drugs, particularly transit traffic in respect of heroin and hashish from the Middle East region destined for Western countries. As a result of this transit traffic, metropolitan

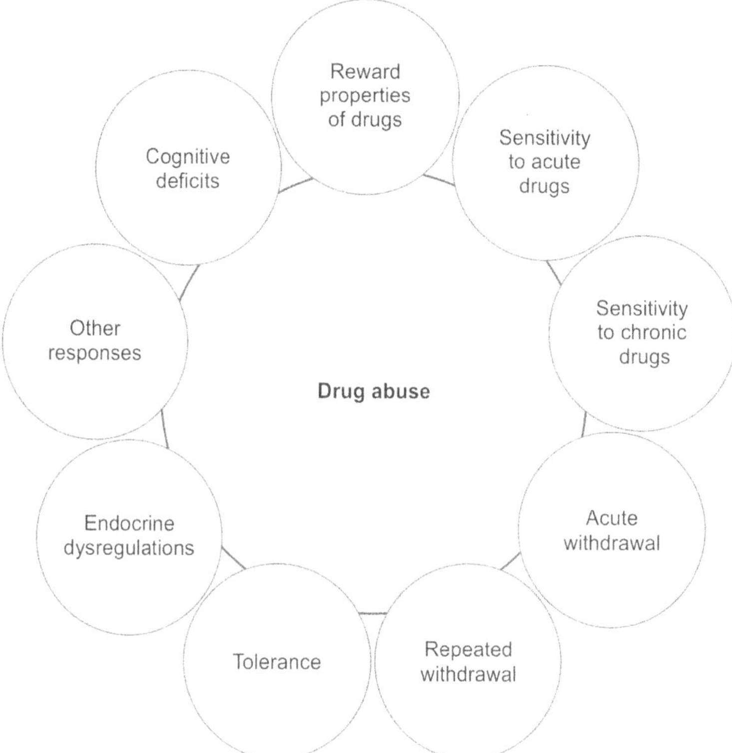

Fig. 10.8: Consequences of drug abuse.

cities such as Mumbai, Delhi, Kolkata, and Chennai have become vulncrablc to drug trafficking.

UTILIZATION OF DRUG TRAFFICKING

The 'profit' generated by drug trafficking is used in many ways:

a. Money IS used for financing politicians and developing lobbies in bureaucracy, judiciary, police, prisons, and media
b. Money is invested in shell corporations that takeover legitimate business organizations

c. Money is laundered in purchasing arms for terrorism.
d. *Terrorist organizations* take the help of drug traffickers to assist in terrorist activity.

TREATING ADDICTS AND PREVENTING DRUG ABUSE

Action Plan on Drug Abuse

The government of India has evolved a four-point action plan on drug abuse:

1. Community-based action for identification, motivation, counseling, treatment, and aftercare.
2. Generation of awareness about the consequences of drug abuse.
3. Training for service providers.
4. Association of NGOs in implementing the program and providing funds to them to establish counseling and de-addiction facilities.

Control Over Drug Abuse

Adoption of the following methods can aid in the control of drug abuse:

- **Imparting education about drugs:** Young college/university students, particularly those living in dormitories and away from their parents' influence, those living in slums, truck drivers, industrial employees, and rickshaw pullers should be the target group for prevention education **(Fig. 10.9)**.
- **Changing physician's attitudes:** A shift in doctors' attitudes on prescribing too many drugs can reduce drug abuse. The doctor must exercise greater caution in not ignoring the negative effects of the drugs, and they must ensure that the patient does not become dependent on the drug.
- An undertaking follow-up study of addicts treated under detoxification programs.
- Parents must play an essential part in preventing their children from using drugs. Because parental neglect, anger, rejection, and marital discord all play a role in the perpetuation of drug addiction. As a result, parents must exercise greater caution in maintaining a pleasant and harmonious home environment.

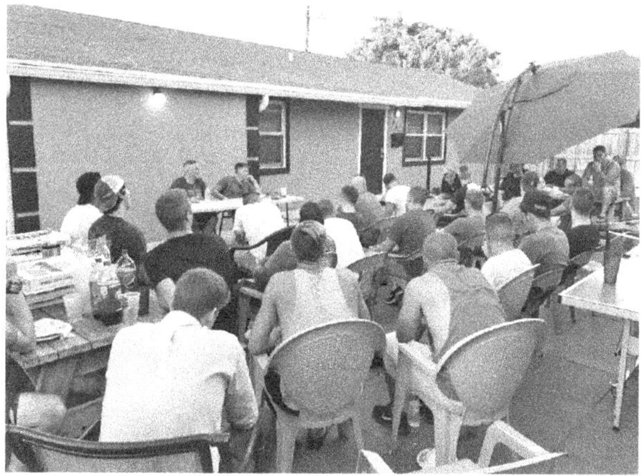

Fig. 10.9: A scene in a drug rehabilitation center.

Because addiction does not happen overnight and involves losing interest in studies, activities, and hobbies, engaging in irresponsible behavior, irritability, impulsive behavior, and having a dazed expression, parents can detect the early signs by remaining vigilant and ensuring that the child breaks the habit.

In preventing drug abuse, the role of the parent could be:
- Communicate openly with the children, listen to their problems patiently, and teach them how to handle them.
- Take an interest in children's activities and their circle of friends.
- Set an example for children by not taking drugs or alcohol.
- Keep track of prescribed drugs at home.
- Learn as much as possible about drugs.

Teachers can also play an essential role in drug abuse prevention:
- They can discuss the dangers of drug abuse with the students by talking informally and openly.
- They can keep themselves interested in their student's interests and activities.
- They can encourage them to volunteer information on drug abuse incidents.
- They can talk about the problems of adolescence and guide students on how to solve them.
- They can help them select career options and set goals.

- They can encourage them to discuss (students') crises (of family, peer group, money, etc.) with them and help them to the best of their abilities in facing these crises.

Drug abuse is a growing human hazard. The high costs to individuals, the environment, and the economy must discourage drug use. Unkempt drug users crowding streets, byways, cinemas, and other public spaces should prompt authorities to eradicate this plague. Government agencies, non-profits, and others must collaborate to educate and prosecute drug addicts.

Social Security

LEARNING OBJECTIVES

☞ Describe the concept and definition of Social Security.
☞ Explain the evolution and the need for Social Security.
☞ What approaches apply to Social Security?
☞ What are the purpose and contingencies of Social Security?
☞ Describe the types of Social Security benefits.
☞ Explain the Social Security Administration in the United States.
☞ Which Social Security Strategies are used in India?
☞ Discuss Protective Social Security Programs.
☞ Describe Social Security for Disabled Persons in India.
☞ Describe the Programs/Schemes required to be designed for Disabled Persons.

INTRODUCTION

Social security is a concept that has evolved over time. In primitive societies, it was humankind's struggle against insecurity to protect himself from the vagaries of nature or find the necessities of day-to-day life. Later, community living came into existence, bringing the family to provide adequate social measures for the needy. With the rapid industrialization, there was a break up of family setup destructing the traditional system resulting in the need for institutionalized and state-cum society regulated social security arrangement.

All the world's industrial countries have developed measures to promote the economic security and welfare of the individuals and their family. These measures have come to be called social security.

DEFINITION OF SOCIAL SECURITY

Social Security is defined by the International Labor Organization (ILO) as *"the protection provided by society through appropriate organization against certain risks to which its members are perpetually exposed. These are contingencies that a person of modest means cannot effectively provide for by his own ability or foresight, or even in private collaboration with his peers. As a result, the mechanics of social security consist in counteracting nature's and economic activity's blind injustice with rationally planned justice tempered by benevolence."*

This ILO definition is clear and focuses on providing assistance to an individual or family to keep them from falling into contingent poverty, which is when an individual is not otherwise poor but for a contingency. According to the ILO, these contingencies include sickness, medical care for the worker, maternity, unemployment, work injury, worker death, invalidity, and widowhood.

The contingencies, however, are work-related, and the individual and his family will be protected only if the individual is working prior to becoming a subject of the contingency. Thus, employment is required before becoming eligible for social security benefits. Ironically, this definition excludes the protection that must be provided for the already poor, and thus Social Assistance programs cover them.

Social security is the protection provided by society to individuals and households to ensure access to healthcare and income security, particularly in old age, unemployment, sickness, invalidity, work injury, maternity, or the loss of a breadwinner.

■ EVOLUTION OF SOCIAL SECURITY

The concept of social security dates back to the dawn of time. Stories of the Bible tell us how, during the years of famine, Joseph tried to tide over the situation by using surplus stocks of grain that he had stocked during the earlier years of plenty. The oldest social security institution is a family that includes the extended family.

The industrial revolution in Europe has seen the growth of urban and industrial centers that affected rural joint families, disturbing the institution of social security in the joint family system. When an individual could not care for his own needs, society realized the importance of protecting the individual and his family. Some evolutionary forms of social security efforts include private savings, mutual aid or mutual benefit associations, private insurance, and life insurance.

■ NEED FOR SOCIAL SECURITY

Modernization and urbanization have resulted in sweeping socioeconomic changes and brought new conflicts and tensions consequent upon the erosion of age-old family and fraternal security. The transition from an agricultural economy to an industrial economy brought in *special accompanied problems* that called for social security.

In India, 90% of families earn a livelihood from the unorganized sector. Most rural and informal sector workers do not have social security measures. In most developing countries, the rural and informal sectors constitute most of the population. They do not have any form of insurance or security (e.g., Maternity benefits, retirement benefits, health insurance, etc.), nor do they have representative organizations that might help them fight for these benefits. The poor are particularly vulnerable to the lack of health security measures. They spend a more significant percentage of their budget on health-related expenditures. During sickness, they need to pay hefty amounts for treatment and cannot earn money while under treatment.

Most poor households reside in remote rural areas where no government or private medical facilities are available, and obtaining treatment at a town or district-level hospital involves travel costs, which are not insignificant. As a Worker/Employee, you are a source of social security protection for yourself and your family. As an employer, you are responsible for providing adequate social security coverage for all your workers.

■ APPROACHES TO SOCIAL SECURITY

There are mainly two types:
1. Social assistance
2. Social insurance

Social Assistance

A method to provide benefits as of right to persons usually of small means in amounts sufficient to meet minimum standards of living from general revenues of the State. The characteristic feature is that the beneficiaries do not contribute towards various benefits that are made available to them. It is a "Non-contributory benefit" towards the maintenance of vulnerable groups such as children, mothers, aged people, disabled, etc. are essential for the effective working of the economic system.

Social Insurance

This is a method to provide benefits as a matter of right for persons of small earnings, in amounts that combine the beneficiaries' contributions with subsidies from the employer and the State. A characteristic feature of this is that the beneficiaries, employers, and the Government contribute to creating a common pool, out of which benefits are paid to the members in the event of any contingencies. The compulsory mutual aid with benefits can be claimed as a matter of right. This is suitable where the class of workers is covered sufficiently well organized, legally regulated, and financially stable.

Purpose and Contingencies of Social Security

The goal of any social security measure is to give individuals and families confidence that their standard of living and quality of life will not be eroded by a social or economic event; to provide medical care and income security against the consequences of defined contingencies; to facilitate victims' physical and vocational rehabilitation; to prevent or reduce occupational ill health and accidents; and to protect against unemployment through job retention and promotion.

As delineated by ILO, the social security contingencies are medical care, sickness benefit, unemployment benefit, old-age benefit, employment injury benefit, family benefit, maternity benefit, invalidity benefit, and survivors' benefit.

Types of Social Security Benefits

Benefits are classified into four categories based on who is receiving them. There are four types of benefits: retirement, disability, survivors, and supplemental.

Retirement Benefits

The majority of people associate Social Security with retirement benefits. People aged 62 and up who have worked for at least ten years are eligible for such payments. Your benefit amount is determined by your pre-retirement wage and the age at which you begin receiving benefits. While it is not intended to be your sole source of income in retirement, it can assist you in avoiding debt. Additionally, even if your spouse or divorced spouse has not paid into Social Security, they may be eligible for retirement payments.

Disability Benefits

Disability benefits assist people who are unable to work due to disabilities. Similar to retirement benefits, you must have worked for a certain number of years to be eligible for Social Security Disability Insurance (SSDI) payments (in the USA). Your monthly benefit amount is determined by your pre-disability pay and the number of hours you need to work. SSDI benefits may be available to your spouse or divorced spouse.

Survivors Benefits

Survivor benefits can assist employees, and retirees' families bridge financial gaps. Widows and widowers, divorced spouses, and children are often eligible recipients.

The level of benefits depends on several factors, including the worker's age at death, the worker's salary, the survivors' ages, and the survivors' relation to the deceased.

Supplemental Security Income Benefits

Supplemental Security Income (SSI) assists persons unable to earn enough money on their own. Adults with disabilities, children with disabilities, and those aged 65 and over are eligible. Individuals with sufficient job experience may be eligible for SSI benefits in addition to disability or retirement benefits. The number of benefits individuals receive varies based on their other sources of income and where they live.

■ SOCIAL SECURITY STRATEGIES IN INDIA

The following are examples of social security strategies:
- Social insurance in which the beneficiary participates in the pooling of risks and resources;
- Social assistance financed from general revenues and granting benefits based on means test;
- Employers liability schemes where there is an identifiable employer and within the economic capacity of the employer;
- National Provident Funds;
- Universal schemes for social security.

■ SOCIAL SECURITY IN INDIA

The responsibility of the State to provide social security to the citizens of this country is stated in Article 43 of the Constitution. All of the above tactics are implemented in India. We can divide the social security systems offered in India into three categories for discussion: preventive, promotional, and protective.

Preventive Schemes

Preventive schemes are those that aim to reduce risk. In the social management strategy of risks, the preventative approach tries to prevent poverty and helps people below the poverty line to come above the poverty line. Preventive healthcare and vaccinations against diseases form part of the preventive strategies. The majority of the schemes are of social assistance in nature.

Promotional Schemes

Promotional social security schemes are mainly of the means-tested social assistance type, which guarantees minimum living standards to vulnerable groups of the population. State and federal governments develop plans that are funded by general government revenues. These are the strategies of risk mitigation. These guarantees:
- **Food and nutritional security** by confirming per capita availability of food grains, access to food, development of agriculture, targeted Public Distribution System, and so on.

- **Employment security** ensures employment by generating employment, redeploying the surplus workforce in any sector, creating rural employment opportunities, and encouraging technological up-gradation.
- **Health security** by ensuring the availability of medical facilities, maintaining sanitation and drinking water standards, eradicating and controlling communicable diseases, timely vaccination of children and childbearing women, health insurance, old age homes, and social insurance for the elderly.
- **Education security** by ensuring the opening of schools, encouraging children to attend classes, making education compulsory up to certain age, opening adult learning centers or formulating schemes like Sakshara, running schemes like mid-day meals, etc.
- **Women security:** empowering women, encouraging women's literacy, banning dowry, and designing widow pension schemes.
- **Assistance to the disabled** by undertaking programs to promote health and education among the disabled, providing rehabilitation services and reservations in services to enable them to participate in social and economic activity.

All of the above are part of promotional social security schemes in which state governments play a larger role than the federal government. Food for work, Jawahar Rojgar Yojana, Rural Landless Laborers Employment Guarantee Schemes, Integrated Rural Development Project, Drought prone area Programs, Sakshara, Integrated Child Development Scheme (ICDS), Public Distribution System, reservations for the disabled in services, special educational institutions for the disabled, and other schemes are examples of promotional social security schemes.

Protective Social Security Programs

The protective social security programs help the poor in removing/reducing contingent poverty. In India, the protective social security programs have been designed to address the contingent poverty or the contingencies defined by the ILO. These programs take care of old-age income needs (Old Age Pension), survival benefits (Provident Funds), the medical need of insured families (Medical Insurance),

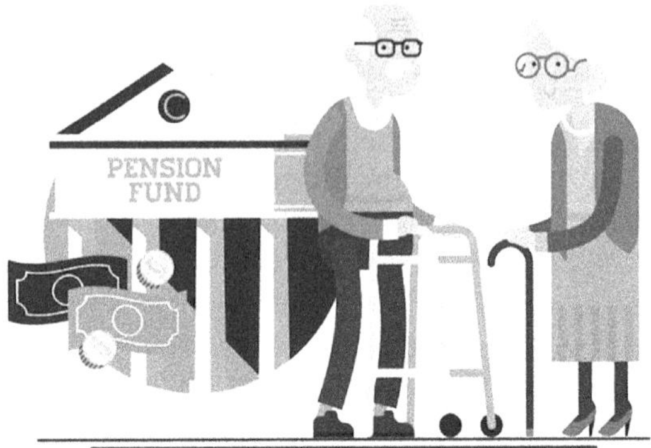

Fig. 11.1: Social security in old age.

widow and children/dependent economic needs (Widow/Children/ Orphan, and dependent pension), maternity benefits, compensation for loss of employment and work injury benefits **(Fig. 11.1)**.

Benefits are only available to the working population, the majority of whom are employed in the organized sector, thanks to legislation such as:

- Employees State Insurance Act of 1948
- Workmen's Compensation Act of 1923
- Employees Provident Fund and Miscellaneous Provisions Act of 1952
- Payment of Gratuity Act of 1972
- Maternity Benefits Act of 1976

SOCIAL SECURITY FOR DISABLED PERSONS IN INDIA

Having discussed the social security concepts, strategies, and programs available for vulnerable groups, the need for Social Security programs for persons with disabilities can hardly be overemphasized. However, we must recognize that the family has always been the primary producer of welfare, even before the contemporary welfare state was established. Later, the community, membership institutions, markets, and the Government offered welfare services. Producing and distributing welfare for society's most disadvantaged segments has long been a political obligation, particularly in democratic democracies. The magnitude of the woes of persons with disabilities is vast, and its impact on the individual, family, and community is severe.

Very young children, women, and the elderly with impairments are among the most vulnerable groups of people with disabilities. In the absence of benevolent markets and communities, and especially when the families of disabled people are unable to provide for their needs, some agency in society must provide for their survival and livelihood. That agency may be the State. Furthermore, a State's ability to assure its citizens is part of social justice.

SOCIAL SECURITY ADMINISTRATION IN THE UNITED STATES

In the USA, the Social Security Administration (SSA) deems a person disabled under Social Security Rules if they cannot do previous employment and cannot transition to a new position due to a medical condition (s). The handicap must also endure for at least one year or result in death. Working families are assumed to have alternative resources, such as workers' compensation, insurance, savings, and investments, to support during short-term disability under Social Security program guidelines.

The Persons with Disabilities (Equal Opportunities, Protection of Rights, and Full Participation) Act of 1995, among other things, aims to encourage disability empowerment. The right to receive support and assistance, while essential in improving the quality of life for people with disabilities, is insufficient. The goal of social security should be to ensure equal access to political, social, economic, and cultural rights.

National Sample Survey Organization (NSSO) 58th Round, undertaken in 2002, estimates that about 1.85 percent of the population suffer from some disability or other. However, detailed data for designing a comprehensive social security system for people with disabilities is now available.

In contrast, detailed statistics on Europe's disabled population are available, which are used to plan and implement social security. Among the fundamental rights enshrined in the European Convention on Human Rights and its Protocols, as well as the Revised European

Social Charter, are the right to work, the right to education, the right to private and family life, the right to health and social security, the right to protection against poverty and social exclusion, and the right to adequate housing. Based on these figures, European countries are working hard to ensure that programs benefit their disabled citizens.

Therefore, the availability of detailed data on the disabled population in India is a prerequisite for better planning and implementation of social security schemes. Data on the disabled people in the country will be helpful in this regard:

- **Parents with disabled children below the poverty line:** This is mandatory to design some additional social assistance schemes.
- **Unemployed, disabled persons who can be gainfully employed:** This is necessary to create special job schemes and employment drives for disabled people, develop income-generating plans for them, and eventually make them eligible for protected Social Security programs.
- **Non-employable disabled persons who always require the support of the Family/Community or the State:** This is necessary to design State assisted/funded schemes and rehabilitate them in the homes for disabled persons.
- **Disabled persons above 60 years of age:** This is essential to aid disabled senior persons in alleviating their miseries through Old Age Pension Schemes, Social Assistance, and State-assisted healthcare.
- **Disabled women:** This is essential to understand whether the disabled women are dependent on their parents or their husbands and the poverty status of their family/parents and to design schemes of Assistance or Insurance Accordingly. This will also help us understand the requirements of the disabled women of the childbearing age and make provisions for their maternity care.
- **Disabled widowers:** This will help planners understand the widows' dependency levels if they are pensioners, their economic status, etc.
- **Disabled persons engaged in agriculture and the informal sector:** This information will allow the government to create skill-upgradation programs for informal and self-employment workers, as well as backward and forward linkages for their economic

activities. It is also possible to grant export concessions and subsidies for products manufactured by the disabled.

- **Disabled veterans of the armed forces who can work again:** This information will allow planners to determine the level of help required for this group of people.

SOCIAL SECURITY PROGRAMS FOR THE DISABLED PERSONS IN INDIA

Assistance and benefits, both monetary and non-monetary, will help improve the situation of disabled people who face significant economic and social costs due to their disability. Benefits for disabled people are necessary but insufficient for their empowerment and general growth. People with disabilities, like everyone else, need love and affection, which is usually best offered by their family. As a result, specific measures and assistance are required to aid these families in overcoming the threat of a variety of potential sources of deprivation and providing a loving home as a far better and more natural alternative to living in large institutions/homes for the disabled. If the family is impoverished, the disabled member may not receive any assistance and may be treated as an additional burden. This essential social understanding should not be disregarded while building the programs proposed below.

Cash benefits in the form of assistance could take the following forms:
- Scholarships for disabled children
- Old-age pension for the elderly and widows
- Educationally Disabled Unemployment Assistance
- Subsidies for self-employment
- Disability pension
- Pension at retirement

The advantages include:
- Concessions and assistance in various activities, as well as concessions in transportation
- Medical attention
- Medical insurance in cases where employer liability schemes are available
- Compensation in the event of a work-related injury that results in disability

- Maternity care for disabled mothers
- Mandatory provision of crèches for the children of disabled mothers in all workplaces.
- Service reservations and concessions
- Special skill development programs
- Special schools and Teacher Education Programs
- Tax exemptions for disabled people and their parents with disabled children

▮ AVAILABLE PROGRAM FOR THE DISABLED

Currently, the country offers reservations in services, concessions in employment, disability pensions under the Employees' Provident Funds and Miscellaneous Provisions Act 1952, medical and maternity benefits under the Employees' State Insurance Act 1948, benefits under the Workmen's Compensation Act 1923, special schools for disabled children, and disability-specific assistance programs, though the coverage is not comprehensive. Employer liability and employment-related benefit schemes are two of the three major Social Security Acts cited above. They are only applicable in the event of a work-related disability.

There are no programs for old age and survivor benefits in the case of the disabled who cannot be employed or disabled persons who are not employed even after crossing the employable age. There are no programs for the disabled, dependent, and aged widows excepting some very meager assistance given by some State Governments, such as an old-age pension of ₹ 800 per month.

▮ PROGRAMS/SCHEMES REQUIRED TO BE DESIGNED FOR THE DISABLED PERSONS

Currently, available schemes or programs do not comprehensively address the problems of disabled persons. The principal Social Security Acts available in India *aim only at employment-related disabilities*. Many disabled persons are outside employment, informal economic activities, or simply dependent on their parents, children, and/or spouses. Some of the Rural Development and other programs have some disabled beneficiaries. However, the coverage is negligible, considering the statutory provision of a 3% reservation for persons with disabilities in all poverty alleviation schemes. This provision needs to be effectively implemented.

Based on the global best practices and the India-specific requirements, the urgent need is to formulate the following types of benefits and programs:

- **Universal old-age defined benefit pension scheme** for the disabled without any means test (As Social Assistance) should be thought of based on the national average wage that guarantees poverty alleviation among the persons with disabilities;
- **Universal medical benefits** *(the possibility of opening separate outpatient windows for the disabled should be seen as a way to alleviate the hardships of disabled patients waiting in general lines in public hospitals), free treatment for disabled people by corporate hospitals could be considered a precondition for corporate hospitals receiving a license;*
- **Universal unemployment assistance** to disabled persons with means test will alleviate poverty among persons with disabilities and employment. However, a system of benefit discontinuation in the event of non-acceptance of jobs should be considered to prevent people from sliding into the unemployment trap;
- Trying up with corporate hospitals to cover medical care at a concessional rate to the disabled, where the disabled can pay, and subsidizing the cost of surgical treatments in the hospitals;
- Social aid for disadvantaged children, including scholarships if they attend school. Pre-examination preparation to enable them to compete with other candidates in competitive tests;
- Special Employment and Skill upgradation programs;
- **Bank credit at a subsidized rate of interest** for the self-employment projects taken up by the disabled persons (NHFDC activities need to be expanded);
- **Reservations in services** and other concessions provided need to be effectively implemented;
- **Incentives** to be given to employers providing employment of disabled persons in consonance with the provisions in the PWD Act, 1995.

FINANCING OF THE SCHEMES

The approach to financing disabled-person schemes, as well as the launch of new social security schemes for people with disabilities, should be broadened, and the following options, including traditional budget allocations from government funds, should be explored:
- Finance from general revenues or taxation as the primary source;
- Collection of cess from industries where employment causes occupational diseases and hazards;
- A special tax on luxury items and items consumed that are harmful to one's health;
- Contributions from employed disabled parents to establish a separate fund for disability welfare;
- Contributions from charitable organizations;
- Assistance from international donors and organizations.

ADMINISTRATIVE ARRANGEMENTS

The current administrative arrangements for delivering support and benefits to persons with disabilities are scattered. Neither a uniform benefit formula nor a single agency administers or guides the program **(Fig. 11.2)**.

It is proposed that the various agencies or departments currently in charge of disability benefits be integrated in order to have a comprehensive program design and implementation policy under one umbrella with a Chief Executive Officer. However, disability-specific branches of that agency may be designed to maintain the professional approach. According to the Act, one of the duties of the office of the Chief Commissioner for Persons with Disabilities is to monitor the use of funds disbursed by the Central Government. This must be guaranteed. A National

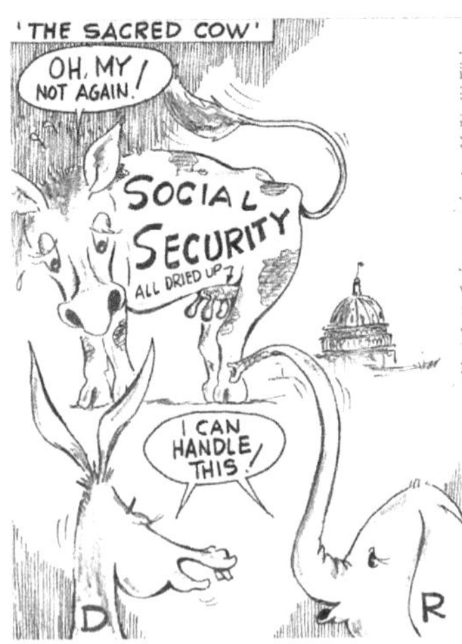

Fig. 11.2: Satire on social security.

Commission was recently established to assist and advise the government on disability and rehabilitation issues, as well as to make recommendations.

Data may be collected through census as also NSSO surveys at regular intervals. A national Unique Identification Number on the National Social Security Number lines may be considered to avoid duplicity in benefit delivery. The State Governments may start, in the right earnest issue of identity cards, preferably, SMART cards, assigning such numbers. All states may appoint independent State Commissioners who, according to the Act, may perform quasi-judicial functions such as supervising and enforcing various provisions of the Act and resolving grievances.

Administrative arrangements may be made to collect and record contributions and donations for developing a fund for social security programs for the disabled. The current collection system of grants under protective Social Security schemes needs not be disturbed; investment of funds and budgetary allocations made for the purpose needs to be enhanced, and effective income-generating schemes may be given attention. Suitable plans and administrative arrangements may be made to deliver medical benefits, old-age pension, and benefits in cash or kind.

CONCLUSION

The current Social Security programs are employment-based and do not prioritize disabled people. To be eligible for benefits, one must become disabled while working. This approach ignores disability and the significant problems of unemployment and poverty among disabled people. Disabled people are the most vulnerable group in India. Unfortunately, disabled people face social exclusion in society regardless of their economic status. Building economic, psychological, and social confidence is thus urgently required. To some extent, Social security disability programs will alleviate the agony of dependency.

Other immediate needs include a comprehensive administrative arrangement, the pooling of funds from various sources, and the provision of the benefit under professional supervision and control. Persons with disabilities are frequently unaware of benefits and schemes due to a lack of information and dissemination, as well as the absence of a single-window approach. More funds from local, state, national, and international agencies, governments, and non-governmental organizations, as well as ensuring that available benefits reach them, must be mobilized.

For example, resources are available through various Departments/Ministries and schemes such as Rural Development, HRD Ministry, Labor Ministry, District Rural Development Agency (DRDA) Programs, grant in aid schemes for special schools, pension schemes, United Nations Development Programs (UNDP), National Handicapped Finance Development Corporation (NHFDC), and international funding organizations such as The Norwegian Agency for International Development (NAID), Action Aid, and a variety of other organizations.

12

Social Work

☞ Describe the meaning and nature of social work.
☞ Describe the scope, goals and definitions of social work.
☞ Describe principles, roles and methods of social work.
☞ What is the role of a medical social worker?
☞ What are the functions of a medical social worker?

▣ MEANING OF SOCIAL WORK

Social work is a term used to describe various organized methods of helping people with some needs they cannot meet unaided.In the 19th century, it was developed as an organized method in the United Kingdom and the USA to help the poor people with material and spiritual welfare. Later it was extended to promote health and mental and emotional well-being. These days social work has become a professionalized activity. Since the later part of the 20th century, several universities have offered specialized advanced social work courses.

Social work is an academic and professional discipline that aims to improve the quality of life and well-being of an individual, a group, or a community by intervening on behalf of those affected by poverty, actual or perceived social injustices, and violations of their civil liberties and human rights through research, policy, crisis intervention, community organizing, direct practice, and teaching.

Social work is a profession that has been developed to administer the extensive and complex human service system put in place by society. It is a scientific discipline but requires a creative and artful approach to work with individuals, families, groups, and communities struggling with problems.

Its seven core functions are described as:

1. Engagement—the social worker must engage the client in early meetings to foster a relationship of collaboration

2. Assessment—data must be collected to guide and direct a plan of action to assist the client
3. Planning—negotiate and create an Action Plan
4. Implementation—promote resource procurement and improve role performance
5. Monitoring/evaluation—continuous tracking and assessment involve documenting the achievement of short-term goals to determine the extent to which the client is adhering to them.
6. Supportive counseling—affirming, challenging, encouraging, apprising, and exploring options
7. Graduated disengagement—looking to substitute the social worker with a naturally occurring resource.

Six other core values of social work are identified:
1. Service—assisting those in need and solving social issues
2. Social Justice—contest social injustices
3. Dignity and worth of the person
4. Significance of human relationships
5. Integrity—behave in a trustworthy way
6. Competence—practice in one's fields of competence and; build and improve professional skills.

Nature of Social Work

Social work is not a science in the same way that physics or chemistry is. Social work, on the other hand, draws on scientific information from various disciplines and increasingly uses scientific methods to construct theoretical frameworks and assess efficacy.

In the following ways, social work might be considered scientific:
- It collects, organizes, and analyses data about people's social functioning.
- It creates new techniques, formulates new practice guidelines, and develops new programs and policies based on observations, experiences, and formal studies.
- It assesses its interventions objectively and their impact on people's social functioning.
- It discusses and assesses the ideas, research, and practices described by others in the field.
  Like many other occupations, the social worker is more of a techie than a scientist. A social scientist is exclusively interested in learning

about the client's reality. As a technologist, the social worker aspires to transform it. As a result, social work can be regarded as a practicing profession that necessitates solid knowledge and competency (in data gathering, analysis, and evaluation).

Scope of Social Work

Social work is concerned with supporting people in need so that they can develop the courage to handle their issues themselves.It is both science and art. Social work is a science because it is obtained from different disciplines, and they use this theoretical knowledge to help people.

A social worker has to create a positive rapport with the clients. They should know how to interview and write reports. They should be able to find out the cause of the problem, and finally, they should work out a solution. The four significant steps involved in social work are *an assessment of the problem, planning for its solution, implementing the plan*, and *evaluating the outcome*. The keen interest of the social worker in helping the client will not solve the problem alone. She should know how to help their clients.

Goals of Social Work

Social work aims to reduce suffering by solving the problems faced by people. Individuals have psychosocial issues concerning their physical and mental health. Apart from this, adjustment problems in children and adults can be dealt with separately.

In other words, social work promotes the social functioning of individuals, groups, and families by providing recreational services, and it can prevent delinquency and crime in society by using leisure time sensibly.

It also links the client system with the needed resources. Social work helps the individual bring about a change in the environment in favor of his growth and development.

Social work provides democratic ideas and encourages the development of goodinterpersonal relations, resulting in proper adjustments with the family and neighborhood. Social work does not believe in 'Social Darwinism.' It does not accept the principle of survival of the fittest. Hence, it works for social justice through legal aid. It also promotes social justice through the development of social policy. Social work improves the operation of the social service delivery network as well.

■ DEFINITIONS

Social work may be defined as an art, a science, and a profession that helps people solve personal, group (especially family), and community problems and attain satisfying individual, group, and community relationships through social work practice.

"Social work is professional service based on knowledge of human relations and skill relationship and concerned with the problem of intra-personal and inter-personal adjustments resulting from an unmet individual, group, or community need." (Mirza R Ahmed)

Social work is "help rendered to any person or group, who is suffering from any disability, mental, physical, emotional or moral so that the individual or group so helped is enabled to help himself or herself." (Moorthy and Rao)

The aim of social work, as generally understood, is to remove social injustice, relieve distress, prevent suffering, and assist the weaker member of society in rehabilitating themselves and their families and, in the short fight the five giant evils of (1) Physical wants, (2) Disease, (3) Ignorance, (4) Squalor, (5) Idleness." (Kher)

"Social work is both a practice and an academic discipline that promotes social change and development, social cohesion, and people's empowerment and liberation. Social work is founded on the principles of social justice, human rights, collective responsibility, and diversity. Social work, which is based on social work theories, social sciences, humanities, and indigenous knowledge, engages people and structures to address life challenges and improve well-being." (International Social Workers Federation)

"Social work is a profession concerned with helping individuals, families, groups, and communities to enhance their individual and collective well-being. It aims to help people develop their skills and ability to use their resources and community resources to resolve problems. Social work concerns individual and personal problems and broader social issues such as poverty, unemployment, and domestic violence." (Canadian Association of Social Workers)

The professional application of social work values, principles, and techniques to one or more of the following ends: assisting people in obtaining tangible services; counseling and psychotherapy with individuals, families, and groups; assisting communities or groups in providing or improving social and health services; and participating in legislative processes. Knowledge of human development and behavior, as well as social, economic, and cultural institutions, is required for the practice of social work." (National Association of Social Workers)

"Social workers work with individuals and families to help improve outcomes in their lives. This may be helping to protect vulnerable people from harm or abuse or supporting people to live independently. Social workers support people, act as advocates, and direct people to the services they may require. Social workers often work in multi-disciplinary teams alongside health and education professionals." (British Association of Social Workers)

PRINCIPLES

The social work profession is guided by a distinct set of abstract values and a code of ethics. These values are transformed into accepted practice principles to inform our intervention with clients. A listing of nine social work principles follows and a brief description of each.

Acceptance: A fundamental social work principle implies a genuine understanding of clients. Acceptance is conveyed in the professional relationship through the expression of genuine concern, receptive listening, intentional responses that acknowledge the other-person's point of view, and the creation of a climate of mutual respect.

Affirming individuality: To affirm a client's individuality is to recognize and appreciate the unique qualities of that client. It means to 'begin where the client is.' Clients expect personalized understanding and undivided attention from professionals. Individualization requires freedom from bias and prejudice, avoidance of labeling and stereotyping, recognition and appreciation of diversity, and knowledge of human behavior.

Purposeful expression of feelings: Clients need to have opportunities to express their feelings freely to the social worker. As social workers, we must go beyond 'just the facts' to uncover the underlying feelings.

Nonjudgmentalism: Communicating nonjudgmentalism is essential to developing a relationship with any client. It does not imply that social workers do not make decisions; rather, it means a non-blaming attitude and behavior. Social workers judge others as neither good nor bad nor worthy or unworthy.

Objectivity: Closely related to nonjudgmentalism, objectivity is the principle of examining situations without bias. Social workers must avoid injecting personal feelings and prejudices into client relationships to be objective in their observations and understanding.

Controlled emotional involvement: There are three components to a controlled emotional response to a client's situation—sensitivity to expressed or unexpressed feelings, an understanding based on knowledge of human behavior, and a response guided by wisdom and purpose. The social worker should not respond in a way that conveys coldness or lack of interest while simultaneously cannot over-identify with the client.

Self-determination: The principle of self-determination is based on recognizing the right and need of clients to freedom in making their own choices and decisions. Social workers are responsible for creating a working relationship in which choice can be exercised.

Access to resources: Social workers are implored to ensure that everyone has the necessary resources, services, and opportunities, to pay attention to expanding choices and opportunities for the oppressed and disadvantaged, and to advocate for policy and legislative changes that improve social conditions and promote social justice.

Confidentiality: This or the right to privacy implies that clients must give expressed consent before information such as their identity, the content of discussions held with them, one's professional opinion about them, or their record.

METHOD SOCIAL WORK

Social work methods fall into three major categories:
- **Social casework:** This is concerned with individuals and their families.
- **Social group work:** Associations with others are the primary therapeutic agent.
- **Community work:** The focus is on developing and utilizing neighborhood and community resources.

ROLES

Social workers may play these roles in different contexts and at other times in their careers, and there may be a conflict between them. The roles are:

- Counselor (or caseworker) who works with individuals to help them address personal issues.
- Advocate on behalf of the poor and socially excluded.
- Partner working together with disadvantaged or disempowered individuals and groups.
- Assess risk or need for several client groups; also associated with surveillance. This role may conflict with Counseling.
- A care manager arranges services for users in a mixed care economy but may have little direct client contact.
- The agent of social control helps maintain the social system against the demands of individuals whose behavior is problematic.

MEDICAL SOCIAL WORKER

Medical social work is a branch of social work. Typically, medical social workers work in hospitals, outpatient clinics, community health agencies, skilled nursing facilities, long-term care facilities, or hospices. They work with patients and their families in need of psychosocial help. Medical social workers evaluate and intervene when appropriate in the psychosocial functioning of patients and families **(Fig. 12.1)**.

Social workers address questions such as: Who should intervene and when should they intervene? Interventions may include referring patients and families to appropriate community services and help, such as preventive care, psychotherapy, supportive counseling,

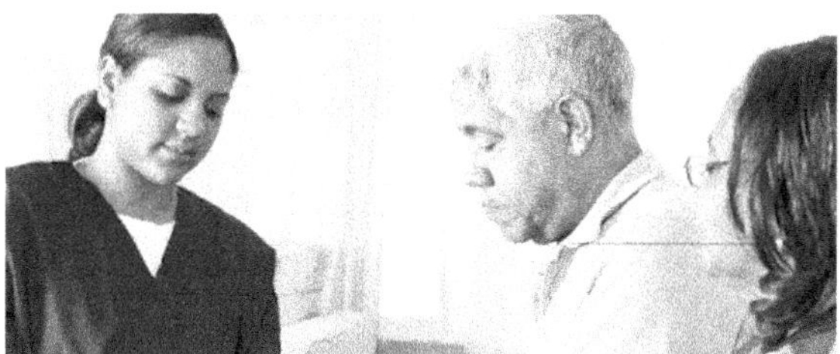

Fig. 12.1: Medical social worker interviewing a patient.

grief counseling; or helping a patient strengthen their social support network.

A medical social worker's role is to "restore balance in the individual's personal, family and social life, to help that person maintain or recover his or her health, and to strengthen his or her ability to adapt and reintegrate into society."

MSWs in this field typically work with other disciplines such as medicine, nursing, occupational therapy, speech therapy, physiotherapy, and recreational therapy.

Role of a Medical Social Worker

The role of the medical social worker (MSW) has been increasingly receiving significant attention in the medical profession in India for the last three decades. In most large cities, MSWs are appointed in hospitals, public health centers, etc. They are also engaged in community health programs. Recently some industrial firms have also started creating positions for social workers in their establishments.

Although most of the MSWs are employed in the hospitals run by the state government, central government, or municipal corporations, many a time, psychiatrists and physicians also employ some MSWs. Social workers in hospitals and medical centers deliver frontline services to patients with conditions spanning the entire healthcare continuum.

Following are the significant areas of role of an MSW:
- **Securing material help for the patient:** The MSW in the hospital helps the patient and their family to procure expensive medicines and treatment facilities. This turned out to be the most helpful service to the hospital as it ensured money and other material help were necessary for proper treatment.
- **Casework service:** Usually, people display specific social and emotional reactions to their disease. Some can cope withit unaided, but others need help and guidance in meeting their social and emotional difficulties. MSW provides this service by considering each case separately. MSWs establish professional relationships with the patient and help the patient with diagnosis and treatment.
- **Discharge of patients:** The MSW follow-up the case even after discharge and helps the patient by catering to physical,

emotional,and economic needs. With the rise of a modern complex society based on an urban industrial setup, the role of MSW is becoming increasingly significant. This is happening because traditional support systems such as joint family, caste, etc., are fast declining in this respect.

- **Group work service:** The MSW serves the patients by conducting recreational, educational, and therapeutic group activities in the wards and hospitals. They also take up such actions for physically or mentally disabled persons.
- **Community planning for health and happiness:** The MSW's role is equally significant in planning for community health in both urban and rural areas.

They also work as motivators in community health programs such as vaccination drives, family planning programs, awareness about health and hygiene, etc.

Thus, the MSW's role is intrinsically integrated with the prevention, diagnosis, treatment, and rehabilitation aspects of patients' healthcare. MSW's immediate task is to help patients and families through casework, group work, and consultation. To keep pace with new knowledge in medical science, the medical social worker must also gain new knowledge to meet the needs of people.

Functions of the Medical Social Worker

Hospital social workers help patients and their families understand a particular illness, work through the emotions of a diagnosis, and provide Counseling about the decisions that need to be made. Social workers are also essential members of interdisciplinary hospital teams. Working with doctors, nurses, allied health professionals, and social workers sensitizes other healthcare providers to a patient's illness's social and emotional aspects. Hospital social workers use case management skills to help patients and their families address and resolve their health condition's social, financial, and psychological problems.

Job functions that a social worker might perform within a hospital include:

- Initial screening and evaluation of patients and families
- Comprehensive psychosocial assessment of patients

- Helping patients and families understand the illness and treatment options, as well as the consequences of various treatments or treatment refusal
- Helping patients/families to adjust hospital admission; possible role changes; exploring emotional/social responses to illness and treatment
- Educating patients on the role of healthcare team members; assisting patients and families in communicating with one another and with members of the healthcare team; interpreting information
- Educating patients on the levels of health care (i.e., acute,subacute, home care); entitlements; community resources; and advance directives
- Facilitating decision-making on behalf of patients and families
- Employing crisis intervention
- Diagnosing underlying mental illness; providing or making referrals for individual, family, and group psychotherapy
- Educating hospital staff on patient psychosocial issues
- Promoting communication and collaboration among healthcare team members
- Coordinating patient discharge and continuity of care planning
- Promoting patient navigation services
- Arranging for resources/funds to finance medications, durable medical equipment, and other needed services
- Ensuring communication and understanding about post-hospital care among patient, family, and healthcare team members
- Advocating for patient and family needs in different settings— inpatient, outpatient, home, and in the community
- Championing the healthcare rights of patients through advocacy at the policy level.

To sum up, the role of the medical social worker includes the following:
- To stimulate socialization among patients through casework and group work, etc.
- To provide emotional support and encouragement to the patients through sharing of experiences with them to help them later in managing their disease or disability

- To motivate patients to follow medical recommendations and their exercise program
- To participate in the education, training, and orientation program of the hospital
- To participate in community planning as related to the interests of the hospital
- To participate in the planning and development of services within the hospital.

13

Social Control

▦ INTRODUCTION

In sociology, the study of social control occupies central importance. The existence and persistence of organized social life are impossible without some minimum degree of control over its members. Social control is needed to maintain social order; what do we mean by 'social order'? Social order refers to a system of people, relationships, and customs, all these together operating smoothly to accomplish the work of a society. No society can function effectively unless human behavior can be predicted. Orderliness depends on a network of roles. The network of reciprocal rights and duties is kept in force through social control.

▦ MEANING AND NATURE

The term 'social control' is broadly concerned with maintaining order and stability. It may be used in the limited sense of denoting the various specialized means employed to maintain order, such as codes, courts, and constables. It also categorizes social institutions and their interrelations as they contribute specifically to social stability, e.g., legal, religious, and political institutions. Social control is one of the most fundamental subjects of sociological discussion. It arises in all discussions about the nature and causes of stability and change.

DEFINITIONS

Social control pertains to the intentional or unintentional regulation of a group based on its beliefs, principles, and values. Its primary objective is to halt or prevent negative deviance, which refers to the breach of established laws and values that may bring harm to others. It is crucial to note that norms, morality, values, ethics, and deviance are relative to different social groups.

Some definitions emphasize social order. McIver and Page define social control as to how the social order maintains itself. Social control is how some see society as maintaining order.

Social control is also defined as conformity to group norms and expectations. The focus is on how a group or society ensures conformity among its members. Social control is how a society reins in errant members. Social control limits deviations from social norms through processes and means.

The main points that emerge from all these definitions about the meaning of social controls are:
- The term refers to means and processes whereby specific goals are achieved.
- The two most important goals sought to be achieved by social control are:
  - Conformity to the norms and expectations of the group.
  - Maintenance of order in society.
- There is an element of influence, persuasion, or compulsion in control. The individual or group is directed to act in a particular way. Conformity is expected of imposed irrespective of whether one likes it or not.
- The scope of social control is vast. It may operate at different levels. One group may seek to control another group; a group may control its members, or an individual may seek to control another individual. The scope of control ranges from the management of deviants to social planning.

■ RELATED CONCEPTS

Here, we discuss some concepts closely related to social control as follows.

Concept of Self-control

Self-control implies that the imposition of external control is not required to compel the individual to do the right thing in a given situation. In this sense, self-control supplements the mechanism of social control in producing conformity. But, it should also be remembered that self-control originates in social control. The processes of social control in still a sense of internal control in the individual. The relation between self-control and social control can be understood in this manner.

The group applies some sanctions (punishment, etc.) on an individual for indulging in deviant behavior. But, many people can visualize the consequences of their actions in advance and restrain themselves. In this sense, self-control is also a form of social control. From this point of view, we can also maintain that self-control and social control are closely related to yet another process—socialization, to which we now turn.

Socialization

Socialization teaches children their group's cultural traits. They can join the group or society. Parents use reward, punishment, and discipline in childhood to enforce their expectations. One acquires many traits by observing others' behavior and anticipating the consequences of one's actions. This develops self-control and morality. Through learning, we conform to group expectations without conscious effort. You perform many minor and major supposed' activities without knowing why. Thus, socialization promotes effective social control. When socialization fails, a person may act against group expectations. Sanctions are needed.

Social control helps socialize. Socialization is a learning process that requires a reward-and-punishment system. Social control and socialization work together to ensure group norm conformity and social order.

■ GOALS OF SOCIAL CONTROL

Some important goals of social control are mentioned below:

Conformity

One of the social control aims is to bring about conformity in society. Social control mechanisms are employed to control, check,or prevent deviant behavior. As we know that deviant behavior is dysfunctional to society in several ways, the objective of social control is to safeguard the group against such dysfunctional consequencesof deviant behavior.

Uniformity

A related objective of social control is to produce uniformity of behavior. This does not mean that all the members have to behave alike. It only implies that coordination should be among the several inter-related activities performed by different people. For example, traffic movement on the road will be impossible if all road users do not follow some traffic rules (keeping to the left, etc.). A game cannot be played if all teams do not follow uniform rules.In every sphere of social life, some uniformity of behavior is expected and essential.

Solidarity

Solidarity is an essential objective of social control. MacIver and Page have noted that social control ensures order and solidarity in society. Society is constituted of several parts of units. These different parts must maintain equilibrium with each other and the whole to ensure social solidarity and stability. The mechanisms of social control are directed at maintaining this equilibrium among the parts and between the parts and the whole.

Continuity

Social control is also necessary to maintain and preserve the accumulated culture of the group. Compelling or inducing individuals to conform to the prevailing norms and values ensures the continuity of these cultural characteristics. For example, when parents insist on their children following family customs or practices, their continuity over generations is sought to be assured.

Social Change

Social control is employed to conserve the existing patterns and sometimes to induce desired social changes. Many persuasion, inducement, and compulsions are used in our country to bring about desired changes in some social customs, attitudes, and behavior. Prescribing the age of marriage, the two-child family norm, removal of untouchability, dowry, etc., are attempting to bring about social change through various means of social control.

Essential Features of Social Control

The following are three main features of social control:
1. It is an influence exerted through social suggestions, public opinion, religion, and appeal.
2. Society exercises influence more bitterly than a single person or individual; such groups may be in the form of a family, union, club, etc.
3. Every control is the influence exercised by a specific society to promote group welfare. Social control is exercised for specific ends and goals to achieve by the individual of a collective group.

These are other essential features of social control:
- **Social regulations are normative in nature:** They are standards that individuals must meet, and failure to do so may be considered a lapse. Every individual, for example, is required to speak the truth, and lies, when discovered, are regarded as acts devoid of social dignity.
- **Social regulations are relative and partial:** Regulations are viewed as relative because, as the authors point out, they primarily protect the interests of dominant social groups. Such groups may be religious or politically powerful, and economic power is a powerful determinant of interests that must be protected in modern times. Codes and regulations are only partially effective because no single category can fully control human thoughts and actions; different social control agencies complement each other's efforts.

- **The codes and regulations that affect social control can emanate from different agencies:** There may be rules and regulations in voluntary associations, such as the club or the church. Violations of each set of rules have been sanctioned, and the severity of the sanctions varies. A club or a professional organization may have specific agreed-upon rules that serve as its code, with a reprimand, suspension, or expulsion as sanctions. Similarly, 'communal' codes may regulate necessary community customs, with ridicule or ostracism as penalties for disobedience or violation.

- **No regulatory code is effective unless it is backed up by sanctions that can be enforced in the real world:** For example, moral and religious codes are less effective today than they were previously because modern men regard concepts of sin and hell as more superstitious than logical; however, the State's intentions are felt in absolute terms when its civil or criminal laws are broken.

Psychologists deny that a person's fear complex causes him to follow the rules. Even when it comes to obeying the law, an individual's motivations are likely similar to those that shape his socialization process. Suggestions and imitation are typical in developing a social being, and with his habituation to specific ideas, he naturally enters the stage of indoctrination.

Even in his own family, he may be indoctrinated and willingly and readily respond to specific codes. The person develops a sense of loyalty to the principles taught to him, and he does not want to question their validity. The average Indian does not believe that young people should have pre-marital sex experiences, and a large majority of young people share this viewpoint.

The Need for Social Control

For an orderly social life, social control is required. Society must regulate and pattern individual behavior to maintain normative social order. Without social control, society's organization is about to be disrupted. If a person has been effectively socialized, the force of habit and his desire to be accepted and approved by others will cause him to confirm the accepted ways.

If he has not been adequately socialized, he will deviate from the accepted ways, but the pressures of social control will force him to conform. "To bring about solidarity, conformity, and continuity of a particular group or society," according to Kimball Young, is necessary. "Only through social control is it possible." Society must rely on its mechanisms to achieve the necessary order and discipline.

The notion put forth by Herbert Spencer suggests that society is a group of individuals who coexist for functional purposes. Individuals participate in society to uphold their identity and opinions. They must have a role in establishing specific rules and institutions to preserve their traits and maintain their individuality. Social control mechanisms play a vital role in safeguarding both individual and societal identity.

The needs for social control are discussed as under:

- **Reestablishing the social system:** Social control's primary goal is to maintain the status quo. In other words, society wants its members to live the same way their forefathers did. Even though enforcing the old order in a changing society may impede social progress, it is necessary to maintain society's continuity and uniformity.
- **Regulation of individual social behavior:** Individual behavior is regulated by social objectives and values, which require social control. This contributes to the preservation of social order. It will be difficult to maintain social organization effectively unless individuals follow the prescribed norms of conduct and their self-seeking impulses are subjugated to the welfare of the whole. As a result, social control is required for society to exist and progress.
- **Obedience to social decisions:** Society takes certain decisions. These decisions are taken to maintain and uphold the values of society. An attempt is made to get the social decision obeyed through social control.
- **To establish social unity:** Unity is not possible without social control. Social control regulates the behavior of individuals by establishing norms that bring uniformity of behavior and unity among the individuals.
- **To bring solidarity:** In people's minds, social control creates a sense of solidarity. In a competitive world, the more powerful group may exploit the weaker group, or equally powerful groups may clash. This has an impact on harmony and order. Some groups may develop antisocial attitudes and threaten society's structure. As a result, different groups and institutions are required.
- **To bring conformity in society:** The goal of social control is to bring about uniformity in the behavior of individual members and various types of conformity in their societies.

- **To provide social sanction:** Any significant departure from the accepted norms is considered a threat to the group's well-being. As a result, the group employs sanctions to manage individual behavior.
- **To check cultural maladjustment:** The society around us is constantly changing. Individuals must adapt their behavior to the changes that are occurring in society. On the other hand, individuals cannot adapt to new situations. Some people may turn out to be deviants. As a result, social control is required to avoid individual maladjustment.

■ METHODS OF SOCIAL CONTROL

Methods of social control can be classified into two types:
1. Informal
2. Formal

The informal type of control is casual and unwritten. It lacks regulation, scheduling, and organization. The informal type consists of casual praise, ridicule, gossip, and ostracism. The formal type is scheduled, organized,codified,or regulated, as in promotion, demotion, satire, monetary payment, mass media, etc. We now discuss each method in detail.

Informal Social Control

Informal social control is also called primary social control because it is more compelling than primary groups. Small, intimate, homogeneous groups are the norm. Loyalty binds group members. Family, playgroups, neighborhoods, rural communities, and primitive societies are compact social groupings. Every person in a totalitarian society is controlled by neighborhood or kinship groups. Nobody is immune to social control.

In such social settings, social control surrounds individuals and groups like 'concentric circles.' It's informal, spontaneous, and unplanned. The group shows its disapproval by ridicule, gossip, opprobrium, criticism, ostracism, and sometimes physical force and coercion. Since the group is small, ties are substantial, members are known, and the individual has few membership options. They can't ignore their group's disapproval, so they must conform.

Such control methods are effective in primitive societies where primary groups and relationships abound, but also in modern complex societies like ours, particularly within secondary groups (such as voluntary associations, clubs, and trade unions), where informal controls are sufficient to achieve the organization's goals.

Formal Social Control

Formal social control is called 'secondary social control' because it is found in larger groups. Our complex society has such social groupings. Such societies have many impersonal groups with specific goals. Examples are the party, union, factory, office, student group, etc. These secondary groups have less intimate relationships. They interact according to laws, rules, and procedures. This does not mean mockery, criticism, or gossip are not informal controls. Informal groups from within formal organizations, according to sociology. In university or college cliques, informal controls are more effective. Informal groups can inhibit or facilitate formal secondary controls, affecting the organization's performance.

Formal control is rare in secondary groups. This type of control uses rewards, honor, punishment, expulsion, etc. Such controls include law, police, courts, prisons, and other law enforcement agencies.

Formal control mechanisms include media propaganda to 'engineer' social control. Large secondary groups' informal controls are weakened by anonymity, mobility, and conflicting norms and values. Members do not care about each other, and intimacy is fading. They frequently switch locations or groups.

They can therefore evade group control. In a complex society, different groups' norms and values conflict; one group may approve of conduct while others don't. In such cases, social control agencies intervene.

MECHANISMS, MEANS, AND CONSEQUENCES OF SOCIAL CONTROL

Mechanisms

Every society has devised various mechanisms to exercise control. Sociologists view social control mechanisms as all those social arrangements that:

a. Prevent such strains as may develop from the individual's place in the social structure
b. Prevent the strains from leading to deviance. Every society has specific means to exercise social control, and there are clear consequences of exercising social control for promoting stability and conformity in societies.

Types of Mechanisms

Mechanisms of social control can be classified into the following four categories:

1. Preventive mechanisms: These mechanisms are designed to prevent such situations from developing, which might lead to deviance. Socialization, social pressures, the establishment of role priorities, and force are some of the mechanisms through which conformity is promoted or prevents the occurrence of deviance.
2. Mechanisms to manage tensions: Institutionalized safety valves such as humor, games and sports, leisure, and religious rituals are considered outlets for the tension generated by social restraints and cultural inconsistencies.
3. Mechanisms to check or change deviant behavior: Sanctions are used by every society to bring about conformity and check or change deviant behavior. Sanctions have been classified into:
   - Psychological sanctions:Negative sanctions are ridicule, non-acceptance, ostracism, etc. Positive sanctions include acceptance in the group, praise, invitation to the innercircle events, verbal or physical pat on the back, gifts, etc.
   - Physical sanctions: These are primarily negative. The most important physical sanctions are expulsion, physical punishment, and extermination.
   - Economic sanctions: These include positive rewards such as the promotion of a loyal, sincere worker, grant of tenders to civic-minded business people, etc., or negative sanctions such as the threat of loss or reduction in one's income (e.g., threat to discharge by employer may prevent the employee from continuing their strike), economic boycott, etc.
4. Propaganda mechanisms: Another important mechanism that can change the desired direction is propaganda or molding

public opinion. Propaganda is a deliberate attempt to control the behavior and interrelationships of members to change their feelings, attitudes, and values—for example,the efforts of the Government to control population growth through family planning propaganda.

Means of Social Control

Sociologists have been fascinated by the operation of social control mechanisms. Social control has always existed, though its operational nature has evolved. The norms, values, and so on have always existed, but their constituents have changed over time.

Informal Means of Social Control

- **Norms:** The institution is the source of norms. They set the bar for acceptable behavior and regulate it. Institutional norms limit individual freedom to pursue cultural goals. These serve as a roadmap for action. The norms give society cohesion. They have an impact on people's attitudes. A social norm in one social system may not be effective in another. Because of the socially defined situation, conformity to norms is qualified. Loss of prestige, social ridicule, or even more severe punishment may await the violator of the norm.
- **Value:** It is made up of culturally defined objectives. It is a legitimate goal for all or variously situated members of society. There are various levels of "sentiments and significance" involved. These could include motivational quotes. Values are "aims worth pursuing." These are the fundamentals, but they are not exhaustive.
- **Folkways:** Folks are people who have a strong sense of belonging to a community. They have a uniform and a way of life in common. This is what the folkway is made up of "Simple habits of action common to the group members; they are the ways of folk that are somewhat standardized and have some degree of traditional sanction for their persistence," according to FB Renter and CW Hart. These are accepted as binding in the interest of communal life and uniformity. Disapproval is elicited by the indifference shown to these.
- **More:** These are value-based folkways that are deeply rooted in community life. Any disregard for these will result in retaliation.

Green defines mores as "common ways of acting that are more strongly regarded as right and proper than folkways and carry greater certainty and severity of punishment if violated..."

- **Custom:** A "rule or norm of action" is defined as "a rule or norm of action." It is the result of a social necessity. It is followed because it involves sentiment that is based on logic. It is self-enforcing; no specific agency is required to enforce it. It is enforced as is, and any disregard for it results in social censure.

  It can't be stretched to meet the demands of the future. It may vanish due to a change in circumstances. It is a force that reflects the social consensus at any given time. It is something that a legislator must think about. He cannot just ignore it. Custom is the result of the passage of time. It evolves as a blueprint for a specific social purpose. It takes time for something to evolve.

  A king, according to Manu, must investigate the rules of families and "establish their particular law." According to him, a king is nothing more than a "distributor of justice." He is not to enact legislation. Customs cannot be ignored when making laws. In group situations, the custom is still a powerful force. However, custom as a social discipline is on the decline. It lacks the automation necessary to adapt to the demands of a rapidly changing society.

- **Belief system:** Man's behavior is heavily influenced by his belief system. It has given social norms legitimacy and influenced the development of culture. It has been effective as a form of informal social control. Some of the beliefs have a significant impact on the social structure. Man has believed in the existence of an unseen power since the dawn of time. He believed he was being watched because of his fear.

  Prayer and meditation appear to be guided by this spirit. It is indicated by raising hands in supplication, kneeling before a religious symbol, or other practices and rituals. Faith in the continuity of life motivates belief in the theory of incarnation. Birth and death were accepted as changes from one body to another in the endless scheme.

  It fueled man's faith in goodness. He believed that wrongdoing would have disastrous consequences. As a result, he did his best to avoid them. As a result, all Indian religious systems consider belief in the theory of Karma to be fundamental. Religious thinking and practices have been primarily motivated by the belief in the soul's immortality.

- **Ideology:** Ideology is the social determinant of thinking. Ideology has always influenced social thinking. Varnashrama Dharma, Punarjanam, and Dhamma have all influenced our social thinking. Politically, the ideology has been the country's unity. In ancient texts, this land is referred to as devanirmitamsthanam—the land fashioned by the gods themselves.

  "Recall and worship the image of his mother country as the land of seven sacred rivers, the Ganga, Yamuna, Saraswati, Godavari, Narmada, Sindhu, and Kaveri, which together cover its entire area," says one of the most common prayers.

- **Suggestions and ideas from others:** Suggestions and ideas from others are essential to social control. Society controls its members' behavior through these suggestions and ideologies. In general, society controls and regulates its members' behavior in various ways, such as through books, writings, spoken words, inculcation of ideas, and so on.

- **Religion:** It includes customs, rituals, prohibitions, conduct standards, and roles primarily concerned with or justified in terms of the supernatural and sacred. Religion is a powerful social control agent. It regulates man's interactions with the physical and social forces surrounding him. The degree to which religion influences men's behavior is determined by how much its adherents accept its teachings.

- **Art:** It is a method of sublimation and redirecting an individual's instinct. It combines religion, morality, ideals, and many things. Art is an indirect and inadvertent that trains the child or an individual for either way of life.

Formal Means of Social Control

- **Education:** Education is a fantastic tool for social control. After the family, there are the classroom, peer group, and leaders who impact a child. The differences between Dvija and Ekaja highlighted the importance of education in ancient society's social structure.

  Individuals are instilled with moral, intellectual, and social values through education. It gives the impression of continuity. It connects one to one's ancestors and gives one a sense of perspective. It gives the individual a social vision of uniformity and prepares him for his social role.

The current character crisis is due partly to an education system that is culturally alienating, socially non-collective, politically fractious, and not rooted in our heritage. Education's increased social importance is receiving more attention at all levels—primary and secondary, literary and technical.

- **Law:** For all practical purposes, the law is "a general rule of external action enforced by a sovereign political authority," as Professor Holland put it. It is the State's general condition, which members of the political body are expected to follow under certain conditions. It is standard and intended for everyone.

  Any disregard for it will almost certainly result in a penalty. However, as Pollock pointed out, it will almost certainly result in a penalty. It "existed before the state had any adequate means of compelling its observance and before there was any regular enforcement process," as Pollock points out.

  The First Law was a custom that was upheld by a recognized authority. It arose from the general usages of the family, tribe, or clans as a prescribed course of action. Some of these faded as circumstances changed, while those passed down from generation to generation gained clout. As a result, the custom became an essential source of law. Religion, equity, judicial decisions, scientific commentaries, and legislation are some of the other sources of law.

  Law is a broad term that encompasses both Common Law, primarily based on custom enforced by the courts, and statutory law, which Parliament enacts. Constitutional law is another branch of law, which is the law outlined in the Constitution. The Constitutional Law establishes the appropriate authority of the Government's organs.

- **Coercion:** Using force to maintain social control is as old as society itself. All societies have used it to varying degrees. Even today, some societies use force to deal with deviants. It has not received much attention in our society. Our political ethics have traditionally been based on nonviolence or minor violence.

  The Asokanstate was the only one to abandon force and coercion as a tool of state policy. Gandhiji used nonviolence as a weapon against the world's most influential British Empire. Penal codes are reviewed in all civilized societies to make criminal law more humane. Force breeds vengeance rather than reform.

Agencies of Social Control

Social control is exercised through many different agencies. The arrangements through which society's values and norms are communicated are called 'agencies' of social control. They are distinct entities that allow institutional norms to function in society. They are 'executive' agencies that ensure that norms are followed. They are the institutions in charge of procedural procedures. Family, school, Government, and public opinion are crucial social control mechanisms **(Fig. 13.1)**.

- **Family:** Family is an essential social control mechanism. On the one hand, it socializes a person while also training him in social behavior. The family establishes rules and regulations that all members must adhere to. Social control includes these rules and regulations. The family instills in the child the need to conform to societal norms. It exerts control over its members to achieve the desired result.
- **State:** The State is the primary social control agency because it is the society's overall regulatory system. It uses legislation, the police, the armed forces, and prisons to maintain control over its

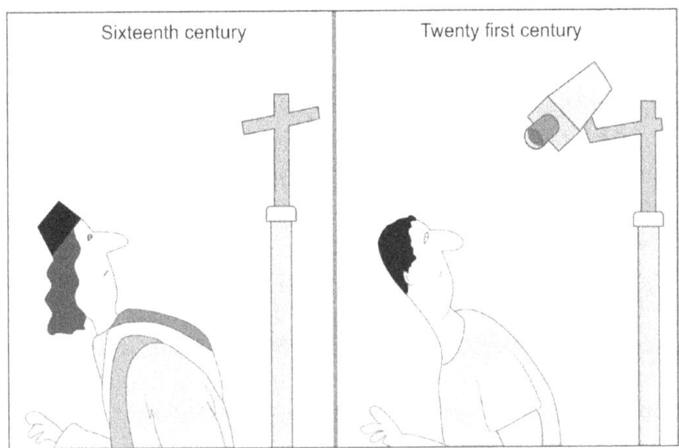

Fig. 13.1: Agents of social control through the ages.

citizens. The State's emergence is a gift of the modern, complex social order.

In such a social order, the State can more effectively exercise control through rules and regulations. The most effective method of man-made social control is the law. "Law means the code upheld by the State, which, because of its inclusive applicability, is thus the guardian of society itself," say Maclver and Page. The State is the agency of society that exercises its social control most effectively.

- **Educational institutions:** Educational institutions—schools – are powerful social control agents, and they are dedicated to shaping citizens **(Fig. 13.2)**. In modern societies, formal education communicates ideas and values that play a more significant role in behavior regulation. Education teaches us to conform to societal norms. Education is a deliberate teaching program that aids society in socializing children for them to absorb its values, beliefs, and norms.

  "The only sense in which education can be used as a means of social control is that by teaching people how to arrive at truth, it trains them in the use of their intelligence and thus expands the scope of control through feelings, customs, and traditions," write Gillin and Gillin.

- **Neighborhood:** The neighborhood reinforces the individual family's role as a social control agent. Group controls in the

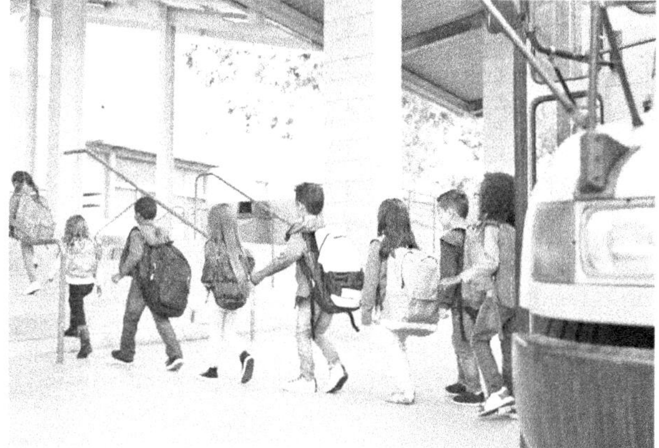

Fig. 13.2: Compulsory education as social control.

neighborhood have traditionally taken the form of mores. The older residents of the community keep them alive and enforce them.

- **Public opinion:** In a democratic setup, the people's opinion is the most important method of social control. Every man tries to get away from society's criticism and condemnation. As a result, he tries to act on public opinion and sentiments. Public opinion is more effective and influential than any other agency in a democratic system.
- **Propaganda and press:** Propaganda is the deliberate effort to control the behavior and relationships of social groups through methods that affect the feelings and attitudes of the individuals who make up the group. Radio, television, press, and literature influence people's ideas and bring about changes in life and way of thinking.
- **Economic organization:** A shift in the distribution of social control among the major institutions has occurred due to the rise of modern industrial organizations and the growth of community size. Economic organizations, education, and the Government have all risen to the forefront of social control. Fear of losing a job motivates people to follow the industry's rules and regulations.

Consequences of Social Control

Social control is necessary for promoting stability and conformity in societies, but it can sometimes become dysfunctional. The following are some of the dysfunctional aspects of social control.

Exploitation: Social control may sometimes become a subtle means of exploitation. Some dominant groups or individuals may simply use it to fulfill their vested interests. These interests may be political, economic, or social. In such cases, the real motivations are hidden under some laudable objectives. A ruling party may try to perpetuate its rule, or a business firm may try to sell its substandard goods using the techniques of social control.

Inhibiting reforms and change: Social control may have limiting consequences in that it may sometimes inhibit creativity and obstruct attempts at constructive reforms and social changes.

Psychological pressures: Social control may also exert enormous emotional and psychological pressures on some individuals. The best example is that of institutions such as prisons and mental hospitals. The strict regime and oppressive atmosphere sometimes create mental tensions and even illnesses. Similarly, where parents have rigorous standards of discipline, their children's personalities do not develop normally. In repressive police states, many individuals likewise suffer from stress and tension. Thus, the individual must pay the price for social control in psychological terms.

Social tension: Social control may also lead to social tensions, particularly in a large, complex society. Here, different groups may have specific interests, norms, and values, which may conflict. Conflict and struggle become inevitable when one or more groups attempt to impose their standards on others.

Limits on Social Control

The effectiveness of social control is limited due to the following factors:

- Each group is organized around norms and values: Social control is intended to check deviation from these standards. Yet, it is not possible to contain the deviation completely. Some deviation from prescribed norms will always be there. Each group or society must determine the tolerance limit of deviant conduct and thus set a realistic limit on social control.
- The effectiveness of social control is also limited by the degree of consistency in the cultural directives. If the cultural prescriptions are uncertain and inconsistent, social control cannot operate successfully. This is why in a rapidly changing society where normative standards become inconsistent, mechanisms of social control are generally weak. Individuals may not know what is expected of them in a particular situation.
- In a complex society, it is not generally possible to impose social control uniformly on all groups, which are divided based on class, caste, religion, race, etc. Sometimes, the uniform application of law also encounters numerous difficulties. Despite constitutional directives to have a uniform civil code in our country, evolving one so far has not been possible.

- Social control implies substantial economic costs to society: The control of deviance requires a disproportionate share of societal attention and resources. Huge expenditure must be incurred on establishing social control agencies such as the police, prisons, mental hospitals, etc. There is a limit beyond which a developing country such as ours cannot afford to deploy such resources at the cost of other developmental programs.

Importance of Social Control in Society

Social control is essential for every society. Without social control, society, as well as individuals, cannot exist. Therefore, the need for social control is vital. For the following reasons, social control is required.

- **To maintain the old order:** Every society or group must maintain its social order, which is only possible if its members act following it. The preservation of the old order is a crucial goal of social control. This goal can be achieved with the help of family. The elderly members of the family exert control over the children.
- **To establish social unity:** Social unity would be a pipe dream without social control. Social control regulates behavior by establishing norms, bringing uniformity to behavior, and fostering unity among individuals. Because its members behave similarly and follow family norms, the family maintains unity.
- **To control or regulate individual behavior:** No two men are alike regarding their attitudes, ideas, hobbies, or habits. Children with the same parents have different attitudes, habits, and interests. Men follow various religions, dress in various ways, eat various foods, marry in various ways, and have various ideologies. There are so many differences in people's lifestyles that a clash between them is possible with every movement. Because man has become too self-centered in modern times, this possibility has grown. Social control is required to protect social interests and meet everyday needs. Society would be reduced to the State of the Jungle if social control were removed and individuals were free to act as they pleased.
- **To provide social sanction:** Social control gives social behavior a social sanction. In today's society, numerous folkways, modes, and customs exist. Everyone must follow them. Individuals who violate

social norms are compelled to observe due to social control. As a result, social control gives social norms legitimacy.

- **To detect cultural misadjustment:** Society is constantly changing. In society, new inventions, discoveries, and philosophies continue to emerge. Individuals must adjust their behavior in response to societal changes. On the other hand, individuals cannot adjust to the new circumstances. Some people become progressive, while others stay conservative. When a villager relocates to the city, he encounters new cultural standards and may incorrectly adjust to the new environment. He may succumb to his passions, frequent bars, and spend nights in nightclubs. He must maintain social control during this transition period, lest he becomes a deviant.

14   Sociology of Stress

LEARNING OBJECTIVES

- ☞ Define stress.
- ☞ Explain reactions to stress.
- ☞ What is homeostasis in the context of stress?
- ☞ How do social factors cause stress?
- ☞ Familiarize yourself with the Holmes and Rahe Social Readjustment Rating Scale.
- ☞ Identify the sources of stress in a person's life?
- ☞ How to deal with stressful situations?
- ☞ Describe stress management strategies.

■ INTRODUCTION

Social influences upon the onset and the subsequent course of a particular disease are not limited to such variables as age, sex, race, social class, and the conditions of poverty as they relate to lifestyle, habits, and customs. It is also important to recognize that interaction between the human mind and body represents a critical factor regarding health. A considerable amount of literature maintains that psychological responses to social events can cause stress.

■ DEFINITION OF STRESS

Stress is the body's reaction to any change that necessitates a response or adjustment. Physical, mental, and the body produces emotional responses to these changes. Stress is an unavoidable part of everyday life. Stress can be caused by one's surroundings, body, and thoughts.

Stress is an emotional-psycho-physiological state of an organism that occurs in a situational context, involving stimuli that serve as cues to elicit fear or anxiety responses. A feeling of emotional or physical tension is referred to as stress. It can be triggered by any event or thought that causes frustration, anger, or anxiety **(Fig. 14.1)**.

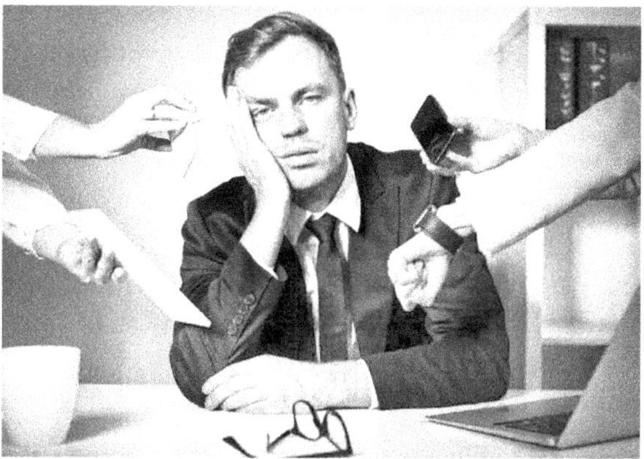
Fig. 14.1: A stressed person.

REACTIONS TO STRESS

Usually, stress is thought to occur when individuals are forced into a situation where their usual modes of behavior are not adequate, and the consequences of not adapting to the problem are perceived as serious. In general, it appears that there are four possible types of reactions to stress:

1. Normal, where an effective defensive reaction follows anxiety.
2. Neurotic, where anxiety is so great that the defense is ineffective.
3. Psychotic, where anxiety is misperceived or possibly ignored.
4. Psycho-physiological, where defense fails and anxiety results in changes in body tissues.

Most studies on stress indicate that most, if not all, stress is socially induced due to interaction between people. There exists a relationship between social interaction and stress. Embarrassment and psychological discomfort can be socially painful, yet the effects of stress can also transcend the social situation and cause physiological damage. Hence, a physiological perspective of stress must be considered.

HOMEOSTASIS: THE PHYSIOLOGICAL ADAPTATION

Walter Cannon believed that the objective measure of health is not the absence of disease but the ability of humans to function effectively within a given environment. This belief was based upon the observation that the human body undergoes continuous adaptation to its environment in response to weather, microbes, chemical irritants and pollutants, and the emotional pressure of daily life. Cannon called this process of physiological adaptation homeostasis, derived from the Greek and meant **'staying the same'**.

Homeostasis refers to the maintenance of a relatively stable condition. For example, when the body becomes cold, heat is produced; when bacteria threaten the body, antibodies are produced to fight the germs; and when an attack from another human being threatens the body, the body prepares itself either to fight or to run.

Real/Symbolic Threats

As an organism, the human body is thus prepared to meet both internal and external threats to survival, whether these threats are real or symbolic. A person may react with fear to an actual objector a symbol of that object, e.g., a bear versus a bear's footprint. In the second case, the fear is not of the footprint, but of the bear that the footprint represents. Symbolic threats in contemporary urban Societies could include stimuli such as heavy traffic, loud noises, or struggle at work, all of which can produce emotional stress related more to a social situation than to a specific person or object.

Physiological Responses to Stress

Whether or not the stressful situation induces physiological change depends upon an individual's perception of the stress stimulus and the meaning that the stimulus holds for them. For example, a person's reaction may not correspond to the actual reality of the dangers that the stimulus represents, i.e., a person may over-react or under-react. Thus, there is considerable agreement that an individual's subjective interpretation of a social situation is the trigger that produces physiological responses. Situations themselves cannot usually be assumed beforehand to produce physiological changes.

Cannon gave the concept of the *'fight or flight'* pattern of physiological change to illustrate how the body copes with stress resulting from a social situation. When a person experiences fear or anxiety, the body undergoes physiological changes that prepare it for forceful effort and the effect of possible injury. Physiological changes in the body due to stress situations primarily involve the autonomic and neuroendocrine systems.

Role of Autonomic Nervous System

The autonomic nervous system (ANS) controls heart rate, blood pressure, and gastrointestinal functions, processes that occur automatically and are not under the voluntary control of the central nervous system (CNS). The ANS is delicately balanced between relaxation and stimulation and is activated primarily through the hypothalamus is located in the central ventral portion of the brain. It comprises two major divisions, the parasympathetic and the sympathetic systems. When there is no emergency, the parasympathetic system is dominant and regulates the body's vegetative processes, such as storing sugar in the liver, constricting the pupil of the eye in response to intense light, and decreasing heart rate. In an emergency, the sympathetic system governs the body's autonomic functions and increases heart rate, so blood flows swiftly to the organs and muscles needed in defense. It also inhibits bowel movements and dilates the eye's pupil to improve sight.

Role of the Endocrine System

Besides the ANS, the endocrine glands perform a critical role in the body's physiological reaction to stress. The neuroendocrine system consists of the adrenal and pituitary glands, the parathyroids, the islets of Langerhans, and the gonads. They secrete hormones directly into the bloodstream because they lack ducts to carry their hormones to particular glands. The two glands that are the most responsive to stressful situations are the adrenal and pituitary glands. The adrenal glands secrete two hormones—epinephrine and norepinephrine, under stimulation from the hypothalamus. Epinephrine accelerates the heart rate and helps to distribute blood to the heart, lungs, CNS, and limbs; also, it makes the blood coagulate more readily so that as little blood as possible will be lost in case of injury. Norepinephrine raises blood pressure and joins with epinephrine to mobilize fatty acids in the bloodstream for use as energy. The function of the pituitary gland is upon stimulation by the hypothalamus, to secrete hormones that, in turn, stimulate other endocrine glands to secrete their hormones.

At first, most medical scientists believed that only the adrenal glands were involved in stress reaction. However, in 1936 **Hans Selye** demonstrated the existence of *a pituitary-adrenal cortical axis* as having known as the general adaptation syndrome. He believed that after an initial alarm reaction, the second stage of resistance to prolonged stress was accomplished primarily through increased activity of the anterior pituitary and adrenal cortex. If stress continued and pituitary and adrenal defenses were consumed, **Selye** indicated that a person would enter the third stage as premature aging due to wear and tear on the body. However, it now seems that the entire endocrine system, not just the pituitary, and adrenal glands, are involved in some stress reaction. Under the acute stimulus, hormone secretions by the endocrine glands increase; under calming influences, secretions decrease.

Consequences of Lack of Physiological Response

Most threats in modern society are symbolic, not physical, and do not usually require a physical response. Today, humans face emotional threats with the same physical system used to fight enemies. Yet modern society disapproves of such physical responses as fighting. Socially, the human is often left with no course of action except verbal insults; this inability to respond externally leaves the body physiologically mobilized for action, a readiness that can damage the body. For example, fat that has been mobilized for energy in defense may not be burned up in response, but instead may be left as deposits in the arteries and contribute to the development of arteriosclerosis.

Several studies have shown that the human's inability to manage the social, psychological, and emotional aspects of life to respond suitably to a social situation can lead to the development of cardiovascular complications and hypertension, peptic ulcers, muscular pain, compulsive vomiting, asthma, migraine headaches, and other health problems. Some research suggests that even the onset of cancer is related to changes and disappointments in social relationships.

■ SOCIAL FACTORS AND STRESS

There is considerable empirical research in medical sociology dealing with stress and stress-related topics. Also, relevant research on group influences and changes in life events is considered.

Stress Situations

Robert Schwab and John Pritchard classified situations that may lead to physiological disorders and chronic diseases. Their classification system was based not only upon the type of situation but also on the duration of the influence of the situation and the degree of stress induced by that situation.

Types of Stress Situations

Stress situations were classified as either:

- **Short-stress situations** in which mild stress occurred, whose effects lasted from seconds to hours. Examples of a short-stress situation are annoying insects, public appearances before large audiences, and door slamming. In other words, these are the so-called minor burdens and annoyances of everyday life, which probably do not produce the onset of stress-related disease.
- **Moderate-stress situations** in which the effects lasted from days to weeks. Moderate-stress situations are characterized by overwork, the temporary absence of loved ones, gastric upsets, or minor psychological setbacks during social interaction.
- **Severe-stress situations** in which the effects lasted from weeks to months and even years. Severe-stress situations include the death of loved ones, severe financial reverses, the perpetuation of intolerable social situations, illness, or perhaps prolonged absence from loved ones.

The moderate- and severe- stress situations (in particular) would be capable of producing a serious physiological response.

Specific Types

Specific types of stress formulated by Schwab and Pritchard were those of:

- Trauma, such as fear in armed combat
- Infection from disease
- Financial reverses and the feeling of frustration
- Death of a loved one
- Fear of an unknown situation such as recovery from surgery
- Fright
- Chronic worry

- Fatigue from overwork
- Fatigue from extensive travel
- Rejection and feeling of isolation
- Disappointment
- Conflict.

Schwab and Pritchard believe that the common element in their typology of stress situations, other than duration, is that of the disruption of social relationships, either threatened or actual.

Stress Adaptations

Mechanic Model

Mechanic attempts to explain the social determinants of stress from the standpoint of the community's social structure rather than from the personal experiences of the individual alone. The outcome or effect of a crisis depends upon how well a person comes to terms with the situation. Therefore, stress refers to difficulties experienced by the individual due to perceived challenges.

Mechanic believes that in social situations, people have different skills and abilities in coping with problems; not everyone has an equal degree of control in managing emotional defenses or the same motivation and personal involvement in a situation. In analyzing any particular situation, an observer must consider whether an individual is prepared to meet a threat and whether or not he is motivated to meet it.

Biosocial Resonation/Moss Model

Moss has conceptualized the biosocial resonation model. The significance of this model lies in its attempt to link sociology with bodyphysiology. Moss defines this as *"the continuing reciprocal influences of physiological and social behavior in social interaction".* He suggests that humans are biosocial resonating beings, living in a social world of communication networks that enable them to perceive the environment.

Moss believes that conformance with the norms of the communication network and participation within that network will reduce an individual's opportunity to contact members of other networks and their information, which might be incongruous.

However, it is difficult in modern society not to come into contact with incompatible networks and inappropriate information. Stress and physiological change are likely to occur when someone experiences information incongruities.

Stress and the Social Group

An individual's perception of an event may be influenced by their intelligence, experience, socialization, and awareness of stimuli, but the influence of group membership is also important. Moss has indicated that the significance of a group or communication network in influencing physiological responses lies in its providing corrective information to counteract incongruities and in isolating members from opposing information perspectives. There is often a tendency among members of small groups to develop a consensus about how social events should be perceived; this minimizes individual differences and maintains group conformity and ideological purity. Conformity to group-approved attitudes and definitions has long been hypothesized in sociology and social psychology as reducing anxiety by ensuring acceptance from persons and groups important to the individual.

For example, research on combat motivation during war time has shown primary group relations to be a decisive factor in determining whether or not a soldier will fight. What motivated him to fight was to show other members of his group that he supported them so that other group members would support him.

Life Changes

Another important factor in the production of stress is the occurrence of significant changes in a person's life. Selye has suggested that any type of environmental change, either pleasant or unpleasant, requiring the individual to adapt can produce a specific stress response. It is seen that unpleasant events such as earthquakes, tornados, and presidential assassinations can induce stress. It has also been shown that rapid urbanization and industrialization are stress-inducing agents.

Thomas Holmes and Robert Rahe devised a social readjustment rating scale that reflects the assumption that change, no matter how good or how bad, demands a certain degree of adjustment on the part of an individual; the more significant the adjustment, the greater the stress. Holmes and Rahe have carried out their analysis one step further suggested that life events change in a cumulative pattern that can eventually build a stressful impact.

The Holmes and Rahe Social Readjustment Rating Scale lists certain life events associated with varying amounts of disruption in the life of an average person. It was constructed by having hundreds of persons of different social backgrounds rank the relative amount of adjustment accompanying a particular life experience.

Death of a spouse is ranked highest, with a relative stress value of 100; marriage ranks 7th with a value of 50, retirement 10th with a value of 45; taking a vacation is ranked 41st with a value of 13; and so forth **(Table 14.1)**.

Holmes and Rahe call each stress value a *'life change'* unit. They suggest that as the total value of life change units mounts, the probability of having a serious illness also increases, particularly if a person accumulates too many life change units in too short a time.If an individual accumulates 200 or more life-change units within a year, Holmes and Rahe believe such a person will risk a serious disorder.

Table 14.1: Life events and weighted values.

Life event	Value	Life event	Value
Death of spouse	100	Son or daughter leaving home	29
Divorce	73	Trouble with in-laws	29
Marital separation	65	Outstanding personal achievement	28
Jail term	63	Wife beginning or stopping work	26
Death of close family member	63	Beginning or ending school	26
Personal injury or illness	53	Revision of habits	24
Marriage	50	Trouble with boss	23
Fired at work	47	Change in work hours	20
Marital reconciliation	45	Change in residence	20

Contd...

Contd...

Life event	Value	Life event	Value
Retirement	45	Change of responsibility at work	29
Change in health of family	44	Change in schools	20
Pregnancy	40	Change in recreation	19
Sex difficulties	39	Change in social activity	18
Gain of a new family member	39	Change in sleeping habits	16
Change in financial state	38	Change in numbers of family get-togethers	15
Death of close friend	37	Change in eating habits	15
Change of work	36	Vacation	13
Change in number of arguments with spouse	35	Minor violations of law	11
Foreclosure of mortgage	30		

■ STRESS MANAGEMENT

Introduction

Managing stress is about controlling one's thoughts, emotions, schedule, environment, and problem-solving style. The ultimate goal is a balanced life, with time for work, relationships, relaxation, and fun—plus the resilience to hold up under pressure and meet challenges head-on.

Identify the Sources of Stress in One's Life

Stress management starts with identifying the sources of stress in one's life. This is not as easy as it sounds. Someone's true sources of stress are not always obvious, and it is all too easy to overlook one's stress-inducing thoughts, feelings, and behaviors. One may know that he is constantly worried about work deadlines. But may be it's his procrastination, rather than the actual job demands, that leads to deadline stress.

To identify true sources of stress, look closely at one's habits, attitude, and excuses:

- Do you explain stress away as temporary ("I've just one million things going on right now") even though you can't remember the last time you took a breather?
- Would you describe stress as an important part of your job or home life ('Things are still nuts around here') or as a part of your personality ('I have a lot of nervous energy, that's all')?
- Do you blame other people or outside events for your stress, or do you perceive it as totally natural and unusual?

Until one accepts responsibility for his role in creating or maintaining it, the stress level will remain outside his control.

Start a Stress Journal

A stress journal can help identify the regular stressors in life and the way one deals with them. Each time one feels stressed, keep track of it in the journal. As you keep a daily log, you will begin to see patterns and common themes. Write down:

- What caused your stress (guess if you're unsure).
- How you felt, both physically and emotionally.
- How you acted in response.
- What you did to make yourself feel better.

Look at How You Currently Cope with Stress

Consider how you currently deal with and manage stress in your life. You can use your stress journal to help you figure out what they are. Are your coping mechanisms healthy or unhealthy, productive or ineffective? Many people, unfortunately, deal with stress in ways that exacerbate the problem.

Unhealthy Ways of Coping with Stress

These coping strategies may temporarily reduce stress, but they cause more damage in the long run:

- Smoking
- Drinking too much
- Over-eating or under-eating
- Zoning out for hours in front of the TV or computer
- Withdrawing from friends, family, and activities
- Using pills or drugs to relax

- Sleeping too much
- Procrastinating
- Filling up every minute of the day to avoid facing problems
- Taking out your stress on others (lashing out, angry outbursts, physical violence).

Learning Healthier Ways to Manage Stress

It is time to find healthier ways to cope with stress if your current ones are not helping you achieve better emotional and physical health. There are numerous healthy ways to manage and cope with stress, but all of them necessitate change. Either you can change the situation or you can change your reaction. When deciding which path to take, keep the four A's in mind: avoid, alter, adapt, or accept.

Because everybody's response to stress varies, there is no "one size fits all" solution to managing stress. Experiment with different techniques and strategies because no single technique or strategy will work for everyone or in every situation. Concentrate on the things that make you feel comfortable and in control.

Dealing with Stressful Situations: The Four A's

Change the situation
1. Avoid the stressor.
2. Alter the stressor.
Change your reaction
3. Adapt to the stressor.
4. Accept the stressor.

STRESS MANAGEMENT STRATEGIES

Avoid Unnecessary Stress

Not all stress can be avoided, and avoiding a situation that needs to be addressed is unhealthy. You might be surprised at how many stressors you can eliminate from your life.

- **Learn how to say "no":** Recognize and respect your personal boundaries. When you're close to achieving your goals, whether in your personal or professional life, refuse to take on additional responsibilities. Taking on more than you can handle is an easy way to get into trouble.

- **Avoid people who stress you out:** Limit the amount of time you spend with that person or end the relationship entirely if someone consistently causes stress in your life and you are unable to change the relationship.
- **Take control of your environment:** Turn off the television if the evening news makes you nervous. If you're worried about traffic, take a longer but less-traveled route. If going to the grocery store is a chore, shop for groceries online.
- **Avoid hot-button topics:** Cross religion and politics off your list of topics to discuss if they make you angry. Stop bringing up the same subject with the same people, or excuse yourself when it comes up in conversation.
- **Pare down your to-do list:** Examine your daily tasks, responsibilities, and schedule. If you have too much on your plate, distinguish between "should" and "must." Tasks that are not necessary should be moved to the bottom of the list or eliminated.

Alter the Situation

Try to change a stressful situation if you can't avoid it. Determine what you can do to change things so that the issue does not recur in the future. Changing how you communicate and operate in your daily life is a standard part of this process.

- **Express your feelings instead of bottling them up:** If something or someone is bothering you, communicate your concerns openly and respectfully. If you don't voice your feelings, resentment will build and the situation will likely remain the same.
- **Be willing to compromise:** Be willing to do the same when you ask someone to change their behavior. You'll have a good chance of finding a happy middle ground if you're both willing to bend a little.
- **Be more assertive:** Don't let your own life slip away from you. Deal with issues head on, doing your best to anticipate and avoid them. If you have an exam to study for and your chatty roommate just got home, say up front that you only have five minutes to talk.
- **Manage your time better:** Poor time management can cause much stress. Staying calm and focused is hard when you are stretched too thin and running behind. But if you plan and make

sure you don't overextend yourself, you can alter the amount of stress you are under.

Adapt to the Stressor

Change yourself if you cannot change the stressor. You can adapt to stressful situations and regain control by altering your expectations and attitude.

- **Reframe problems:** Try to see things more positively when you are in a stressful situation. Instead of being annoyed by a traffic jam, consider it an opportunity to regroup, listen to your favorite radio station, or enjoy some alone time.
- **Look at the big picture:** Consider the situation from a different angle. Consider how crucial it will be in the long run. Will it make a difference in a month? Is it really a year? Is it worth getting worked up about? If the answer is no, you should devote your time and energy to something else.
- **Adjust your expectations:** Perfectionism is a major source of stress that can be avoided. Stop expecting perfection and setting yourself up for failure. Establish reasonable expectations for yourself and others, and learn to accept "good enough."
- **Concentrate on the positive aspects of your situation:** Take a moment to introspect on all the things you appreciate in your life, including your positive qualities and gifts when stress is getting to you. This straightforward strategy can assist you in keeping things in perspective.

Adjusting Your Attitude

The way you think has a big impact on your emotional and physical health. Your body responds as if it were in the midst of a tense situation whenever you think negatively about yourself. If you see yourself in a positive light, you are more likely to feel good about yourself; conversely, if you see yourself in a negative light, you are less likely to feel good. Words like "always," "never," "should," and "must" should be avoided. These are telltale signs of negative self-talk.

Accept the Things You can't Change

Stress is unavoidable in some situations. Stressors like the death of a loved one, a serious illness, or a national recession are impossible to avoid or change. Acceptance is the best way to deal with stress in these situations. Acceptance may be difficult, but it is preferable to railing against a situation you can't change in the long run.

- Don't try to control what you can't control. Many aspects of life are beyond our control, particularly the actions of others. Rather than getting stressed out about them, concentrate on the things you can control, such as how you respond to problems.
- Keep an eye out for the bright side. "What does not kill us makes us stronger," as the saying goes. When confronted with major obstacles, try to see them as opportunities for personal development. Reflect on your poor choices if they contributed to a stressful situation, and learn from them.
- Express your emotions. Make an appointment with a therapist or talk to a trusted friend. Even if there is nothing you can do to change the stressful situation, expressing what you are going through can be very cathartic.
- Acquire the ability to forgive. Recognize that we live in an imperfect world where people make mistakes. Allow yourself to be free of rage and resentment. By forgiving and moving on, you can free yourself from negative energy.

Make Time for Fun and Relaxation

Beyond a take-charge approach and a positive attitude, you can reduce stress in your life by nurturing yourself. If you regularly make time for fun and relaxation, you will be better at handling life's stressors when they inevitably come.

Healthy Ways to Relax and Recharge

- Go for a walk.
- Spend time in nature.
- Call a good friend.
- Sweat out tension with a good workout.
- Write in your journal.
- Take a long bath.
- Light scented candles
- Savor a warm cup of coffee or tea.
- Play with a pet.
- Work in your garden.

- Get a massage.
- Curl up with a good book.
- Listen to music.
- Watch a comedy

Don't get caught up in the hustle and bustle of life to the point where you forget to look after yourself. Self-care is a requirement, not a luxury.

- **Make time for relaxation:** Make time for relaxation in your daily routine. Allow no other obligations to interfere. This is your chance to disconnect from all responsibilities and re-energize.
- **Make connections with other people:** Spend time with people who will make your life better. You will be protected from the negative effects of stress if you have a strong support system.
- Every day, do something you enjoy. Make time for your favorite pastimes, whether it is stargazing, playing the piano, or riding your bike.
- Maintain a sense of humour. This includes the ability to make yourself laugh. Laughter aids your body's stress-reduction efforts in a variety of ways.

Learn the Relaxation Response

You can control your stress levels with relaxation techniques that evoke the body's relaxation response, a state of restfulness that is the opposite of the stress response. Regularly practicing these techniques will build your physical and emotional resilience, heal your body, and boost your overall feelings of joy and equanimity.

Adopt a Healthy Lifestyle

Strengthening your physical health can help you become more resistant to stress.

- **Exercise regularly:** Physical activity is essential for reducing and preventing the negative effects of stress. Make time to exercise for at least 30 minutes three times per week. For releasing pent-up stress and tension, nothing beats aerobic exercise.
- **Eat a well-balanced diet:** Be mindful of what you eat because well-nourished bodies are better prepared to cope with stress. Start your day with breakfast, and keep your energy and mind clear throughout the day with balanced, nutritious meals.

- **Limit your caffeine and sugar intake:** Caffeine and sugar's temporary "highs" are frequently followed by a slump in mood and energy. You will feel more relaxed and sleep better if you reduce your intake of coffee, soft drinks, chocolate, and sugary snacks.
- **Stay away from booze, cigarettes, and drugs:** Self-medicating with alcohol or drugs may provide a quick fix for stress, but the effects are only temporary. Deal with problems head-on and with a clear mind, rather than avoiding or masking them.
- **Get adequate rest:** A good night's sleep fuels both your mind and your body. You will be more stressed if you are tired because it may cause you to think irrationally.

Sociology of Education

LEARNING OBJECTIVES

☞ Define education.
☞ Describe the goals of education.
☞ What are the different aspects of education?
☞ What are the social functions of education?
☞ How does education bring social change?
☞ How does education influence modernization?
☞ How does education influence culture?
☞ How does education help in social control?

INTRODUCTION

Individuals and society benefit from education; without it, all of history's accumulated knowledge and standards of conduct would be lost. A person must learn the society's culture or the accepted ways of doing things. He must be socialized into the current culture and taught the rules of conduct and future expectations.

As a result, rather than leaving learning to chance, society designs its instructional programs to meet personal and social needs. Education is a deliberate teaching program that aids in instilling values, norms, and social skills that enable an individual to develop his personality while sustaining the social system.

Education comes from the Latin word 'Educare,' which means 'to bring up,' and is linked to the verb 'Educare,' which means 'to bring forth.' Education aims not just to impart knowledge in a few subjects to students but to help them develop habits and attitudes that will help them face the future with confidence.

"A large part of our social and technical skills are acquired through deliberate instruction, which we call education," according to Peter Worsley. It is the primary source of waking activity for children aged 5 to 15 and frequently beyond. Some sociologists have become increasingly interested in education in recent years. As a result, the sociology of education has emerged as a new branch of sociology.

Education is a milestone in a country's development because it develops its economy and society. Education imparts knowledge and skills to the general public and shapes the personalities of a country's youth.

Education is essential for a person's long-term success. It has a significant impact on the quality of human life opportunities. Education is widely regarded as the bedrock of society, bringing economic prosperity, social stability, and political stability.

Individuals' economic and social status are influenced by their educational attainment, as education contributes to their ability to manage their quality of life. It can assist an individual in avoiding poverty while also promoting harmony and democratic society.

Education can also empower them to express their opinions, expose them to their full potential, help them grow as people, and broaden their horizons in a specific area.

Education is the key to moving in the world, seeking better jobs, and ultimately succeeding in life. Education is the best investment for the people because well-educated people have more opportunities to get jobs that satisfy them. Educated individuals enjoy respect among their colleagues and can effectively contribute to their country's and society's development by inventing new devices and discoveries.

The primary purpose of education is to educate individuals within society, prepare and qualify them for work in the economy, integrate people into society, and teach them the values and morals of society. The role of education is a means of socializing individuals and keeping society smooth and remain stable.

Education in society prepares youngsters for adulthood so that they may form the next generation of leaders. One of the essential education tasks is to enable people to understand themselves. Students must be equipped with the knowledge and skills needed to participate effectively as a member of society and contribute to the development of shared values and common identity.

■ DEFINITIONS

Education means a change in man's conduct in life. It means upgrading a man's ability to choose the best alternative available in any circumstance he faces. It means the person's development prepares him to adopt the best approach to a problem at any given time.

Education is the 'adjustment ability to a changing situation and environment.' Education is more than an economic investment: it is an essential input upon which life, development, and man's survival depend. We all know that it is the responsibility of everyone in a country to educate; whether we are parents, adults, children, or teachers, in the public or private sector, education is the responsibility of everyone.

But however we see the needs and problems, most of us would agree that the role of education is to help provide the opportunity for all people to develop as fully as possible. Education should be a means to empower children and adults alike to become active participants in the transformation of their societies. Learning should also focus on the values, attitudes, and behaviors which enable individuals to learn to live together in a world characterized by diversity and pluralism.

Education, therefore, has a crucial long-term role in developing a knowledge and understanding of human rights, the values base they represent, and the skills required to strengthen democratic culture.

Education, according to Durkheim, is defined as the socialization of the younger generation. They say that it is a never-ending effort to impose on the child ways of seeing, feeling, and acting that they could not have come up with on their own.

Sumner defined education as the attempt to transmit the mores of group to the child to learn what behavior is acceptable and what is not. What they should believe and reject, and how they should act in various situations.

According to Green AW, education has traditionally meant the deliberate preparation of children for later adoption of adult roles. However, according to modern convention, education has come to mean formal training by specialists within the formal organization of the school.

Socrates defined education as, 'Education means the bringing out of ideas of universal validity, which are latent in every man's mind.'

Vivekananda states, 'Education is the manifestation of perfection already reached in man.'

Kant defined education as, 'Education is the development, in the individual, of all the perfection he is capable of.'

Rabindranath Tagore said, 'Education means to enable the child to find out ultimate truth... making truth its own and giving expression to it.'

Goals of Education

Sidney Hook has described the goals of education as:
- To develop the powers of critical, independent thought;
- To induce sensitiveness of perception, receptiveness to new ideas, and imaginative sympathy with the experiences of others;
- To produce an awareness of the mainstream of our cultural and literary, and scientific traditions;
- To make available essential bodies of knowledge concerning nature, society, ourselves, our country, and its history;
- To cultivate an intelligent loyalty to the ideals of the democratic community;
- To equip young men and women with the general skills and techniques and the specialized knowledge, which, together with the virtues and aptitude already mentioned, will make it possible for them to do some productive work related to their capacities and interests; and
- To strengthen those inner resources and traits of character, which enable the individual, when necessary, to standalone.

Aspects of Education

Several sociological aspects of education can be identified.

Firstly, learning is a creative process where individuals respond creatively to stimuli. Thus, education is an act of creativity for the student.

Secondly, there are two types of education: informal and formal. Informal education serves as a mechanism for lifelong learning and reinforcement of previous knowledge.

Thirdly, formal education is a socially designed technique to put students in situations where they can learn. However, individuals only receive formal education for a short period.

Fourthly, education is a way of life and also a way of preparing for life. Preparation for life includes the ability to earn a living, appreciate cultural heritage and inner resources, and function effectively as a member of society and citizen of the State.

Finally, education entails mastery of learning tools such as reading, writing, and arithmetic, as well as mastery of oneself, neighbors, and the universe.

Education is defined as "narrow" and "broader." Education is a planned, organized, and formalized process in a narrow sense. It is delivered at a specific location (School, College, or University) and at a specific time. It has a formal curriculum as well. Education is restricted to the classroom in a strict sense. Education, in a broad sense, is unrelated to schooling or teaching.

Every individual receives some education, even if he has never attended a school, because his acquired characteristics result from educational experiences and activities. In a broad sense, education is used to teach people all the characteristics that will allow them to function in society.

Education is a 'process' that never ends. Human education begins at conception and continues until death. Throughout his life, he learns. There's no way to stop it. Schooling is only a small part of education. The child then goes on to reconstruct his entire life's experiences. Instruction comes to a close in the classroom, but education lasts for the rest of one's life.

FUNCTION OF EDUCATION

The concepts of socialization and learning are related to, in fact, often inseparable from the idea of education. The primary function of the educative process is to pass down knowledge from generation to generation—a process essential to cultural development.Formal education is primarily designed to inculcate crucial skills and values central to the survival of the society or to those who hold effective power. Inherent in education, in all periods of man's history, it is a stimulus to creative thinking and action, which accounts in part for culture change, itself being a powerful stimulus to further innovation (**Fig. 15.1**).

Social Functions of Education

Education is an important social institution in our society. Within and outside of the school system, education serves a multifaceted purpose. Its purpose is to socialize the individual in preparation for various social roles and personality development. It is also an essential part of society's control mechanisms. Education is required

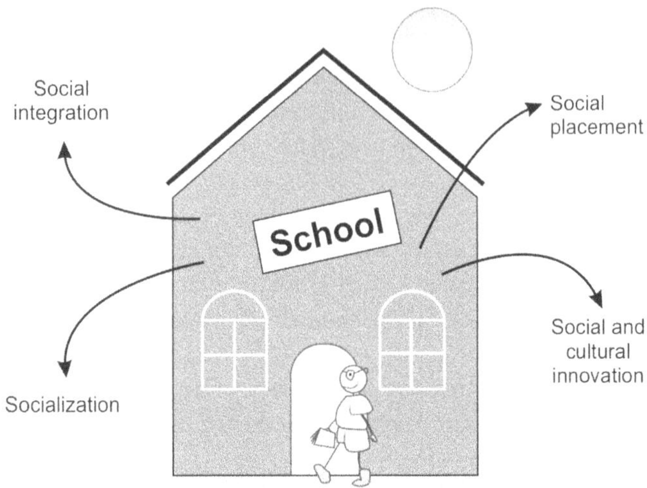

Fig. 15.1: The functions of education.

for a simple society to evolve into a modern complex industrial society.

The Socialization Process

Socialization is an essential function of education. Children are unaware of their society's culture. They must learn about them and understand how their society works. As a result, children must be exposed to the culture they will encounter as they grow older. As a result, society provides a conscious teaching program to instill values, norms, and social skills that are appropriate for individuals' adult roles in society.

Through schools and colleges, students gain academic knowledge that they will need later on, as well as practical and technical knowledge that will prepare them for a specific job. Simultaneously, schools and colleges instill social values and norms in them **(Figs. 15.2 and 15.3).**

People learn a lot from their parents, clubs, and friends, but they learn more about their society's culture through the educational system. Because the young are exposed to social norms and values outside of those available for learning in the family and other social

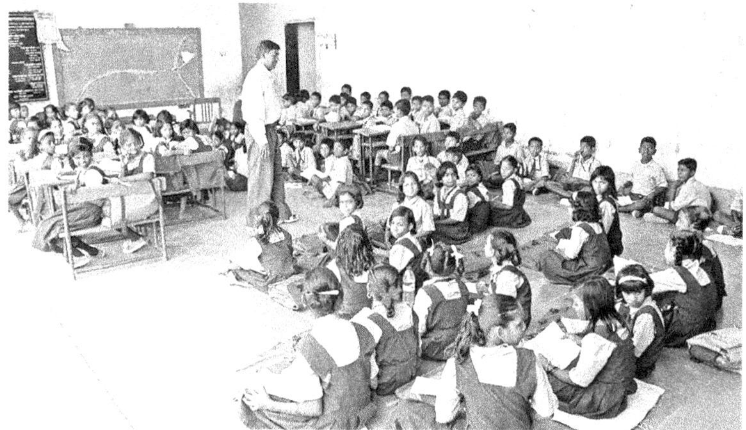

Fig. 15.2: A rural school in India.

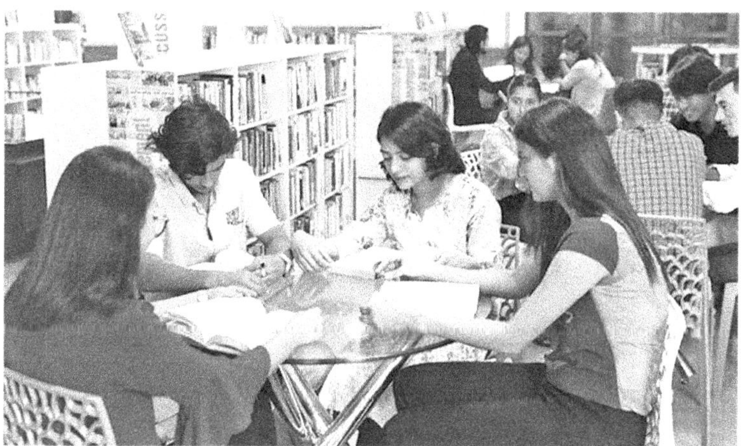

Fig. 15.3: A modern college facility.

groups, they are exposed to them in educational institutions. The child can develop reasoning in social relationships, cultivate social virtues, and become socially efficient due to education.

Personality Development

Education is crucial in developing a person's personality. "To awaken and develop in the child those physical, intellectual, and moral states which are required of him both by his society as a whole and by the milieu for which he is specially designed," Durkheim said. Education aids in the development of a person's physical, mental, and emotional characteristics, as well as his temperament and character.

The core of a person's personality develops due to a child's interactions with others. As a result, the educational process shapes an individual's habits, traits, attitudes, and ideals. His personality is indirectly developed when a learner is encouraged to form his attitudes and values by studying notable people in history and literature. Furthermore, their peers and teachers influence a learner's outlook and attitudes.

Social Control

Education is critical for regulating individual behavior by transmitting a way of life and passing on ideas and values to future generations.

"In the early socialization of the child," says Bottomore, "education contributes to the regulations of social conduct." All societies develop educational systems to train their younger generations to transmit their social heritage and survive as a social order. To keep society running, the young must be consciously prepared for adult roles. Society regulates its members' behavior and enforces conformity to its norms through education.

In modern societies, formal education communicates ideas and values that help to regulate behavior. New generations are taught to follow social norms, which can result in punishment if they are broken.

Social Integration

Education helps people integrate into society by instilling values. Specific values and social skills such as cooperation or team spirit, obedience, and fair play are communicated through the school's curriculum, extracurricular activities, and informal relationships between students and teachers.

Establishing Status

Establishing an individual's status is an essential function of education. From the lower working class to the upper class, education is a good indicator of socioeconomic status; education leads to economic opportunity. Young people obtain higher-status jobs due to their education than their parents. They associate with people of higher status as their income rises. As a result, education is a pathway to a better socioeconomic status.

Provides a Path to Social Mobility

Educational qualifications are increasingly being used to assign people to social statuses and mobility. Due to educational attainment, there has been a steady progression from one status to the next. In an industrial society like the United States or the United Kingdom, the attainment of both skills acquired in primary, secondary, and higher education, as well as educational credentials obtained for a job, is becoming increasingly important.

The educational system is expected to provide opportunities for social and economic mobility by identifying and training the most capable and hardworking youth for positions of higher social status.

Those with more abilities and training are placed in higher positions in the educational system, while those with fewer abilities and training are placed in lower positions. As a result, education tends to increase their earning power and prepare them for higher-status occupations than their parents, resulting in vertical social mobility.

Social Development

The economy and occupational structure are directly related to the skills and values learned in school. Individuals are taught skills that are in demand in the workplace through education. In a modern planned economy, skilled workers' output must consciously align with society's economic and social priorities. This explains why education is so important in social development. Because literacy promotes economic and social development, all developing countries have implemented large-scale literacy programs. Poor people's political consciousness grows due to literacy, and they now organize themselves into various forms of organization.

Equality of Educational Opportunity

The equalization of educational opportunities is essentially linked with the equality notions in the social system. The social system,which intends to provide equal opportunities for the advancement of all, also has provisions for equal educational opportunities. In modern industrial society, education has become the primary agency for socializing newborns into law-abiding citizens and productive members of society. Formal education has become almost indispensable because to participate in economic production; one needs to learn specialized skills, which cannot be acquired through family or any other agency. Due to the indispensability of formal education in advanced industrial societies, education is provided by the State as a matter of right for all its citizens. Formal institutions such as schools, colleges, and universities are organized for this purpose.

Today in most societies, legislations guarantee equality of the right to education. The welfare states make special efforts in industrial societies to provide compulsory education to the socially deprived, to realize this ideal of equality of education.

Inequalities of educational opportunities arise due to:
- Poverty—the poor cannot afford to meet education expenses.
- Children studying in rural schools must compete with children in urban areas, where well-equipped schools exist.
- In places where no primary, secondary or collegiate educational institutions exist, children do not get the same opportunity as those with all these in their neighborhood.
- Wide inequalities also arise from differences in home environments—a child from a rural household or slum does not have the same opportunity as a child from an upper-class home with educated parents.
- There is wide sex disparity in India—a girl's education is not given the same encouragement as boys.
- Education of backward classes, including SC and ST, and economically backward sections are not at par with that of other communities or classes.

Education and Social Change

The role of education as an agent of social change and development is widely recognized today. Earlier educational institutions and teachers used to show students a specific way of life, and education was more social control than an instrument of social change. Modern educational institutions do not emphasize transmitting a way of life to the students. The traditional education was meant for an unchanging, static society not marked by change. But, today, education aims at imparting knowledge. Education was associated with religion; it has become secular today and is an independent institution.

Education and Modernization

Modernization is a process of socio-cultural transformation. It is a thorough-going process of change involving values, norms, institutions, and structures. Political dimensions of modernization involve the creation of a modern nation-state and developing key institutions such as political parties, bureaucratic structures, legislative bodies, and a system of elections based on universal franchise and secret ballot.

Cultural modernization involves adherence to nationalistic ideology, belief in equality, freedom, humanism, and a rational and scientific outlook. Economic modernization involves industrialization accompanied by monetization of the economy, increasing division of labor, use of management techniques and improved technology, and expanding the service sector. Social modernization involves universalistic values, achievement motivation, improving social and geographic mobility, increasing literacy and urbanization, and declining traditional authority.

Education and Culture

Education has as one of its fundamental goals the imparting of culture from generation to generation. Culture is a growing whole. There can be no break in the continuity of culture. The cultural elements are passed on through agents such as family, school, and other associations. All societies maintain themselves through their culture. The culture here refers to beliefs, skills, art, literature, philosophy, religion, music, etc., that must be learned. This social heritage must be transmitted through social organizations.

Education has this function of cultural transmission in all societies. The curriculum of a school, its extracurricular activities,and the informal relationships among students and teachers communicate social skills and values. The school imparts values such as cooperation, team spirit, obedience, discipline, etc., through various activities. Education unites society by spreading shared values. The school helps children integrate into society's culture by teaching them skills.

Career Selection

Education plays a crucial role in helping individuals to contemplate the careers they wish to pursue in the future, and it also prepares them for upcoming endeavors. It equips them with the essential knowledge and skills needed to excel in both their professional and social lives. Education provides individuals with all the necessary information and tools required to navigate the complexities of society and make informed decisions about their personal and professional goals.

Techniques of Learning Skills

Education teaches individuals various techniques for learning professional skills. There are different educational institutions for learning other professional skills. For example, if a person wants to pursue a career in engineering, there are engineering colleges and universities which will equip them with the skills required for their career.

Rational Thinking

Education helps us a reason and conclude any event, situation, and issue with a reasonable explanation.

Adjustment in Society

Education grooms the personality of an individual, which helps them adjust to any environment, group, community, and society.

Patriotism

Love for nation and country is instilled in people from a very young age through educational institutions. They learn their duties and obligation towards the government and their country.

16 Social Welfare Programs of India

LEARNING OBJECTIVES

Briefly discuss:
- Swachh Bharat Abhiyan
- Pradhan Mantri Jan Dhan Yojana
- Saansad Adarsh Gram Yojana (SAGY)
- The Government Introduced Labor Reforms
- Beti Bachao, Beti Padhao Yojana
- Housing for All by 2022
- Soil Health Card Scheme for Every Farmer
- Deendayal Upadhyaya Gram Jyoti Yojana
- Vanbandhu Kalyan Yojana
- National Heritage City Development and Augmentation Yojana
- Shyama Prasad Mukherji Rurban Mission
- Neeranchal Scheme
- Pashmina Promotion Program

SWACHH BHARAT ABHIYAN

On October 2, 2014, Prime Minister Narendra Modi launched the 'Swachh Bharat Mission,' also known as the 'Clean India Campaign,' from the Valmiki Basti in New Delhi. This campaign aims to realize Mahatma Gandhi's vision of a "clean India" by October 2, 2019, Mahatma Gandhi's 150th birthday. The mission's urban component will be implemented over five years, beginning on October 2, 2014, in all 4041 statutory towns.

The urban component includes eliminating open defecation, converting unsanitary toilets to pour flush toilets, eradicating manual scavenging, municipal solid waste management, and bringing about a behavioral change in people regarding healthy sanitation practices.

The total expected cost of the Program is Rs 62,009 crore, out of which the proposed central assistance will be Rs 14,623 crore. The "Nirmal Bharat Abhiyan" (NBA) is restructured into the "Swachh Bharat" Mission (rural).

PRADHAN MANTRI JAN DHAN YOJANA

The core development philosophy of this program is "Sab Ka Sath, Sab Ka Vikas". Under the scheme, account holders have been provided with a zero-balance bank account, a RuPay debit card, and an accidental insurance cover of Rs 1 lakh. Those who opened accounts until 26 January 2015, over and above the Rs 1 lakh accident cover, were also given life insurance cover of Rs 30,000. Six months after the bank account opening, holders can avail Rs 5,000 loan from the bank.

SAANSAD ADARSH GRAM YOJANA (SAGY)

The scheme was launched on 11th October 2014, on the occasion of the birth anniversary of Lok Nayak Jai Prakash Narayan. The program's goal is to develop three Adarsh Grams by March 2019, of which one will be achieved by 2016. After that, five such would Adarsh Grams (one per year) will be selected and developed by 2024.

Under the scheme, each MP will develop physical and institutional infrastructure in three villages by 2019. The MP would be free to identify a suitable Gram Panchayat for developing it into an Adarsh Gram other than his/her village or that of his/her spouse.

A Gram Panchayat would be the basic unit. It will have a population of 3,000-5,000 in plain areas and 1,000-3,000 in hilly, tribal, and difficult areas.

THE GOVERNMENT INTRODUCED LABOR REFORMS

- **The Deendayal Upadhyaya Shramev Jayate program** was launched to emphasize labor dignity, especially those performed by blue-collared workers, referring to them as "shram yogi".
- **The Universal Account Number (UAN) scheme or 'Shram Suvidha'** for all Provident Fund (PF) contributors will allow the portability of PF benefits and online tracking of PF benefits. The UAN is provided for all 4.17 crores PF users.
- To support the graduates from Industrial Training Institutes (ITIs) across the country, who undergo vocational training after completing class X, the government will reimburse 50% of the

stipend paid to apprentices during the first two years. There are 2.82 lakhs apprentices undergoing training against 4.9 lakh seats. The program will aim to increase this to 24 lakhs apprentices.

- **The Rashtriya Swasthya Bima Yojana (RSBY)** ensures families of unorganized sector workers for up to Rs. Thirty thousand medical care must be transferred from the Ministry of Labour and Employment to the Union Health Ministry.

BETI BACHAO, BETI PADHAO YOJANA

The government has introduced a new scheme called Beti Bachao, BetiPadhao, which will help generate awareness and improve the efficiency of the delivery of welfare services meant for women with an initial corpus of Rs 100 crores. Under the scheme, the government would focus on campaigns to sensitize the people of this country towards the concerns of the girl child and women.

HOUSING FOR ALL BY 2022

To provide housing for all by 2022, the government will soon launch an urban housing mission named after Sardar Patel by merging and improving existing housing schemes. The mission's focus is Low-Cost Affordable Housing to be anchored in the National Housing Bank to increase the flow of cheaper credit for affordable housing to the urban poor. Currently, several schemes include Jawaharlal Nehru National Urban Renewal Mission, Rajiv Awas Yojana, Indira Awas Yojana, and Rajiv Rinn Yojana, which provide housing facilities to economically weaker sections.

SOIL HEALTH CARD SCHEME FOR EVERY FARMER

In a Mission mode, the government has launched the Soil Health Card Scheme to provide every farmer with a Soil Health Card. The card will include crop-specific recommendations for nutrients and fertilizers needed for farms, allowing farmers to boost productivity by using the right inputs. The Soil Health Card is used to assess the current state of soil health and to track changes in soil health that are influenced by land management over time. A total of Rs. 100 crores have been allocated. A further Rs. 56 crores have been set aside to establish 100 mobile soil testing laboratories.

■ DEENDAYAL UPADHYAYA GRAM JYOTI YOJANA

"Deendayal Upadhyaya Gram Jyoti Yojana" for feeder separation will be launched to augment rural areas' power supply and strengthen sub-transmission and distribution systems. Its long-term aim is to provide all homes a 24×7 uninterrupted power supply.

The government has earmarked Rs. 43,000 crores for the Deendayal Upadhyaya Gram Jyoti Yojana for feeder separation to supply electricity through separate feeders for agricultural and rural domestic consumption, providing round-the-clock power to village households.

■ VANBANDHU KALYAN YOJANA

The Union Ministry of Tribal Affairs, on 28th October 2014, launched Vanbandhu Kalyan Yojana (VKY) for the welfare of Tribal people and particularly to lift the human development indices of tribal people. The scheme was launched on a pilot basis in one block in each of the States of Andhra Pradesh, Madhya Pradesh, Himachal Pradesh, Telangana, Orissa, Jharkhand, Chhattisgarh, Rajasthan, Maharashtra, and Gujarat.

Under the scheme, the Union Government will provide ten crores rupees for each block to develop facilities for the Tribal people. These blocks have been selected on the recommendations of the concerned states and have a meager literacy rate.

■ NATIONAL HERITAGE CITY DEVELOPMENT AND AUGMENTATION YOJANA

The Heritage City Development and Augmentation Yojana (HRIDAY) program is to be launched to conserve and preserve the cities' heritage characteristics. The beginning program is launched in Mathura, Amritsar, Gaya, Kanchipuram, Vellankani, and Ajmer. A sum of Rs. 200 crores are set aside for this purpose. The Project will partner with the government, academic institutions, and the local community combining affordable technologies.

SHYAMA PRASAD MUKHERJI RURBAN MISSION

Shyama Prasad Mukherji Rurban Mission will be launched to deliver integrated project-based infrastructure in rural areas. The scheme will also include the development of economic activities and skill development. The preferred mode of delivery would be through PPPs while using various scheme funds.

NEERANCHAL SCHEME

A new program called "Neeranchal" with an initial outlay of ₹2,142 crores in the current financial year, has been launched to boost watershed development in the country.

PASHMINA PROMOTION PROGRAM

P-3 and a program for developing other crafts of Jammu and Kashmir are being started. For this, a sum of Rs. Fifty crores are set aside.

Sociology of Aging

LEARNING OBJECTIVES

☞ How is aging connected with the life cycle?
☞ What are the indications of aging?
☞ Describe the problems faced in old age.

▓ INTRODUCTION

Several health-related factors, including improved medical care, nutrition, sanitation, and housing, have combined in the 21st century to help and promote longer lives for most Indians. The present century in India can be described as a period of the exceedingly rapid growth of the aged population.

The increasing longevity of people has helped foster a growing interest among social and medical scientists in the biological and behavioral aspects of the aging process and the social role of older adults. Accordingly, the study of gerontology has increased in scope and importance in recent years; many medical sociologists specialize in social gerontology, i.e., the study of aging as asocial and psychological experience.

Aging is a biological and sociological process wherein human beings experience and accomplishes stages of biological and social maturation. Aging may be seen as a relatively objective biological process whereby one becomes older, and experiences varied biological developments. Aging may also be seen as a subjective series of social processes whereby people interpret, negotiate, and make sense of biological development with existing conceptualizations of what it means to be a certain age.

▓ AGING IS BOTH BIOLOGICAL AND SOCIOLOGICAL

An example of the bio-social and objective/subjective nature of aging may be helpful. Take, for example, a social being born in the

United States in 1980. This person will likely experience a biological development characterized by the addition of years from birth and by biological understandings of the time (e.g., a being born in 1980 would have a life expectancy, medical and legal definition, and contextual series of economic, educational, and other possibilities based upon birth at this time). As such, a person born in the United States during the 1980s can be expected to follow relatively stable patterns of biological development that will be interpreted similarly to others born at the same time.

However, this child born in the United States in 1980 will experience social development characterized by many factors. For instance, was this child raised in a family or an orphanage? What kind of education did this child receive, public or private, and what educational funding and other educational opportunities did this child receive? Was this child born lower, middle, or upper class? Did this child begin full-time work and adopt adult responsibilities as an adolescent, young adult, or never? Given the many possible answers to these questions, this person can be expected to follow relatively varied patterns of social development that will be interpreted in different ways by others born at the same time. As a result, this child's biological age (how far from birth one is) may or may not match this child's subjective age (how old they feel and what responsibilities develop at what age). Additionally, this child may not align with societal age norms by not doing what society expects the child to do at certain ages.

Aging is a complex process of subjective biological and social realities intertwined with relatively objective biological and social standards that shift within and between historical and cultural periods.

AGING AND THE LIFE CYCLE

In India, the age of 62 has generally marked that point when a person is 'officially' old—primarily because of its arbitrary selection by the administration as the age of eligibility for old-age benefits. Except for its bureaucratic significance; however, being 62 has no other particular relevance. This is because chronological age is an inconsistent indicator of the aging process. Just as physical and intellectual capabilities mature at different points in time for different people. It is possible to be a 'young' 62 or an 'old' 55-year-old person.

One way to 'explain' the social and psychological aspects of the aging experience is to categorize that experience into phases or stages, denoting the human life cycle. Although the life cycle stages are based upon chronological age and do not account for variations among individuals, they nevertheless indicate the general life course most people follow. Implicit in the idea of a life cycle is a standard set of social experiences through which all members of a society are expected to pass. For instance, childhood is when a person generally receives a primary education; adolescence and young adulthood are usually the time of courtship and marriage; the period of later maturity is typically the time of retirement.

Age as a Dimension of Social Organization

As Bengtson points out, age is a dimension of social organization because the life cycle's divisions are prescribed by the society's culture to lend stability and predictability to the typical sequence of life events. This arrangement implies that individuals also change behavior as they pass from one stage of life into a subsequent stage. Infants, children, young adults, middle-aged adults, and older persons are all expected by other people to behave in a manner characteristic of their age group. Social judgments of their maturity depend on how close their behavior approximates the corresponding age-related norm. Furthermore, at each stage of life, a person takes on new social roles and the responsibilities that accrue to those roles, while the person's status and relationships with other people are modified accordingly.

Stage of Human Life Cycle

The typical stages of the human life cycle and the approximate ages are shown in **Table 17.1**. Although a person can be regarded as aging from the moment of conception or the moment the individual reaches full maturation (there is some disagreement on this point), for our purpose, the stages of middle age, later maturity, and old age are most relevant.

The Onset of Old Age

As previously noted, the onset of old age varies among individuals. Although aging is known to occur due to changes in the body's cells, the exact cause of the process is still a mystery. The two most

Table 17.1: Typical stages of the human life cycle.

Stages	Approximate age
Infancy	2
Preschool	2–5
Childhood	5–12
Adolescence	12–17
Early maturity	17–25
Maturity	25–40
Middle age	40–55
Later maturity	55–75
Old age	> 75

widely accepted theories state that aging may be primarily due to deterioration in the integrator homeostasis between cells of the same tissue and those of other tissues, or it may be the result of some form of the present genetic program for cell aging. Whatever the cause, the interaction of biological, genetic, and social–psychological factors seems to be involved. Aging can also be of a primary or secondary nature. Primary aging occurs over time, while secondary aging occurs through disease or trauma and may be temporally premature.

Indication of Aging

The most apparent indication of aging is the appearance of the skin, which tends to dry out and wrinkle **(Figs. 17.1 and 17.2)**. The person's capacity for sight and hearing is reduced, and the brain begins to shrink, losing about 100,000 cells a day. Muscles also shrink and become weaker, joints stiffness and swelling, while the heart, lungs, kidneys, and bladder operate at reduced levels of effectiveness, and the body's output of hormones begins to diminish. The body becomes increasingly susceptible to stress, infection, degenerative diseases, cancer, arteriosclerosis, and diabetes.

Middle Age

According to Atchley, middle-age is the period of life when a person initially becomes aware that they are aging. Middle age is when the

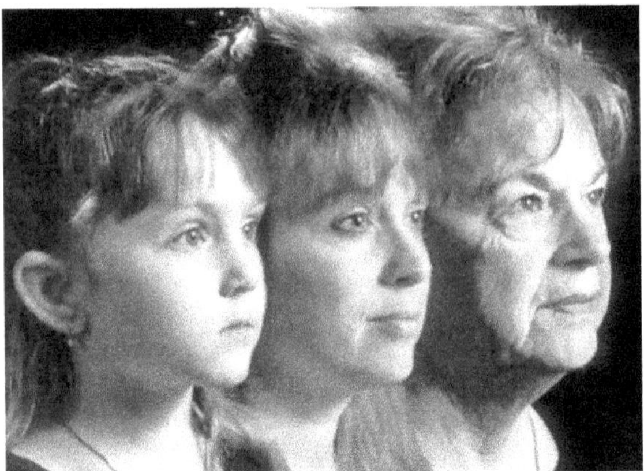

Fig. 17.1: Aging in females.

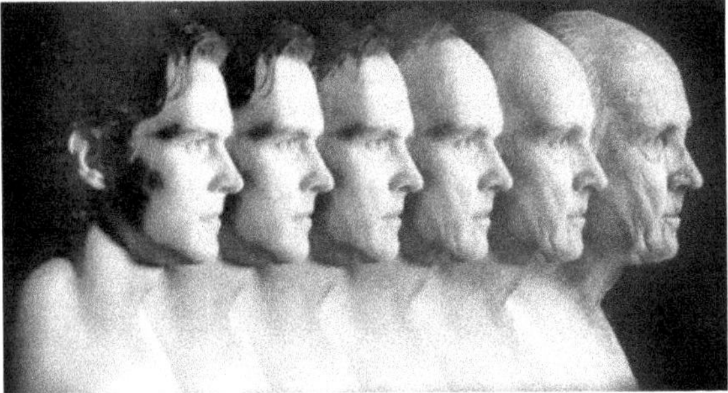

Fig. 17.2: Aging in males.

person recognizes a reduction of energy and often begins to favor intellectual activities over physical endeavors. Usually, the person's work career more or less reaches a plateau, and the great majority of a couple's children will have left home to lead their own lives. As Atchley explains, middle-age is when most people realize that they are aging and that death is real, not just something that happens to somebody else. Kastenbaum suggests that most people are past-oriented by age 40, and virtually all people are by age 55.

Later maturity is characterized by a marked reduction in energy, vision, and hearing. Chronic health disorders are commonplace and poor health can join with reduced income, retirement, and the deaths of friends/relatives to curtail social interaction. By the time they are in their mid-60s, most women are widows. But, as Atchley notes, the period of later maturity can be pleasant for those who plan for it, retain a good measure of physical vigor, and perhaps wish to enjoy a time of lessened responsibilities. Also, the aged individual may continue to be a highly productive member of society. Bowden and Burstein point out that the myth that age necessarily involves an inability to produce is challenged by the number of second careers and examples of influence maintained by prominent individuals late into their lives.

Kastenbaum has found that a characteristic of old age is a foreshortened time perspective. The older person avoids thoughts of the future because of the limited time left and instead dwells on the past.

Old Age

In contrast to other stages of life, old age is more likely to be a rather unpleasant period as there is a higher probability of loneliness, boredom, and loss of self-esteem. Also, it can be a time when mental processes are diminished. Whereas it seems clear that the aged brain takes longer to respond to a stimulus and the recall of recent events may be impaired (probably due to the tendency toward increased distractibility on the part of the older person), remote memory of past events is usually quite good. If there is considerable memory loss, it can be a sign of organic brain damage. But it should be realized that, while such brain damage may be likely to occur with increasing age, it does not occur in all elderly persons. Besides reduced mental activity in very old age, another problem peculiar to the elderly is that of physical frailty and the possibility of being disabled such that physical mobility is highly restricted or defined.

Physical and mental infirmities and the reality of being tired, ill, and less able to cope with problems are all set in a framework of the recognition of impending death, which can and do produce severe problems of adjustment and depression for the elderly. With reduced resources, the older adult is less able to cope with stress, and adapt to new conditions. Old age is thus a period in life that many people fear and wish to avoid, yet as in the period of later maturity, the key to success in old age is to maintain an optimal level of physical strength and mental awareness.

Problems Faced in Old Age

In most cases, a man's life is divided into four stages: childhood, adolescence, adulthood, and old age. An individual finds himself in different situations and faces different problems at each stage. Old age is considered an unavoidable, unwelcome, and troublesome stage of life. After the age of 65, aging problems are more common.

These problems may be divided into five heads:
1. Physiological
2. Psychological
3. Social
4. Emotional
5. Financial

Physiological Problems

The term "old age" refers to a period of physical decline. Even if one does not lose one's eyes, teeth, or everything right away, one's physical abilities begin to deteriorate. The physical condition is influenced by hereditary factors, lifestyle choices, and environmental factors. Living vicissitudes, poor diet, malnutrition, infectious diseases, intoxications, gluttony, insufficient rest, emotional stress, overwork, endocrine disorders, and environmental conditions such as heat and cold are common secondary causes of physical decline.

The jaw shrinks, and the skin sags **due to** tooth loss. Wrinkles cause the cheeks to become pendulous and the eyelids to become baggy, with the upper lids overhanging the lower. Due to poor tear gland function, the eyes appear dull and lustrous **and** frequently have a watery appearance. Denture loss affects speech, and some people even appear to lisp.

The skin becomes rough and brittle, and its elasticity is lost. Wrinkles form and the veins on the skin become more visible. As people age, their perspiration becomes less frequent, and new skin pigmentation appears. Hair becomes thin and gray, and nails thicken and become rigid. Hand tremors, forearm tremors, head tremors, and lower jaw tremors are typical. Bones harden, become brittle, and are susceptible to fractures and breaks as they age.

The nervous system has a significant impact on the brain. The spleen, liver, and soft organs all show signs of atrophy. Gradually, the ratio of heart weight to body weight decreases. Because of an increase in fibrous tissue caused by cholesterol and calcium deposits, the valves' softness and pliability gradually change. Heart disease, other minor ailments, and chronic diseases are all common among the elderly.

Body temperature is affected as a result of the weakened regulatory mechanism. As a result, the elderly are more sensitive to climate change than others. They have digestive issues as well as insomnia. They are unable to chew or swallow due to dental issues.

Because of their slow reaction to dangers, the elderly are more likely to be involved in accidents. As sense organs fail and mental abilities deteriorate, their capacity to work decreases. The eyes and ears are severely harmed. Vision is affected by changes in the brain's nerve center and retina, and sensitivity to specific colors gradually decreases. Because of their deteriorating eyesight, most of the elderly suffer from farsightedness.

As people get older, their sexual potency decreases, as do their secondary sex characters. Nervousness, headaches, giddiness, emotional instability, irritability, and insomnia are common symptoms of menopause in women between the ages of 45 and 50. The elderly have fewer coordinates in their movements. They are easily fatigued. They lose interest in learning new skills and become sedentary due to a lack of motivation. Visiting the doctor has become a routine task for them.

Psychological Problems

Mental illnesses are frequently associated with advanced age. Psychotic depressions are more common in the elderly. Senile dementia (associated with cerebral atrophy and degeneration) and psychosis with cerebral arteriosclerosis are the two most common psychotic disorders in older people (associated with either blocking or rupturing the cerebral arteries). It has been estimated that these two disorders account for roughly 80% of psychotic disorders among the elderly in civilized societies.

Senile Dementia

Senile dementia affects the elderly. They develop symptoms such as poor memory, intolerance of change, disorientation, insomnia, failure of judgment, the gradual formation of delusions and hallucinations, extreme-mental depression and agitation, and severe mental clouding in which the individual becomes restless, combative, resistive, and incoherent, and severe mental clouding in which the individual becomes restless, combative, resistive, and incoherent. In the worst-case scenario, the patient becomes bedridden, his disease resistance is reduced, and his days are numbered.

Psychosis with Cerebral Arteriosclerosis

Physiological symptoms include acute indigestion, unsteadiness in gait, and small strokes that result in cumulative brain damage and gradual personality changes. Seizures that are conclusive are relatively common. Symptoms include weakness, fatigue, dizziness, headache, depression, memory loss, periods of confusion, decreased work efficiency, increased irritability, and a tendency to be suspicious about minor matters. One of the most common psychological issues associated with aging is forgetfulness. In old age, general intelligence and independent creative thinking are usually harmed.

Emotional Problem

They become dependent as their mental abilities deteriorate. They have lost faith in their abilities and judgments but still want to maintain control over the younger ones. They want to be involved in every aspect of family life and business. Young people do not listen to their suggestions and advice because of the generation gap. They begin asserting their rights and power instead of developing a sympathetic attitude toward the elderly. This may make them feel that their dignity and importance have been taken away.

Another risk is the death of a spouse in old age. The loss of a spouse can leave you feeling lonely and isolated. More emotional problems arise due to family members' negligence and indifference toward the elderly.

Social Problems

With age, older people suffer significant social losses. Their social lives have been limited by the loss of work, the deaths of relatives, friends, and spouses, and their poor health, which prevents them from participating in social activities. Their social lives become confined to interpersonal relationships with family members as the home becomes the focal point of their social lives. They are likely to be lonely due to the loss of most of the social roles they once played, and isolated severe chromic health problems allow them to become socially isolated, resulting in loneliness and depression.

Financial Problem

Retirement from service usually means a loss of income and the pensions that the elderly receive are often insufficient to keep up with the rising cost of living. They are relegated to the role of "chief breadwinner to mere dependent" due to their reduced income, despite spending their provident fund on children's marriages, the purchase of new property, children's education, and family maintenance. The diagnosis and treatment of their disease added to their financial woes as they grew older.

Old age is a time of physical decline and, in some cases, social alienation, including losing a spouse, friends, job, property, and physical appearance. Physical strength deteriorates as people age, mental stability deteriorates, financial power dwindles, and eyesight deteriorates. It is a time of disappointment, depression, illness, repentance, and isolation.

Grandparents, on the other hand, provide an additional source of affection and experience in child care and family business. Regardless of the various problems associated with old age, one must remain actively engaged for one's well-being as well as for the good of society.

Economic Security Schemes for Elderly

Under standardized economic security policy, the government covers retirement benefits for those in the organized sector, economic security benefits for those in the unorganized sector, and old-age pension for rural elderly. The government pension bill in 2001 was more than 1% of GDP or 15% of the revenues. The employees' provident funds, though gradually extended from 5 to 179 industries, the increase in the labor force coverage has barely risen from 1% to 5%. Though little evidence is available on poverty among the elderly and the impact of cash transfers, several studies have raised concerns about the target population, administrative efficiency, and other issues. Given the high growth rate among the elderly and high longevity, planners need serious thinking to evolve suitable programs and schemes and bring reforms to the existing pension programs.

As per the National Policy on Aging (1999), one-third of the elderly population (1993-94) is below the poverty line, and about one-third are above it but belong to lower-income groups. The policy document also states that the coverage under the Old Age Pension Scheme for poor persons, which is 2.76 million (as of January 1997), will be significantly expanded with the ultimate objective of covering all older persons below the poverty line. NOAP scheme (National Old Age Pension Scheme), which the Central Government initiates, provides for a pension of Rs.75/- per month to the older adults living in the conditions of destitution. The budgetary allocation for the NOAP scheme, which was Rs.450 crores in 1999, was increased to Rs.465 crores in 2002. The NOAP scheme is in operation all over India, and the reports indicate that the most vulnerable sections of Indian society, like women and lower caste individuals, have benefited from this scheme.

All-State Government and Union Territories have their schemes for old age pension and the criterion of eligibility and the quantum of pension amount vary among these States. The average old-age pension, nearly Rs.150 per month, was below the average per capita income per Indian. The percentage of elderly who benefited from the old-age pension scheme varies across states, with a minimum of 0.3% to 68%. As of 1999, a total amount of Rs.227 million was spent to benefit 49 lakh beneficiaries among the elderly.

The combined national budget allocation for the NOAPS comes to 0.6%, only as compared to 6% of Central Government revenue expended on pension for its employees (Irudaya Rajan, 2001). The Central government announced in the year 1999 another social security program called the 'Annapurna Program' for the elderly destitute. Under the program, all older persons eligible for the NOAPS are given 10 kg. rice/wheat monthly, free of cost, through the existing public distribution system and the expected beneficiaries for the program is estimated to be 6.6 million. The total number of beneficiaries during 2000-2001 for the National Old Age Pension Scheme in the country is approximately 68.81 lakh. This would imply that 13.76 lakh beneficiaries would be eligible for coverage under the

"Annapurna" Scheme. An amount of Rs.100 crores has been provided in the scheme's budget for 2000-2001.

The Ministry realizes that poverty alleviation programs directed at the aged alone cannot provide a solution to the income and social security problems of the elderly and has so commissioned the National Project titled OASIS (Old Age Social and Income Security) as a result of growing concern for old age social and income security; especially for the 330 million young workers in the unorganized sector (including farmers, shopkeepers, professional, taxi-drivers, casual/contract laborers, etc.) out of the total 370 million workers in India. According to this project, every young worker can build up enough savings during their working life, which would serve as a shield against poverty in old age. The need arose because of a lack of adequate instruments to enable workers in the unorganized sector to provide for their future old age.

National Policies for the Elderly

Many national policies for the elderly operate in India. Article 41 of the Indian Constitution provides that the State shall make adequate provisions for securing the right to work, education, and public assistance in unemployment, old age, sickness and disablement, and other similar cases within the limits of its economic development. Besides, the Maintenance and Welfare of Parents and Senior Citizen Act 2007 was enacted in December 2007 to ensure need-based maintenance of parents and senior citizens and their welfare.

To ensure that the elderly live longer and lead a secure, dignified, and productive life is a significant challenge for policymakers in India. To address the issue, an Integrated Program for Older Person (IPOP) has been implemented since 1992 with the sole objective of improving the quality of life of senior citizens by providing basic amenities like shelter, food, medical care, and entertainment opportunities. The National Policy on Older Persons (NPOP) was announced in January 1999 to reaffirm the commitment to ensuring the well-being of the elderly. These policies envisage government support to ensure financial and food security, healthcare, shelter, and other needs of older persons and the availability of services to improve the quality of their lives. The draft National Policy for Senior Citizens (Chairperson: Mohini Giri) discusses housing, productive aging, multigenerational bonding, healthcare, and various other schemes but is yet to be finalized and adopted by the government. The Maintenance and Welfare of Parents and Senior Citizens Act, 2007, assigns responsibility and obligation to the heirs to provide care and support to the elderly. There also is an inter-ministerial committee on older persons to address aging issues. Various ministries like the Railways, Rural Development, and Finance also offer special concessions to the elderly. Also, several financial schemes initiated by the government are primarily focused on BPL households.

To cater to the rising elderly population, the government has also been undertaking pension reforms. Pension Fund Regulatory and Development Authority was established in 2003 and had been making efforts to improve social security in India. Despite such efforts and introducing the New National Pension Scheme that includes Swavalamban and launching an extensive financial education program, only about 20% of the elderly population is covered, mainly those who have retired from the organized sector, including government and public sector Employees. In India, with the Insurance and Regulatory Authority in 1999, life insurance companies have increased from one, LIC, to 24 in 2013, with increasing participation from the private sector. Despite this, life insurance penetration is less than 4% in India by many different estimates.

The survey by UNFPA (2011) reveals that the utilization of all schemes for BPL households were abysmally low. Only less than 20% of the elderly belonging to BPL are beneficiaries, while still, a few utilize the 'Annapoorna Scheme' and IGNWPS. It would be alarming to note that substantial wrong targeting of the schemes was apparent, with up to 9% of non-BPL cardholders benefiting from IGNOAPS and 15% from IGNWPS. Awareness of concessions and benefits regarding train travel, bus reservation, phone connections, the high-interest rate on small savings, income tax benefits, and privileges under NREGA was also found to be poor.

■ CONCLUSION

The elderly population is expected to rise from about 8% of the total population in 2011 to about 20% by 2050. Population aging is already taking place, though gradually, in India-funded health and pension schemes before the full consequences of population aging make themselves apparent in the fiscal. The role of partnerships between the public and private sectors in health, education, and caring for the elderly also needs to be carefully explored. In the case of health, measures should be taken to minimize the fiscal impact of relatively expensive modern medical techniques through telemedicine. In education, private sector involvement could provide significant benefits. Timely action in a phased manner is required as evidence shows that in some developed and many developing countries, scope for increased public expenditure on health and education seems limited, with public finances already overstretched.

Learning from the developed world's experiences, India should be able to develop funded health and pension schemes before the full fiscal consequences of population aging become apparent. Partnerships between the public and private sectors in health, education, and elderly care must also be thoroughly investigated.

In the case of health, telemedicine should be used to reduce the financial impact of relatively expensive modern medical techniques. Private sector involvement in education could have significant advantages. Evidence shows that in some developed and many developing countries, the scope for increased public expenditure on health and education appears to be limited, with public finances already overstretched.

The family institution must be protected and strengthened, and support services must be provided to enable families to cope with their responsibilities of caring for the elderly. Along with proper and effective professional welfare services that must be developed to provide counseling services to the elderly and their family members, it is also critical to provide financial assistance to low-income families with one or more elderly members. The rapid aging of the population will inevitably result in social and economic change.

To effectively solve the emerging problems of the elderly, a holistic approach to population aging that considers social, economic, and cultural changes is required. Given the various aspects of the aging process, it is reasonable to conclude that greater attention should be paid to raising awareness of aging issues and their socioeconomic consequences, as well as promoting the development of policies and programs to deal with an aging society.

18 Social Stratification

LEARNING OBJECTIVES

☞ What is social stratification? Its meaning and nature.
☞ What are the meaning and types of social stratification?
☞ Describe the functions and characteristics of social stratification.
☞ Describe the features of social stratification.
☞ Describe the origin and features of the Indian caste system.
☞ What are the features of caste in India today?
☞ Describe the social class system and status.
☞ What is social mobility? Its meaning and types.
☞ Explain race as a biological concept.
☞ What are the criteria for racial classification?
☞ What are race and racism?
☞ What is the influence of class, caste, and race on health and health practices?

■ INTRODUCTION

The term "social stratification" is used by sociologists to describe the system of social standing. Social stratification is the division of a society's population into socioeconomic tiers based on factors such as wealth, income, race, education, and power.

Social stratification ranks individuals and groups in a more or less permanent status hierarchy. Every society is divided into two social units: upper and lower. Every society is divided into groups that are more or less distinct. Social stratification existed in even the most primitive societies. Some individuals and groups are rated higher than others based on opportunities and privileges. In India, doctors, and engineers, for example, are rated higher than teachers. The formers have a higher social status as a class. The social order, or stratification, is formed by the prestige of various positions.

Stratification tends to limit interaction, with more interaction of a particular type occurring within a stratum than between strata. In some stratification systems, certain types of interaction are restricted more than others. There may be more restrictions in finding a marriage partner, choosing a profession, and making friends than in the flow of automobile traffic. Inequality resulting from the actual functions performed by the people involved, the superior power and control of resources possessed by specific individuals or groups, or both, is referred to as social stratification.

Meaning and Nature of Social Stratification

The arrangement of any social group or society in which hierarchically divides positions is referred to as stratification. The positions are unequal regarding power, property, evaluation, and psychic gratification. We include the word "social" because positions comprise socially defined statuses.

Stratification is a phenomenon that exists in all surplus-producing societies. The process by which members of society rank themselves and one another in hierarchies based on the number of desirable goods they possess is known as stratification.

The problem of social inequality has existed for centuries as a result of stratification. In societies with closed stratification systems, such inequalities become institutionalized and rigid. A person is born into a particular economic and social stratum or caste stays in that stratum until he dies. Most modern industrial societies have a system of open or class stratification. Social mobility is possible in open stratification systems, though some population members do not have the opportunity to reach their full potential.

Individuals and groups are ranked in a more or less permanent hierarchy of status through the process of stratification. It refers to stratifying a population-based on specific characteristics such as inborn qualities, material possessions, and performance.

The creation of structural forms—social classes—results from the layering process in a society. The social structure resembles a pyramid, with society divided into social classes. The lowest social class is at the bottom of the structure, with other social classes arranged in a hierarchy above it.

As a result, stratification entails two phenomena: (1) individual or group differentiation, in which some individuals or groups come to rank higher than others, and (2) individual ranking based on some criterion of value.

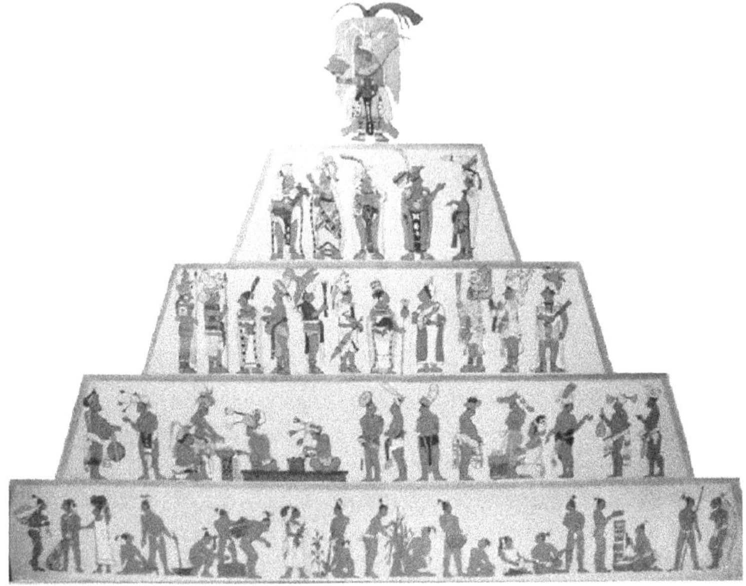

Fig. 18.1: Social stratification in ancient era.

Society compares and ranks individuals and groups based on the values it assigns to various roles. We have social stratification in a hierarchy of status levels based on the inequality of social position when individuals and groups are ranked according to some commonly accepted basis of valuation **(Fig. 18.1)**.

Functions of Stratification

a. Stratification provides a sense of competition, and thus all try to go up and find a higher place in society.
b. It makes people responsible for the nature of the work that they are doing.
c. It helps decide the roles and functions of each category of people living in society.
d. It is also needed to recognize those who are able and capable so that all are not clubbed together with the inefficient.
e. It is also essential for locating the status of a person in society. Without stratification, it will be difficult to locate people and the degree of their wisdom, initiative, and knowledge.

f. It provides for the placement and motivation of individuals to affect the performance of their necessary social duties.

g. It provides a system of rewards and inducements to members for carrying out various duties associated with various positions. The rewards are usually economic. Prestige and leisure are built into social positions so that, being unequal, they result in inequality of positions.

Characteristics of Stratification

The following are the characteristics of social stratification:

1. **It is social:** Stratification is social because it does not represent biologically based inequality. Indeed, characteristics like strength, intelligence, age, and sex are frequently used to determine status. However, such distinctions are insufficient to explain why some social statuses receive more power, wealth, and prestige than others.

   Biological characteristics do not determine social superiority and inferiority until they are socially recognized. An industry manager, for example, achieves a dominant position through socially defined traits rather than physical strength or age. Education, training skills, experience, personality, character, and other factors are more important than biological characteristics.

2. **The stratification system is old:** The stratification system is old. Even the most minor wandering bands had stratification. The main criteria for stratification are age and gender. Almost all ancient civilizations had disparities between rich and poor, powerful and humble, and free and enslaved people. Social philosophers have been deeply concerned with economic, social, and political inequalities since Plato and Kautilya.

3. **It is global:** Social stratification is a global phenomenon. The divide between the wealthy and the poor, referred to as the 'haves' or 'have nots,' is visible everywhere. Stratification can be found even in non-literate societies.

4. **It comes in various forms:** Social stratification has never been uniform in all societies. The Patricians and the Plebians were the two strata of ancient Roman society. The Brahmins, Kshatriyas, Vaishyas, and Shudras were the four Varnas of Aryan society; the ancient Greek society was divided into freemen and enslaved

people; and the ancient Chinese society was divided into mandarins, merchants, farmers, and soldiers. Class and estate appear to be the most common forms of stratification in the modern world.

5. **It has implications:** The stratification system has ramifications. Because of stratification, the most important, most desired, and often scarce things in human life are distributed unequally. The system has two outcomes: (i) life chances and (ii) way of life.

   Infant mortality, longevity, physical and mental illness, marital conflict, separation, and divorce are all possibilities in life. The mode of housing, residential area, education, means of recreation, parent-child relationship, modes of transportation, and so on are all examples of lifestyles.

6. **Inequality or higher-lower positions:** Social stratification refers to the division of society into layers arranged in a hierarchical order in social relationships. While some positions or levels, referred to as higher levels, come with more benefits, privileges, and respect, others have lower positions and status. In this way, stratification contributes to social inequality, considered natural and necessary for a well-ordered, systematic, and healthy society.

7. **Social stratification is a source of competition:** Stratification causes multiple levels in society to emerge. Higher-level individuals are aware of their superior status and strive to maintain and improve it. People from lower levels are constantly striving for higher positions.

   This creates a social competition that promotes social advancement. When competition becomes unhealthy and widespread, however, it can lead to social conflict, struggles, jealousies, and rivalries.

8. **Every social position and status has its prestige:** Every social position and status has prestige. This distinction, however, must be logical. It must not be founded on nefarious practices such as casteism, religious superstitions, or rituals. Because religious ceremonies were held in such high regard in ancient India, the Brahmins were born into a superior position.

   However, people's belief in the Brahmins' superior status grew shaky over time. Persons from other social classes have risen to higher positions in society, and every social class has the right to a life of dignity and respect. There may be a difference in degree, but it is not organic or irrational.

9. **Stratification entails a stable, long-lasting, and hierarchical social division:** In society, stratification creates a stable, long-lasting hierarchical, and permanent division. In every society, there has always been a divide between the rich and the poor. Caste-based social stratification has been so strong in India that it still exists today. Caste-based stratification has been rigid and permanent, and no one from one caste can join another.

10. **Interdependence of different statuses:** Social stratification is the division of society into various classes and statuses. Each social status or class has its place in the social hierarchy. All of the statuses, however, are linked and interdependent. Changes in social stratification always result in shifts in the status of people from different classes.

11. **Stratification is based on social values:** Social stratification is based on social values and traditions in every society. In India, social stratification has traditionally been based on caste. In western societies, however, social stratification has been based on class. Every society's class structure is based on prevailing social values.

12. **Social stratification limits interactions:** People stratified into different levels or classes engage in interactions in every society. On the other hand, inter-class or inter-level interactions are always constrained and defined by social norms.

    People who belong to the same level have similar social styles and do not fully interact with people from other levels. Interactions between people of different social statuses, levels, or classes are defined and limited by social stratification.

13. **Circulation or change in position of various classes of persons:** Possibility and Chances: Social stratification is undeniably long-lasting, if not permanent; however, it allows for social mobility and change. Social elites are constantly shifting. New members are admitted, and some old members are ejected as positions are lost over time.

    Furthermore, social classes are based on economic position in every society: the wealthy, middle class, and poor; however, members of these classes can earn changes in their economic positions. A mixed stratification based on the relationship between Ascribed and Earned Statuses allows members of the wealthy class to become poor by losing money.

Definitions of Social Stratification

P Gisbert: Social stratification is the division of society into permanent groups or categories linked with each other by the relationship of superiority and subordination.

Melvin M Tumin: Social stratification refers to the arrangement of any social group or society into a hierarchy of unequal positions about power, property, social evaluation, and/or psychic gratification.

Types of Social Stratification

Social stratification is based upon a variety of principles. The significant types of stratification are: (i) Caste, (ii) Class, (iii) Estate, and (iv) Slavery.

   i. **Caste** is a hereditary, endogamous social group in which a person's rank and accompanying rights and obligations are ascribed based on his birth into a particular group. For example— Brahmins, Kshatriyas, Vaishyas, and Sudra Caste.
  ii. **Class**—Stratification based on class is dominant in modern society. In this, a person's position depends greatly upon achievement and his ability to use to advantage the inborn characteristics and wealth that he may possess.
 iii. **Estate** system of medieval Europe provides another system of stratification that emphasized birth, wealth, and possessions. Each estate had a state.
  iv. **Slavery** had an economic basis. In slavery, every enslaved person had his master to whom he was subjected. The master's power over the enslaved person was unlimited.

■ CASTE SYSTEM

Introduction

The word caste is used in everyday life, and we use it to distinguish one person from another. We say that such and such a person belongs to a particular caste. In saying this, we generally mean to convey that he is born of parents or is a member of a family said to belong to a particular caste. The word caste is derived from the Spanish word *casta*, which means 'breed.' Caste is a unique social institution of Indian society that originated from the Varna system, described in the Vedas.

The caste system has been the predominant form of social stratification in India, and even today, it exerts considerable influence on our lives and social interactions. Caste is a social phenomenon found in almost all human societies but nowhere had it taken such a well-defined and rigid form as it did in India. It is an institution most highly developed in India and has profoundly influenced the life of the Hindus. One's place of residence, mode of life, personal association, the type of food which one can eat, and from whom one can accept food and water, one's occupation, and the group in which one has to find one's mate, are determined by one's birth.

Social interaction between castes is strictly limited, and inter-caste marriages are prohibited. The caste system is always safeguarded by social laws and sanctified by religion. It is very conservative and lends excellent stability to society. It serves to handover skills and secrets of craftsmanship from one generation to another. However, it also acts as a deterrent to the introduction of new and improved methods of production in industry and agriculture and results in an economy dependent on the interplay of a large number of segregated, sometimes conflicting, interests.

Features of the Caste System

Kingsley Davis has mentioned certain standard features or tendencies which together distinguish Indian caste from other types of groups as follows:

- The membership in the caste is hereditary.
- This inherited membership is fixed for life.
- The choice of a marriage partner is strictly endogamous, for it must take place within the caste group.
- The contact with other groups is further limited by restrictions on touching, associating with, dining with, and eating food cooked by the outsiders.

- The consciousness of caste membership is further emphasized by the caste name.
- The caste is united by a common traditional occupation.
- The relative prestige of the different castes in any locality is well established and jealously guarded.

The Indian Caste System—Origin and Features

The word "caste" comes from the Spanish and Portuguese words "race, lineage, or breed." When the Portuguese applied the term casta to hereditary Indian social groups known as 'jati' in India, they used it in the modern sense. 'Jati' comes from the root word 'Jana,' which means 'to give birth.' As a result, the caste is preoccupied with birth.

"Caste is that extreme form of social class organization in which individuals' position in the status hierarchy is determined by descent and birth," wrote Anderson and Parker.

Origin of Caste System in India

Many theories like traditional, racial, political, occupational, evolutionary, etc., try to explain India's caste system.

1. **Traditional theory:** The caste system, according to this theory, has divine origins. It claims that the caste system is an extension of the varna system, with the four varnas deriving from Brahma's body.

   The Brahmins, who descended from Brahma's head and were primarily teachers and intellectuals, were at the top of the hierarchy. His arms produced Kshatriyas, or warriors and rulers. His thighs were used to create Vaishyas or traders. The Shudras descended from Brahma's feet and were at the bottom. The mouth is used for preaching, learning, etc.; the arms are used for protection; the thighs are used to cultivate or do business, and the feet are used to help the entire body, so the Shudras must serve everyone else. Sub-castes arose later as a result of intermarrying between the four varnas.

2. **Theory of race:** Varna, which means color in Sanskrit, is the Sanskrit word for caste. The chaturvarna system—Brahmins, Kshatriyas, Vaishyas, and Shudras—gave rise to caste stratification in Indian society. The caste system was born after the arrival of

Aryans in India, according to Indian sociologist DN Majumdar in his book "Races and Culture in India."

The Arya and non-Aryans (Dasa) are distinguished in the Rig Vedic literature by their complexion, speech, religious practices, and physical characteristics.During the Vedic period, the Varna system was primarily based on the division of labor and occupation. The Rig Veda frequently mentions the three classes of Brahma, Kshatriya, and Vis. Brahma and Kshatriya were the poet-priest and warrior-chief, respectively. All of the ordinary people were included in Vis. The name 'Sudra,' for the fourth class, appears only once in the Rig Veda. The Sudra class represented domestic servants.

3. **Theory of politics:** According to this theory, the Brahmins created the caste system as a clever device to elevate themselves to the top of the social hierarchy.

4. **Occupational theory:** The caste system is based on the occupation. Those who practiced better and more respectable professions were considered superior to those who practiced dirty professions.

5. **Theory of evolution:** According to this theory, the caste system did not emerge anywhere or at a specific time. It is the result of a long social evolution process.

Principal Features of Caste System in India

Its principal characteristics are as follows:

1. **Social segmentation:** Society is divided into various small social groups known as castes. Each of these castes is a well-developed social group, with membership determined by birth. The children are of the same caste as their parents.

   Caste membership is an unchangeable fact that entirely determines a man's position in the social structure. Even if a person's status, occupation, education, wealth, or other circumstances change, his membership does not change.

2. **Hierarchy:** A hierarchical structure is a command ladder in which the higher rungs encompass the lower rungs in regular succession. The castes teach us a crucial social principle: hierarchy.

   Castes are arranged in descending order of superiority and inferiority. The Brahmin caste is at the top of this hierarchy, and the untouchable caste is at the bottom. In the middle are the intermediate castes, whose relative positions are not always precise, and as a result, disputes among members of these castes over the social precedence of their respective castes are not uncommon.

3. **Endogamy:** Endogamy is the most fundamental feature of the caste system. According to all thinkers, endogamy is the most important feature of caste, i.e., members of a caste or sub-caste should marry within their caste or sub-caste. The violation of the endogamy rule would result in ostracism and caste loss. Although endogamy is the norm for a caste, Anomie and Pratiloma marriage, i.e., hypergamy and hypogamy, were also common in rare cases.

4. **Hereditary status:** In general, caste membership is determined by birth, and a man inherits the status of the caste into which he is born. In this regard, Ketkar has written that the caste is restricted to only those born into it. Thus, membership in the caste is hereditary, and membership does not change even if his status, occupation, education, wealth change, etc.

5. **Hereditary occupation:** A hereditary occupation is a feature of the traditional caste system. Members of a particular caste are expected to follow the caste's occupation. Traditionally, a Brahmin could serve as a priest. In some cases, the caste name is based on the occupation, such as *Napita (barber), Dhobi, Mochi, Mali*, etc.

6. **Food and drink restrictions:** There are rules governing what type of food or drink a person can accept and from which caste. Typically, a caste will not accept cooked food from any other caste lower on the social scale than itself. A person from a higher caste believes that even the shadow of a person from a lower caste pollutes him, as does accept food or drink from him.

7. **Cultural differences:** Because each caste has its own set of rules and regulations regarding endogamy, pollution purity, and occupational specialization, each caste develops its subculture because its caste's requirements govern the individual's behavior. According to the doctrine, a person should follow the 'dharma' (religious obligation) of his caste, no matter how low, before following the 'dharma' of another caste, no matter

how illustrious. As a result, different castes have a different "way of life." "As a result," Prof Ghurye writes, "castes are small and complete social worlds in themselves, clearly distinguished from one another while existing within the larger society."

8. **Social segregation:** One aspect of caste differentiation is social segregation. "Segregation of individual castes or groups of castes in the village is a most obvious mark of civil privileges and disabilities," writes Ghurye, "and it has prevailed in a more or less definite form throughout India."

   The South has greater segregation than the North. Impure castes are segregated and forced to live on the outskirts of villages in some parts of the country, including Marathi, Telugu, and Kanarese-speaking regions. Different castes frequently occupy distinctly different quarters in the Tamil and Malayalam regions. The village is divided into three parts occupied by the dominant caste or by Brahmins, allotted to the Shudras, and the third reserved for the Panchamas or untouchables.

9. **The Pollution concept:** The concept of pollution is critical in maintaining the required distance between different castes. "A high caste man is not allowed even to touch a low caste man, let alone accept cooked food and water from him." Where the two castes involved are at opposite ends of the hierarchy, the lower caste man may be required to maintain a minimum distance between himself and the high caste man." The pollution distance varies according to caste and location.

10. **Unique name:** Each caste has a unique name that we can identify. An occupation is sometimes associated with a specific caste. With the help of the caste name, we can learn about the profession or occupation of the caste.

11. **Jati Panchayat:** Each caste's status is carefully guarded, not only by caste laws but also by conventions. The community openly enforces these. Every Indian region has a governing body or board known as a Jati Panchayat. These Panchayats are named differently in different regions and castes, such as Kuldriya in Madhya Pradesh and Jokhila in South Rajasthan. Adultery, violation of any prescribed taboos, killing sacred animals (the cow), and insulting a Brahmin are some of the offenses dealt with, and the punishments awarded are outcasting, fines, feasts to be given to caste men, and so on.

12. **Taboo:** Another essential feature of the caste system is the taboo (prohibition) by which the superior castes attempt to maintain their ceremonial purity and neutralize the evils believed to exist in everyone. These potentialities are said to become more active and harmful to others during specific life crises.

    The following are the most recent taboos, whose observance by orthodox Hindus frequently entailed several cumbersome observances: the food taboo, which limits the types of food that a man can eat. The cooking taboo, which limits who can cook the food. The eating taboo may establish the mealtime ritual. The commensal taboo refers to the individual with whom one may share food. Finally, the nature of the vessel (earthenware, copper, or brass) used for drinking or cooking is forbidden.

Features of Caste System in Indian Rural Society

The nine features of the caste system in Indian rural society are as follows:

1. Rules of Endogamy and Exogamy
2. The interdependence of Occupations
3. Importance of Caste in Various Stages of Life
4. Caste Associations
5. Dominant Caste
6. Village Economy and Caste
7. Social and Occupational Mobility
8. Hierarchical Relations are based on caste
9. Caste and Joint Family System

The caste system in India is only analyzedbased on structural and cultural aspects. Endogamy, caste hierarchy, and caste occupations are some of the structural properties of the caste system, whereas values refer to the cultural aspect. Though the caste system is found both in rural and urban areas, it has some specific features to perform in rural society.

Some of these features are as follows:

a. **Rules of Endogamy and Exogamy:**Many rules exist concerning marital relations. One cannot marry a person who belongs to the same gotra. A man also cannot marry a girl who is related by blood. In specific tribal communities, village exogamy also exists, as tribals consider marrying within their village a loss of status.

b. **The interdependence of Occupations:**The division of labor-based on caste is an essential feature of the caste system in rural societies. The economy of the village was earlier based on the jajmani system. In this system, the occupational castes render services to their jajmans on an exchange basis, either in cash or in kind.

Generally, most of their payments are made in kind. Thus, the village economy is interdependent on caste occupations. Though the jajmani system in the present day is losing its significance, there are still some villages in which occupational services are rendered on cash payment.

c. **Importance of Caste in Various Stages of Life:**The life of an individual passes from various phases, such as birth ceremonies, marriage, and death. Each of these phases is associated with a set of rituals. A Brahmin officiates all such rituals.

d. **Caste Associations:**Though the power of caste is losing its prominence, caste associations are becoming much more substantial, especially in political matters. The caste war in Bihar today is due to the power gained by these caste associations. The caste associations make most of the political decisions in rural society.

e. **Dominant Caste:**The caste with greater numerical strength than the other castes, which holds the majority of the land and makes critical decisions about the village, is the 'dominant caste.' This concept explains clearly that a single caste exercises authority over the whole village. M. N. Srinivas gave this concept of 'dominant caste.'

f. **Village Economy and Caste:**In rural society, caste determines the economic life of people. Though the village economy is diversified, the traditional village occupations determine the status and wealth of rural people. The clusters of the caste also determine the habitation pattern.

g. **Social and Occupational Mobility:**In any rural society, social and occupational mobility is being analyzed-based on caste. The economic mobility of a person or a family is determined by the caste they belong to. Though some castes have given up their traditional occupations, others follow their caste occupations rigidly.

h. **Hierarchical Relations are based on Caste:** Caste is a system of hierarchical relations, where the Brahmins occupy the highest position and Shudras as the lowest. The Rajputs, artisans, and other caste groups are between these castes. All the interactions among the village members are based on caste status.

His birth determines the status of the individual in a particular caste. Each caste member has a caste occupation, which he must follow. These occupations are divided into pure and impure, based on purity and pollution—the Harijans, regarded as untouchables, followed occupations that are considered impure.

i. **Caste and Joint Family System:** It is generally argued that caste and joint family systems are related. In a village, the caste determines the nature of the family. The caste in the village in India is essentially a cluster or group of joint families.

Significant Changes in Caste and Class in India

The emergence of new associations and institutions in the rural society also marks a watershed in the transformation of post-independence, the latter characterized by planned development. The institutions are castes and class, which assumed new definitions and formations in rural society. We shall discuss some of the significant changes observed in caste and class.

1. **Caste:** Sociology has enough research material to indicate changes in the rural caste system. We shall restrain ourselves only to changes observed in the rural caste system.Some of the changes are as below:

    i. Caste barriers to economic mobility gradually gave way to secular occupations. Traditional occupations in the village, such as oil pressers (Teli) and weavers (Julaha), are now mobile. Village people have taken over all occupations, regardless of caste or religion. As a result, the occupational changes have revolutionary implications.

    ii. There has been an evident migration of rural people to cities and towns. People are moving to cities for a variety of reasons. The burden on land has grown. People have an education that can lead to new job opportunities in cities and towns. Then there's the rural people's fascination with city living. Urban life also provides various facilities, such as health and education.

    iii. Even though caste has taken on new functions in rural society, it remains a source of identity among the village people.

iv. Without a doubt, caste as a system is weakening in rural life; it has taken on new political dimensions. Due to various factors, rural stratification is closed rather than open due to the caste system. There is some correlation between caste and landholding. For example, the Rajputs and Jats have more significant land holdings than the intermediate and lower castes.

v. The empowerment of women and the formation of the Panchayati Raj are two very structural changes that have occurred in rural society. Panchayati Raj is an attempt to develop the village through decisions made by the people. The formation of Panchayati Raj results in power decentralization. The traditional caste associations have been significantly weakened due to this formation. Though caste associations have taken over marriage, succession, and family matters, the ultimate authority to be approached is a court of law.

2. **Class:** Sociologists have recently discussed the caste-class relationship. The claim that the caste is evolving into a class is incorrect. Caste and class are not binary concepts. There is a connection between the two. The caste system is both a cultural and an economic organization. Both caste and class variations are visible in rural society.

The emergence of new classes is a significant feature of class formation in rural society. The green and white revolutions have resulted from planned development. These two revolutions have resulted in rural class polarization. As a result of planned development and seat reservations for scheduled castes and tribes, a new class has emerged from these groups. There are now classes for scheduled castes and tribes.

These classes are integrated into the classes of higher castes, and thus the entire rural society is divided into two classes:

a. classes emerging out of the higher castes who have benefited from rural development programs, and

b. classes belonging to weaker sections who have cornered a more significant portion of the benefits from the programs of rural development.

3. **Associations and Organizations:** The rural primordial associations and institutions have now given way to new associations and institutions such as cooperatives, educational societies, religious

organizations, and political parties. Besides, a new crop of non-governmental organizations (NGOs) has also spread its network in rural society.

There are also peasant organizations of various ideological orientations. Though these peasant organizations claim to be non-political, they have some implicit alliances with some political parties. These organizations advocate programs of rural social change.

SOCIAL CLASS SYSTEM

The word class is by no means an unusual word. It is said that classism is increasing or that new classes are coming into India. The word class lends itself to various uses: the landlord class and business class at one end and the Brahmin class and capitalist class at the other. Every society has many classes, the individual interests of all of which do not coincide. Each social class has its status in society, which receives prestige.

A social class is an aggregate of people who have the same status, rank, or common characteristics (lifestyle). This aggregate of people is identified based on their relationship to the economic market who have differential access to wealth, power, and certain styles of life. Ownership of wealth and occupation are the chief criteria of class differences, but education, hereditary prestige, group participation, self-identification, and recognition by others also play an essential part in class distinction.

Different Bases of Social Class

Occupational basis: Richard Centers considers occupation the basis of class division. According to him, individuals in superior occupations are treated as superior while those in inferior occupations are treated as inferior.

Basis of manual labor: Torstein Veblen looks upon manual labor as the basis of class consciousness. People involved in manual labor are considered inferior, while those in superior classes are engaged in administration, sport, war, religion, and other activities.

Various factors: Raymond B Cattell believes class consciousness to be the total of five factors—prestige, mean IQ, average income, education of some years, and the number of birth restrictions.

But class-consciousness is not based on these five factors only. It continually changes according to circumstances.

Principles of Class System

- The class of an individual is determined by his occupation, power, and wealth. One caste escapes from a class or falls into it.
- The class of an individual is based on the achievement of the individual and the social labor, that is, the right amount of award and appreciation he got for his hard work.
- In the class system, there is no restriction on marriage outside one's class.

Definition of Social Class

RM McIver: A social class is a portion of a community marked off from the rest by social status.

P Gisbert: Social class is a category or group of persons with a definite status in society that permanently determines its relation to other groups.

Max Weber: Social classes are aggregates of individuals who have the same opportunities of acquiring goods and the same exhibited standards of living.

Characteristics of Social Class

Class a status group: Social class is related to social status. There are different statuses in society because of different vocations and activities being done by different kinds of people. Considering the class as a status group makes it possible to apply it to any society with many strata.

Elements of prestige: We have seen that social class is related to the status, and status is associated with prestige. Therefore, social class is related to the prestige attached to status. Thus, the status and prestige enjoyed by the running classes or wealthy classes in every society are superior to that of the class of commoners or the poor.

Universal: Class system is found almost everywhere. It has become an inherent future of modern complex societies across the world.

Social class an open group: Social classes are open groups. They represent an open social system. This means there are no restrictions, or at most only very mild ones, imposed on the upward and downward movement of the individuals in the social hierarchy.

Class consciousness: Class consciousness is the statement that characterizes the relations of men towards the members of their class and those of other classes.

Mode of feeling: In a class system, we may observe three modes of feeling: (1) there is a feeling of equality among the members of one's class; (2) there is a feeling of inferiority concerning those who occupy a higher status in the socioeconomic hierarchy; and (3) there is a feeling of superiority about those who occupy a lower status it.

Achieved status and not ascribed status: In a class system, status is achieved and not ascribed. The status of an individual is not determined by the family he was born in but by what he has achieved. Factors such as income, occupation, wealth, education, lifestyle, and so on decide the status of an individual.

Social class is not merely an economic group: Indeed, social classes have an economic basis primarily. But to say that social classes are mere economic groups or divisions would be simplistic. Besides economic criteria such as wealth, property, and income, other criteria such as education and occupation are equally important.

Mode of living: Lifestyles include such matters as the modes of dress, the kind of house and neighborhood one lives in; the means of recreation one resorts to; the cultural products one can enjoy; the relationship between parents and children; the kinds of book, magazine, and TV show to which one is exposed; one's friends; one's mode of conveyance and communication; one's way of spending money; and so on. They are important determinants of social class.

The element of stability: A social class is a relatively stable group. It is neither transitory nor unstable like a crowd or a mob.

Divisions of Social Classes

Castes are clearly defined status groups, but classes are not. The social status of people varies on a scale. The various social classes can be thought of as points on a continuum. As a result, neither the number of social classes nor the boundaries that separate them are fixed.

Earlier social class researchers divided the status spectrum into upper, middle, and lower categories. Later scholars found this division inadequate and used a six-fold classification system that divided each of these classes into upper and lower sections.

In western societies, Giddens developed a four-part classification system. There is an upper class (which includes the wealthy, employers, and industrialists, as well as top executives); a middle class (which includes most white-collar workers and professionals); and a working-class (which includes most blue-collar workers and professionals) (those in blue-collar or manual jobs). Until recently, a fourth class—peasants (people engaged in traditional agricultural production)—was also crucial in some industrialized countries, such as France or Japan.

In addition to these four classes, the underclass, which includes the ethnic majority and underprivileged minorities, exists. The underclass has worse working and living conditions than most of the population. We can include 'Dalits' in this category in the Indian context.

Social Mobility

Meaning of Social Mobility

The word "mobility" means "shift," "change," and "movement." It could be a change of location or a shift in position. Furthermore, change has no intrinsic value, i.e., it cannot be said whether it is for the better or, the worse. When we combine the words social' and 'mobility,' we are implying that people or individuals in one social position or status move to another.

This upward or downward movement on the social ladder can be inter-generational or intra-generational. In a nutshell, social mobility refers to a shift in an individual's or a group's position from one status to another.

Barber defines social mobility as the movement between social classes or full-time, functionally significant social roles.

This is a long-term process, with people shifting roles and social classes based on social interactions. As people adapt to changing social roles, social mobility emerges.

Mobility "provides the individual with some of his economy's and society's benefits." Sons of rickshaw drivers and clerks become lawyers and doctors. In each case, changing the father-son relationship benefits the son.

Lawyers, doctors, and engineers need initiative, training, and sacrifice. Higher status and greater rewards motivate people to seek new roles. People must compete, conflict, and collaborate to obtain life's good things.

Contrary to the popular belief that social mobility is positive and an open society is preferable, it is not always the case. In a closed society with little social mobility, individuals are shielded from failure and not prone to overconfidence. Additionally, such a society helps individuals to adjust to new environments with ease. On the other hand, in a mobile society, individuals must adapt to new classes, norms, and values. Closed-society members lead a comfortable life with fewer challenges. Thus, mobility in an open society does not guarantee happiness.

A closed, immobile society is unlikely to become a world leader. A capable and wise father does not guarantee his son's abilities. A society that does not allow talented people from lower strata to advance won't last.

Mobility can be described in multiple ways, including:
a. A change in occupation results in a change in status.
b. Advancement within the same occupational group
c. The accumulation of experience within a specific occupation.
d. A shift in occupation from one generation to the next, such as from father to son.

Types of Mobility

Change of social position of an individual or group of individuals takes different forms and shapes. There would be one type of mobility in one period, and in another, it can be another. Each of the following types is not exclusive, but they may overlap; it is only for convenience and analysis that they are given different labels.

1. **Horizontal mobility:** In this type of social mobility, a person's occupation changes, but their overall social status does not. Certain occupations, such as a doctor, engineer, and professor, may have

the same status, but an engineer who changes his occupation from engineer to teaching engineering has moved horizontally from one occupational category to another. However, there has been no change in the social stratification system.

2. **Vertical mobility:** Vertical mobility refers to any change in an individual's or a group's occupational, economic, or political status that results in a shift in their position.

   Simply put, vertical mobility refers to a change in social position, either upward or downward, that can be classified as ascending or descending. When a well-known businessperson suffers losses and is declared bankrupt, he is regarded as a low-status individual. On the other hand, if a small business owner with money and manipulation skills rises through the ranks to become an industrialist, he rises the social ladder. As a result, his position in the hierarchy improves.

3. **Upward mobility:** Upward mobility occurs when a person or group moves from a lower to a higher position; for example, when a person from a lower caste who previously held a lower position becomes a Minister and holds a higher position after winning elections. He may not be able to change his caste, but he may be able to rise through the ranks due to his economic and political clout. Yadavs in India, for example, are living proof of this.

4. **Downward mobility:** Downward mobility refers to losing one's higher position in favor of a lower one. Consider the case of an Engineer who holds a respectable position in society due to his occupation, education, and possibly caste.

   If he is caught accepting a bribe or has committed a sin or done something wrong, he may be sentenced to prison or outcasted by members of his caste, and as a criminal or an outcaste, he may be placed in a lower position than he was previously. If a lady from the higher Brahmin caste married a man from the lower Shudra caste, not only the man and woman were outcastes, but their children were also labeled as 'chandals.'

5. **Intergenerational mobility:** This type of mobility occurs when one generation's social status differs from the previous generation's. This mobility, however, can be upward or downward; for example, people from lower castes or classes may provide opportunities for their children to receive higher education, training, and skills.

With these skills, the younger generation may be able to advance in their careers. Intergenerational upward mobility occurs when a shoemaker's son becomes a clerk, doctor, or engineer after receiving an education.

Similarly, a *Brahmin* family may be engaged in the traditional occupation of teaching and performing rituals, but the younger generation is neither intelligent nor follows in the family's footsteps. They turn into daily bets, and the younger generation experiences intergenerational mobility downward.

6. **Intragenerational mobility:** This mobility occurs within a single generation's lifespan. This can be further broken down into two categories:

   a. A shift in a person's position over the course of his life;

   b. A change in one brother's position but no change in another brother's position.

   A clerk can begin his career. He improves his knowledge and abilities. He eventually rises through the ranks to become an I.A.S. officer or a Professor. As a result, he rises through the ranks and now holds a higher social position than when he began his career. His brother may have also started his career as a clerk, but he never advanced in his career and remained in the same position throughout his life. As a result, one brother changes his position within the same generation while the other does not.

7. **Occupational mobility:** Occupational mobility refers to switching jobs. Because the incumbents of different occupations receive different economic rewards and enjoy different power, prestige, and privileges based on the economic returns, authority, and prestige, they are organized hierarchically.

   These occupations are organized in a hierarchical or stratified manner. Upward vertical mobility occurs when a person or group moves from a lower-status occupation to a higher-status one. Similarly, when an individual or group from higher-status occupations switches to lower-status occupations, this is called Downward Vertical Mobility.

   Upward vertical occupational mobility occurs when a person progresses from a clerk to an officer; similarly, downward vertical occupational mobility occurs when a person progresses from a clerk to a peon or a smuggler. We must remember that society bestows recognition, prestige, and power not only based on monetary gains from a job or profession but also the skills of the individual most valued in society. Although a smuggler earns more than a clerk, society does not recognize his means of subsistence.

As a result, he is positioned at the bottom of the social ladder. Politicians with political power now hold a higher position, regardless of the means used. As a result, people aspire to be in positions of power. In a nutshell, occupational mobility is transitioning from a lower status to a higher-status occupation and vice versa.

Factors Responsible for Social Mobility

The following factors facilitate social mobility:

1. *Motivation:* Everyone wants to improve their social standing as well as their standard of living. It is possible to achieve any status in an open system. People are motivated to work hard and improve their skills to achieve a higher social status due to this openness. Social mobility is impossible without such motivation and effort on the part of the individual.

2. *Achievements and Failures:* An achievement is an exceptional, usually unexpected performance that draws the attention of a larger audience to a person's abilities. Not all accomplishments will lead to social advancement. Only exceptional accomplishments have an impact on one's status. A poor man who gains wealth or an unknown writer who wins a literary prize, for example, will improve his status.

   Failures and misdeeds similarly affect one's ability to move downward. A member of the upper classes who files a fraudulent bankruptcy will be removed from blue books, receive no dinner invitations from his peers, and become ineligible as a marriage partner. His wife may divorce him if he is already married. He will have to resign from all of his clubs and positions. He will not fall into the lowest stratum, although finding a new association will be difficult.

3. *Education:* Education not only aids in acquiring knowledge but also as a passport to a higher-status occupational position. A bachelor's degree in science is required to become a doctor. Similarly, you must be at least a graduate to sit for an IAS competitive examination.

Individuals can only aspire to higher positions after receiving a minimum formal education. In modern India, members of Scheduled Castes and Scheduled Tribes have not only been able to change their traditional occupations but have also begun to hold positions of higher prestige, thanks to education. Education is a must in today's industrial society, where status is attained through hard work.

4. ***Skills and Training:*** Every society provisions for the younger generation to receive skills and training. It takes a lot of time and money to acquire skills and training. Why are these people wasting their money and time? The reason for this is that such people are rewarded by society. When they complete their training, they will be eligible for high-level positions far superior to those they would have been eligible for if they had not received such training.

   Those with this training have a higher social status and more economic rewards and privileges. People participate in this training in the hopes of moving up the social ladder due to these incentives; in other words, skills and training aid in advancing a person's position, resulting in social mobility.

5. ***Migration:*** Social mobility is aided by migration. People migrate from one location to another due to pull and push factors. A location may lack the resources and opportunities to improve. As a result, people are forced to migrate to other locations to make a living. Different openings and opportunities may exist in new places where they migrate.

   These individuals take advantage of these opportunities and improve their social standing. People from the Scheduled Castes of Uttar Pradesh and Bihar, for example, have migrated to the states of Punjab and Haryana to make a living. They work as farm laborers here.

   They return to their villages and buy land after acquiring or accumulating money. They cultivate their land and become landowners. As a result of their traditional work as scavengers or Chamars, they gain status and become cultivators. Asians migrating to various European countries and the United States of America face a similar situation.

   People are drawn to the pull factors because they lack those amenities at their current residence, and the new location entices them by providing these amenities so that they can advance in their careers after learning new skills and knowledge.

People migrate from villages to cities because cities have higher-status institutions and more job opportunities. People migrate to cities to obtain higher education and skills and advance their careers than their parents and brothers, who remain in villages. In this way, we can see how both push and pull factors contribute to migration, facilitating social mobility.

6. ***Industrialization:*** The Industrial Revolution ushered in a new social system in which people were classified based on their abilities and education. Their caste, race, religion, and ethnicity were all ignored. As a result of industrialization, mass production became more affordable. The artisans were forced to leave their jobs as a result of this. They moved to industrial towns in search of work.

   They received new vocational training and were placed in various industries. They progressed up the social ladder due to their experience and training. Statuses are achieved in the industrial society, whereas statuses are ascribed according to birth in traditional societies such as India. As a result, industrialization allows for greater social mobility.

7. ***Urbanization:*** There are more people in cities, and they have formal relationships. People do not have a deep understanding of one another. Anonymity is prevalent in urban areas. Only their friends and relatives are close to them. The caste and background of an individual are kept hidden in urban settlements. Rather than his background, an individual's position is primarily determined by his education, occupation, and income.

   Regardless of caste, an individual with higher education and income is employed in a higher-status occupation and has a high social status. By removing the barriers to social mobility, urbanization facilitates social mobility.

8. ***Legislation:*** New laws can help people move up the social ladder. When the Zamindari Abolition Act was passed, most tenant cultivators became owner cultivators, indicating a change in status from tenants to owners. Similarly, the legal provision for job reservation and advancement for Scheduled Castes and Scheduled Tribes has aided social mobility.

Many people from Scheduled Castes and Scheduled Tribes are trying to improve their status by requesting admission to professional colleges, job reservations, and promotions. The Mandal Commission report was accepted by the V.R Singh government, which included job reservations for the Other Backward Classes (OBCs).

Similarly, the judicial system's ability to bypass certain judgments may aid social mobility. The Hindu Marriage Act has improved the status of women in various ways. In the same way, the Hindu Succession Act has given the daughter equal rights in the family property. The American Racial Anti-Discrimination Act has aided the social mobility of both men and women of the African-American race. We discover that legal provisions facilitate social mobility in this way.

9. ***Politicization:***People have become more aware of their rights due to increased education, exposure to mass media of communication, and increased contacts. People are also educated about their rights by political parties. People band together to demand that the authorities accept their demands to achieve their rights. These individuals may use agitations, strikes, and other tactics to achieve their objectives.

   To gain votes, the political party makes many concessions. They improve their social status with the help of these new concessions and provisions. Only a few people can become political leaders, ministers, cabinet ministers, or state chief ministers.

   In today's Indian politics, there are numerous examples of this. As a result, they have been able to move up the social ladder. Similarly, with increased political awareness among representatives in the State Assembly and Parliament, the government may be able to enact laws that benefit the poorer segments of society.

10. ***Modernization:***Modernization entails the application of scientific knowledge and modern technology. It also refers to rationalism and living a secular lifestyle. People engaged in low-status occupations such as scavengers are abandoning their traditional occupations in favor of occupations that are not dirty and do not pollute the environment due to technological advancements.

They change their position upward in this way. Similarly, a country's level of development influences whether or not social mobility is possible. The old stratification system and accretive statuses persist in less developed and traditional societies.

While developed and modern societies have paved the way for more opportunities and competition, only developed countries have a greater chance of achieving certain statuses. To put it another way, modernization promotes social mobility.

Aspirations for advancement can lead to frustration and various mental and psychological issues. An individual is taught that he can achieve any level of success. However, in reality, his social background, birth into a race, and ethnicity all help or hinder his chances of social mobility. Similarly, countries that lack opportunities for social mobility suffer from stagnation and underdevelopment. In a nutshell, social mobility has both positive and negative implications.

Meaning of Race

The race is one of those terms that has a lot of different connotations. The Greeks divided humanity into two groups: Greeks and Barbarians, neither of which is a racial group. The terms 'race' and 'nationality' are sometimes interchanged; French, Chinese, and German are all referred to as races. The Germans and the French are two separate countries.

Individuals with similar physical characteristics do not necessarily make up a nation. It has been frequently confused with language and religion, for example, when speaking of the Aryan race. However, there is no Aryan race or language. The fact that the Negroes speak English does not make them English.

The term 'race' has been used to describe the classification of humans based on the color of their skin, such as a black or white race. Race, on the other hand, cannot be equated with skin color. We sometimes use the term race broadly, referring to the human race as a whole, including all human beings.

Race a Biological Concept

This misunderstanding arises from failing to recognize that race is a biological and anthropological concept, not a sociological term. It denotes a biological classification. *"A race is a large, biological human grouping with several distinctive inherited characteristics that vary within a certain range," writes AW Green.*

Language and religion are cultural concepts, so a physiological concept based on them cannot be accurately defined. Men's ethnic differences are a matter of blood. They are passed down through the generations, along with physical characteristics like eye, skin, and hair color. Anthropologists define race as a group of people who share hereditary characteristics that distinguish them from other groups.

"A group of individuals is said to belong to a race when all of its members share certain significant physical traits that are transmitted biologically through the mechanism of heredity," according to HT Mazumdar.

As a result, race can be defined as a large group of people who share a physiological similarity due to biological inheritance.

The characteristics that distinguish one race from another should be hereditary and relatively constant despite environmental changes. Furthermore, these characteristics must be shared by a large number of people.

Determinants of Race

In determining race, physical traits are examined, but it is often challenging to be sure that the differences in traits are due to heredity and not to environmental modifications.

Among the physical traits that are generally taken into consideration, the following are the important ones:

i. The form, color, and distribution of the hair on the head, the face, and the body; hair forms are grouped as:
    a. Leiotrichy (soft straight hair) as of the Mongols and Chinese;
    b. Cymotrichy (smooth curly hair) as of the inhabitants of India, Western Europe, Australia, and North East Africa and
    c. Ulotrichy (thick curly hair) as of the Negroes.
ii. The principal diameter of the body, stature, chest, and shoulders;
iii. The form of the head, especially the length and breadth of the skull, the face, and length and breadth of the nose; heads are classified into;
    a. Dolichocephalic
    b. Mesocephalic
    c. Brachycephalic

iv. The facial characteristics such as the nasalform, lipform, the form of eyelids, cheekbones, chin, ear, and jaws. Nasal forms are classified into three types:
   a. Leptorrhine
   b. Mesorrhine, and
   c. Platyrrhine
v. The complexion of the skin and eyes.

Of the color of the skin, three distinctions are made:
   i.   Leucoderm,
   ii. Xanthoderm,
   iii. Melanoderm.
   vi. The length of the arms and the leg.
   vii. Blood types: There are four types of blood, OAB, and AB. Blood type O can be successfully mixed with A, B, and AB, but the other three cannot be generally mixed.

No Single Trait is Fundamental

The combination of these characteristics is used for different racial groups. Curly hair, dark skin, a large head with a small nose, and thick lips are all characteristics of a Negro. He stands out compared to a Chinese with straight hair, a flat nose, and a yellow complexion. However, as previously stated, it can be challenging to determine whether differences in traits are hereditary or environmental.

Because the environment can significantly influence physical characteristics like stature, weight, and skin color, they are of little use in identifying races. Hair color and shape are thought to be more stable genetic factors. However, no single characteristic can be considered fundamental.

Because the skull reaches full growth early in life and is not affected by environmental changes, it was thought that head form was the best race criterion when anthropology first developed. However, since Boas discovered that the cephalic index could be significantly influenced by the environment in which a person is born, this trait is no longer considered the most critical criterion of race. As a result, anthropologists have classified races based on various criteria.

One character or combination of characters is now considered fundamental, while another is not. Some anthropologists believe that color is the most appropriate basis, while others believe that hair form, head shape, or other factors are more appropriate. It is also worth noting that physical traits can differ between races, or people of different races can share the same physical trait.

Classification of Social Races in India

The term "race" has been used to categorize people based on specific physical characteristics. Members of different social groups differ in pigmentation, hair form, and other visible characteristics. Anthropologists have proposed numerous classification schemes that differ greatly from one another.

Some anthropologists follow Huxley's scheme of five major types, namely Negroid, Australoid, Mongoloid, Xanthochroid, and Melanochroid, while others use a four-fold division into Caucasian, Mongol, Negro, and Australian, with the Caucasian further subdivided into Nordic, Alpine, and Mediterranean.

Genealogical Classification

Anthropologists disagree on how to classify races. Due to a lack of proper technique and conception, there are as many race classifications as there are writers. Denikar defines race as a collection of population characteristics. Ripley is looking for pure ideal types.

Races are mixed. Physical anthropologists struggle because individuals rarely exhibit all their type's traits. Race will never be precise. Tribes and nations have always migrated across the globe, and people have mated with strangers, resulting in hybridization.

Racial characteristics are now mixed among human groups, making one wonder if there was ever a pure race. "Race mixing has occurred throughout recorded history," Dunn and Dobzhansky write. "Incontrovertible evidence from studies on human fossil remains shows that mixing of different stocks (at least occasionally) occurred even in prehistory."

Professor Fleure says, "Mankind is a mishmash." "Most Britons are neither all or none." Because races mix, it is hard to agree on a classification scheme.Racial classifications are unrelated to social structure or culture. High cheekbones are linked to reddish-brown skin and brown-black hair.None of these are linked to intelligence, caste, musical ability, religion, polygyny, or anything else but each other. Physical traits used to classify races do not affect social behavior.

Many classifications have been harmful because they led men to believe some races are mentally superior to others and that physical traits are related to intelligence. As we'll see, this assumption is often wrong. This does not preclude categorizing humanity by physical traits.

Three Main Races

The division of races into Negroes, Mongoloids, and Caucasians appears to have gained widespread acceptance. Although no clear-cut lines separate them and considerable overlap, each stock is distinguished by specific characteristics that are more or less shared by all its members.

The Melanesians, who have lighter skin and a slightly different nose than the Negroes, are Negroes with black skin, projecting jaws, broad noses, and curly hair. Lighter skin, prominent cheekbones, olive-shaped eyes, and straight black hair characterize the Mongoloid or yellow race. American Indians are included in this group. Some anthropologists consider whites a separate race, while others consider them an offshoot of the Mongoloid race. Caucasians mix with people of other races.

Each of these three racial divisions can be subdivided further into sub-races, though there is no agreement on what these sub-races should be. Caucasians are divided into sub-races such as Nordics, Mediterraneans, Alpines, Hindus, etc.

Races in India According to Sir Herbert Risley, India has seven racial types:

    i. Pre-Dravidian type is still found among hill and jungle tribes like the Bhils.

   ii. The Dravidian type can be found from the southern Peninsula to the Gangetic valley.

  iii. Kashmir, Punjab, and Rajputana are Indo-Aryan states.

  iv. In the Gangetic Valley, the Aryo-Dravidian type.

   v. The Cytho-Dravidian type runs east of the Indus River.

vi. The Mongoloid type is found in Assam and the eastern Himalayan foothills.

vii. The Negrito races, according to JH Hutton, were the original occupants of India. The Protoaustraloids, whose ancestors could be traced back to Palestine, followed the Negritos. The Mediterranean race came next, giving birth to the Austroasiatic languages. The Alpine race reached India by the end of the fourth millennium BC Around 1500 BC, the Indo-Aryan race arrived in India.

RACISM

Heredity determines the racial characteristics of all the community. Human society has been divided into different stocks based on bodily traits. This division started at the beginning of the 19th century, when the evolutionary theory originated, which started the difference between superior and inferior among the different racial groups.

Meaning of Racism

Racism includes the belief that people of some races are inferior to others and the behavior that results from such beliefs. According to Paula Rothenberg, racism means the dominance of white-colored or skinned people over dark-skinned or blacks. They believe that blacks or non-whites are not qualified and never accepted them, but we cannot describe racism in such a manner as history shows that white people held power and position for a long time.

Definition

According to Jacobs and Stern, racism means each society is characterized by a cluster of values inherited with specific physical, mental, and criticizing features that may be superior or inferior to the ethnic subdivision, and the hereditary factors determine each phase of the cultural life of the people in the society. The people in the society believe that some races are inferior or superior to others, and the behavior of the people changes according to their belief in racism.

Concept of Racism

Institutionalized racism means that each person's thoughts are entwined on cultural ideology with different ideas on racism in our society. Each person has different thoughts, ideas, and concepts about industrialized racism in society. The thought of racism has not only severely affected the minds of all people in society but has also brought certain kinds of conflicts. Industrialized racism has different impacts on society. It benefits particular groups in the society with the power and potential, carrying the multiple generational effects from one generation to another from past to the present, which is called' past in present' discrimination.

The structure of racism features two types of privileges towards the people:

1. To show the difference towards people based on their skin color, for example, to misbehave with black-skinned people; white-skinned treat black-skinned as their subordinates.
2. More societal benefits to the whites than to the blacks. Privileges seem to be an unearned advantage, as per Molly Ivins, who explains that in the United States of America, although the black-skinned people had lots of skills and abilities to improve their status in the society, whites never allowed or appreciated their skills to come up in their lives. Whites dominated blacks and took more privileges.

Consequences of Racism

Certain inherited traits and environmental influences determine the superior and inferior division or the stratification in human society. According to Franz Boas,strong dislikes, antipathy, and antagonism are shown by people of different races because of cultural practices. Bodily appearances never allowed them to accept and appreciate people of different races and castes. Instead of having the beliefs of scientific facts, the primary importance is given to the ideas and feelings. The whites believed they were dominant and superior and described blacks as recessive and inferior. According to Paul AF Walter, racism has given wrong popular ideas and concepts that described and differentiated the people into superior and inferior based on the races they belonged to. The racism created a nationality feeling that white people, for example, disagreed that the black formed ethnocentrism against the blacks in the United States of America, which formed to be a universal tendency of each cultural group. Whites have a strong thought that being with blacks is abnormal.

Criticism of Racism

There is no solid base for describing the concept of racial superiority and inferiority. No scientific fact proves that all the superior races were more potent and intelligent than inferior races. It has not been proved.

There always exists substantial confusion about race and language; substantial confusion still exists among the people about race and the languages they speak. A particular race does not speak one single language, so we cannot categorize that one race people speak only one particular language. They are superior to others is a wring thought as some races can speak different languages, for example, English is the common language spoken by all. There is a vital concept that the superior race is pure and serene, and the lower race is impure. It is not so. Purity cannot be determined based on race. The wrong of certain people created intense conflicts among the people in the community.

Classification of Indian Races

India is a multi-racial melting pot. It is a museum dedicated to ethnology. Most of the current population's ancestors came to India via the Himalayas from neighboring countries. The population of India is made up of people from all over the world. In India, we encounter people of various races.

Classification of BS Guha

Dr Guha has divided the population of India into the following races:
1. **The Negrito:** The presence of the Negrito race in India, he claims, is a contentious issue. However, it is claimed that the Indian population contains a Negrito element and that a Negrito element can be found in the blood of Andaman Islanders. It is also worth noting that the Negrito element can be found in the blood of some South Indian tribal peoples, such as the Kadar and Nagas.

Some argue that there is no solid evidence to support the existence of a Negrito population among Indians. According to them, whatever evidence is available is insufficient to prove the presence of a Negrito element in the Indian population.Despite the debate, it is possible to state that the Negrito race existed in the past and left little trace in India.

2. **The Proto-Austroloid:** The Pre-Dravidian race is another name for the Proto-Austroloid. According to Dr Guha, this racial element dominates the tribal population of central India. The Santhals, Mundas, Juangas, Soaras, and Kondhs are just a few of the many tribes that belong to this racial category.

3. **Mongoloid:** North-Eastern India is home to most people of this racial ancestry. Dr. Guha categorizes this race into two groups: (a) Palaeo-Mongoloids and (b) Tibeto-Mongoloids.

   a. Palaeo-Mongoloid: This racial type is further subdivided into two types, one with a long head and the other with a broad head. The Palaeo-Mongoloid race's Angami Nagas are of the long-headed type. The broad-headed type of the Palaeo-Mongoloid race is said to inhabit the Himalayan foothills from Kashmir to Assam.

   b. Tibeto-Mongoloid: The Tibeto-Mongoloid branch of the Mongoloid race is said to include the people of Sikkim and Bhutan.

4. **The Mediterranean:** This is one of India's most common races. There are three types of Mediterranean.

   a. The Palaeo-Mediterranean: The Tamil and Telugu Brahmins of the South represent this racial type.

   b. Mediterranean: It is thought that people of this racial type built the Indus Valley civilization.

   c. Oriental: Oriental and Mediterranean types are very similar.

5. **Western Brachycephals:** This race is of three types, namely:

   a. The Alpendoid: People of this race are found in Sourashtra, Gujarat, and Bengal.

   b. The Dinaric: This strain is found among the people of Bengal, Orissa, and Coorg.

   c. The Armenian: This racial type is represented by the Parsees of Bombay.

6. **Nordic Race:** During the 2nd millennium BC, people of this racial origin arrived in India from North and South-East Asia and settled

across Northern India. Mixed with the Mediterranean, this race is mainly found in North India. This ancestry is thought to have contributed significantly to Indian culture.

The tribal population comprises the first three races: Negrito, Proto-Austroloid, and Mongoloid. The other three races, namely the Mediterranean, Western Brachycephals, and Nordic, make up India's overall population.

It is possible to say that the Indian population is made up of essential races from around the world. Intermarriages have caused all India's races to become mixed over the centuries. As a result, there is no such thing as a completely pure race in India anymore. As a result, no rigid separation of these races is possible in a true sense.

As a result, we can say that India has been a melting pot of races, earning it the moniker "museum of races." India has been a melting pot of conflicting races and civilizations since the dawn of time, marked by a process of assimilation and synthesis.

■ CASTE AND HEALTH

The caste system significantly impacted health due to many social restrictions and social stratifications common among the Hindus, Christians, Sikhs, and Muslims. Although the Indian Constitution demands equality of outcomes, there is more focus on the educational institutions and employment but not on the parity in the distribution of healthcare facilities. The critical barrier to streamlining healthcare is caste inequality due to sociocultural issues. With the systematic difference in lower caste, culture, tradition, and religion, such matters should be tackled to provide equal healthcare.

Some of the critical principles given by WHO are as follows:

a. To improve the socioeconomic conditions of daily life.

b. To tackle inequality in the distribution of money, human resources, and resources.

c. To raise public awareness on such issues.

d. To measure and evaluate the interventions done to solve those issues.

e. To provide good supplemental nutrition and better psychosocial stimulation to improve the physical and psychological growth of underprivileged and stunted children.

f. To provide compulsory primary and secondary education and accessible healthcare regardless of ability to pay cardinal issues.

g. To improve the underdeveloped urban areas with affordable housing, safe drinking water, and sanitation.

h. There should be better employment opportunities with the fair universal public distribution system.

i. They are improving the mid-day meal schemes, Sarva Shiksha Abhiyan, implementing the Right to Education Act, National Rural Employment Guarantee Act, Food and Security Act, and following all the goals of the National Rural Health Mission.

j. There should be no difference in providing equal healthcare for lower or higher caste people. There should be gender equality and no difference in approaches for the poor or rich. All should be treated equally in providing accessible healthcare in policy decision-making.

k. A better food distribution policy, when implemented, can eradicate poverty with a good focus on food production and trade.

▓ RACE AND DISEASES

Many studies have proved on a large scale that certain races and ethnic groups show a high level of disease expression in their families. One study examined 4197 genes and compared the Mongolian race with the Whites. It showed that around 1097 genes had different kinds of genetic expressions. According to Cheung, those differences highlighted that 11 particular genes have a specific regulator that determines the presence or absence of diseases in the genes; for example, in comparing the Caucasian with the Asian population, the genetic regulator and genetic expression regarding the presence of diseases are found more frequently in the Caucasians than the Asians.

According to biologists, race and ethnicity are essential concerns that predispose some diseases due to differentially expressed genes. Much consideration was not given during the earlier periods to detect genetic disorders. Many studies proved that genetically bounded diseases in particular ethnic groups were more prevalent. Those groups were given more importance and care to prevent the conditions early. Genetic disorders occur due to changes or mutations in the DNA of a particular ethnic group. Many reasons, such as exposure to radiation, teratogens, harmful chemicals, and so on, change or manipulate the genetic coding and expression.

ETHNIC HEALTH INEQUALITIES

There are always inequalities in health status in every society. Many factors interfere health status of the individuals in the society, such as the lifestyle they adopt, which may be sedentary, additive, low financial status; educational level achieved; job insecurity; bad housing conditions; lots of psychosocial stress, and availability of unequal distribution of health services.

Inequalities in the availability of health services have a collective effect on the entire life of any individual since this problem has become a primary issue in the healthcare scenario. Equal distribution of healthcare services has been the main goal of primary healthcare services in India. These inequalities in healthcare issues have been passed over from one generation to another, affecting the growth and development of the children in every family. Many illnesses found to be frequent are discussed in the following.

Cardiovascular Illness

Global statistics say that men in South Asia have 50% more chances of getting a heart attack or myocardial infarction, angina, or coronary diseases when compared with others in the general population. The next highest are Bangladeshi, then Pakistanis, and then Indians. Interestingly, the Caribbean population is at high risk of cerebrovascular accidents or stroke but has less death rate due to cardiovascular illness. Many factors interfere in causing the disease, whichare classified into modifiable and non-modifiable factors:

a. **Modifiable:** Smoking, betel (pan) chewing, alcoholism, obesity, hyperlipidemia, and increased stress in work, which can be modified and treated.

b. **Non-modifiable:** Increased age after 50, increased blood pressure, hypertension, diabetes mellitus, and genetic illness cannot be cured but can be controlled. Therefore, the highly risky populations can be identified, and those families should be informed and given special care to prevent such illnesses through counseling.

Cancer

Global statistics show that smoking is the leading cause of lung cancer. Death rates are higher in Ireland and Scotland due to lung cancer but very low in South Asia, the Caribbean, and Africa. The breast cancer rate is higher in women residing in England and Wales than the women who have migrated from other countries. This shows that many risk factors interfere with causing cancer in women, and all these issues are under research.

Mental Health

Mental illness and ethnic influence are interrelated. Research studies show that psychosis is more prevalent among the black Caribbean than the white British. Many factors interfere with psychiatric illness in the community, such as social isolation and discrimination against a particular ethnic group in receiving healthcare. Research proves that most black Caribbean and Africans receive psychiatric care as they are treated differently by the people in the society. Even psychiatric doctors treat them based on their ethnic group, and this kind of social discrimination increases the incidence of illness in a particular ethnic group.

19 Social Organization and Social System

LEARNING OBJECTIVES

- ☞ What is a social organization? Define social organization.
- ☞ What is the meaning of social organization?
- ☞ Discuss elements of social organization.
- ☞ Describe the characteristics of social organization.
- ☞ What is the purpose of the social organization?
- ☞ Describe the features of social organization.
- ☞ Discuss the types of social organization
- ☞ What are voluntary associations and their meaning?
- ☞ Describe the characteristics of voluntary associations.
- ☞ Which factors motivate voluntary actions?
- ☞ What is the social system?
- ☞ Discuss the meaning and elements of the social system.
- ☞ What are the characteristics of the social system?
- ☞ Describe the functions of the social system.

■ WHAT IS A SOCIAL ORGANIZATION?

A *social organization* is an arrangement of relations between and among individuals and social groups. Social organization characteristics include sexual composition, spatiotemporal cohesion, structure, leadership, division of labor, communication systems, etc **(Fig. 19.1)**.

Because of these social organizational characteristics, people can monitor their daily work and involvement in other controlled forms of human interaction.

Such interactions include affiliation, collective resources, replaceability of individuals, and recorded control. These interactions come together to create standard features in basic social units such as family, clubs, enterprises, states, etc. These can be termed social organizations.

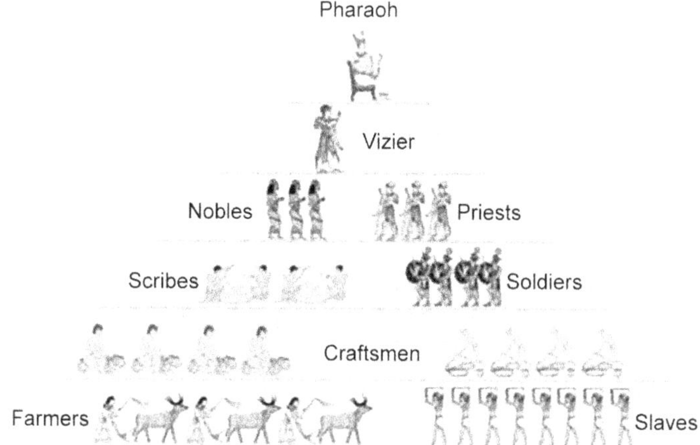

Fig. 19.1: Social organization of ancient Egypt.

Definitions of Social Organization

Edward B Reuter and Clyde W Hart: By social organization is meant the totality of cultural institutions and their inter-relationships together with the body of the unorganized activities characteristic of the group.

Ralph Piddington: The most important bases of social organization are sex, age, kinship, locality, social status, political power, occupation, religion and magic, totemism, and voluntary associations.

MA Elliott and FE Merrill: Social organization is a state of being, a condition in which the various institutions in a society are functioning following their recognized or implied purpose.

▨ MEANING OF SOCIAL ORGANIZATION

It is a social system where people are interrelated with each other. The size and the type of work they do may vary from each other's group, and each group varies according to its nature of work in the society. Although there are differences in their work, people are related to each other and work in unity. Hence, it will be good to refer to the social organization as a social system because sociologists believe it explains the importance of how society is organized.

Although the social organization is complex, the activities of such a society are controlled by policies framed by the government that rules the country; for example, even a small body of organized police can control a large group of people. Some associational groups in our society, such as schools, corporations, banks, prisons, army-related institutions, and so on, are referred to as social organizations.

A state is called a political organization because it is a group of members representing and controlling the state. School is called an educational organization where all the children receive education and form a social organization. According to Ogburn and Nimkoff, a society forms a vast representation of a whole society, representing an organized group of individuals interacting with each other. All the people in the society are interrelated and possess history and civilization.

Social organization in sociology creates a stable structure of relations within a group, which provides a foundation for order and guides relationships for new members. These organizations stress the significance of the arrangement of parts in society and how these different parts affect the whole society.

An organization is defined in sociology as humans' planned, coordinated, and purposeful action to construct or compile a standard tangible or intangible product. Formal membership and form are usually used to frame this action (institutional rules). In sociology, organizations are classified as formal or unplanned informal (i.e., spontaneously formed). Sociology examines organizations first and foremost from an institutional standpoint. The organization, in this sense, is a permanent arrangement of elements. These elements and their actions are governed by rules, allowing a specific task to be completed through a system of coordinated division of labor.

An organization is defined by its elements (who belongs to the organization and who does not?), its communication (which elements communicate and how do they communicate?), its autonomy (which changes are executed autonomously by the organization or its elements?) and its rules of action with external events (what causes an organization to act as a collective actor?).

Elements of Social Organization

In everyday life, social organizations are there. Many people are members of diverse social structures — institutional and informal.

They include clubs and professional and religious organizations. Having a sense of identity with the social organization helps build a sense of community by being closer to each other.

While organizations connect many like-minded people, the differences in thought can also cause a separation from others not in their organization.Social organizations are designed where there is a hierarchical system.

A hierarchical structure in social groups affects how a group is structured and how likely the group will remain together.A group must have a durable affiliation within itself. Being associated with an organization means connecting and accepting within that group. Affiliation means an obligation to return to that organization. To be affiliated with an organization, the organization must know and recognize that you are a member.

Through the collective resources of these affiliations, the organization gains power. Often affiliates have invested something in these resources that motivate them to keep improving the organization.

On the other hand, the organization must bear in mind that these individuals are replaceable. While the organization needs the members and the resources to thrive, it must also be able to replace those left to keep the organization running. Because of these characteristics, managing within the organization can often be tricky. It is where recorded control emerges because writing down issues makes them more precise and structured.

The essential elements are summarized as follows:
a. A social group usually forms a unique society.
b. Each society has an interrelated hierarchy level of groups and status.
c. Each member of the society values the groups and lives and works in cooperation.
d. There is an excellent level of integration and association among the members of the society who follow policies and social practices to avoid conflicts.
e. A specific code of conduct and ethics is framed in the society to be followed by all, and it is customary to follow relationships.

CHARACTERISTICS OF SOCIAL ORGANIZATION

Many characteristics exist in a society framed as per the purpose of human welfare. They are as follows:

a. Every social organization has been framed with a definite purpose.
b. Every individual has definite goals, forming a definite interaction pattern.
c. Each organization runs efficiently since all members cooperate, unite, and have a mutual understanding.
d. An organization can bring different kinds of people to work together and do different kinds of jobs.
e. The organization makes the individuals takeover different roles and obtain social status.
f. The organization runs smoothly since the members accept the roles and responsibilities and enact their roles well.
g. The organization evaluates the code of conduct and controls the individual's behavior.

Purpose of the Social Organization

a. Usually, the social system has all the constituents of society, forming strong interrelationships among them. Institutions such as schools, churches, banks, and prisons inform associated groups.
b. A society is called organized and systematic only if all the constituents in the society are functioning smoothly and perform their functions properly.
c. As per the views of ME Jones, social organization is the whole part of a social system in the society, and each part of the system is interrelated to each other.
d. Every activity of the society is organized to maintain suitable production activities, which promotes the social status of the society and helps attain the objectives of the societal works.

■ FEATURES OF SOCIAL ORGANIZATION

a. **Unanimity among the members:** Social organization demands unanimity among the members of society. If there is no unanimity, it will give rise to conflict, which in turn will lead to social disorganization.
b. **Readiness to accept roles:** If unanimity has to be maintained among the members of a society, then they must be ready to accept their status and respective roles within the social organization. Society has a great variety in terms of sex, age, status, physical

capability, skills, and duties. A combination of these factors leads to everyone having a definite social status. Now, this social status forms the basis on which roles are apportioned. Society will lose its organic character if everyone covets the same role.

c. **Control of society:** There will be no grudges regarding the role apportioned to the members as long as the society controls them. Habits, customs, traditions, mores, rituals, and institutions are agents of social control.

Types of Social Organization

There are two types of social organization:

Formal Organization

A formal organization is a social system with specific goals and several interrelated groups or subsystems. Formal organizations are governed by clearly stated and enforced norms.

The formal organization is a goal-oriented entity that accurately measures individuals' efforts and refers to the structure of jobs and positions with clearly defined functions, responsibilities, and authorities. According to Chester Barnard, "an organization is formal when the activities are coordinated towards a common objective." For many tasks within modern societies, people require groups they can deliberately create to achieve specific goals. Amitai Etzioni classified organizations based on people's reasons for entering them: voluntary, coercive, and utilitarian. This notion mainly deals with the standardization of organization operation & personnel behavior regarding the organization. "Formal organization is a group that restricts membership and uses officially designated positions and roles, formal rules and regulations, and a bureaucratic structure." This notion deals with an organization with specific rules and organization regulations regarding the structure. For example, Corporations, the Catholic Church, court systems, military organizations, and university administrations are formal organizations.

Informal Organization

The informal organization consists of roles rather than statuses. The relationship between the members is more personal than the status relationship. Interaction and communication in informal organizations are direct, face to face, and intimate. It is more flexible than a formal organization. It is smaller in size, and the structural arrangement is less complex—examples: gangs, friendship groups, peer groups, Bands, etc.

Whenever a set of people get together and start interacting on a long-term basis, they start to form an informal group. An informal group is more than just a collection of people. Groups have an internal social structure based on dominance and friendship relations. There are social leaders. There are hangers-on. These factors influenced the development of the informal organization.

Here some examples of Social organizations are given:

Family: The family is the basic unit in all societies. It is a group of biologically related individuals living together and eating from a common kitchen

Religion and caste: The caste system in India is an example of a closed class; that is, there is no mobility in caste or shifting from one class to another, and the members remain throughout their life wherein they are born. Each caste is governed by rules and sanctions relating to endogamy, food taboos, ritual purity, etc. Each caste group within a village is expected to give certain standardized services to the families of other castes.

Temporary Social Groups

Crowd: When a group of people comes together temporarily for a short period, groups motivated by a common interest or curiosity are known as a crowd.

Mob: A mob is a crowd, but it has a leader who forces the members into action. There may be a symbol in the shape of a flag or slogan. A mob is more emotional than a crowd

Herd: This is a crowd with a leader. Here, the members of the group have to follow the orders of the leader without question; for example, a tourist group under a guide.

Permanent Social Groups

Band: It is the most elementary community of a few families living together. Here the group has organized itself and follows a pattern of life; for example, gypsies in India.

Village: A village is a small collection of people permanently settled down in a locality with their homes and cultural equipment.

Towns and cities: From a sociological point of view, a city or town may be defined as a relatively large, dense, and permanent settlement of socially heterogeneous individuals. The community is subdivided into smaller groups based on wealth and social class.

Government and Political organizations

Government is an association, of which law is the institutional activity. There is no society which lacks government. It is the supreme agent authorized to regulate the balanced social life in the interests of the public.

Voluntary Associations

The state is not the sole organization operating in society, as numerous voluntary associations carry out diverse functions for the betterment, integration, and solidarity of society. Due to its nature, the state is a limited agency, and there are specific functions that it cannot perform advantageously.

Meaning of Voluntary Association

Voluntarism is derived from the Latin word 'voluntas,' which means "will" or "freedom." Harold Laski, an eminent British political scientist, defined "Freedom of association" as a recognized legal right on the part of all persons to combine for the promotion of purposes in which they are interested. Article 19 (1) (c) of the Constitution of India confers the Indian citizens' right 'to form an association.' Freedom of association is rightly regarded as taking high rank among the liberties of man.

It is the liberty of the broadest scope for men who may wish to associate for any purpose that two or more of them may have in common. They may wish to do something together or get something done to further their or other people's interests, resist oppression or injustice, or pursue great or small, general or public objects. In the UN terminology, voluntary organizations are called non-governmental organizations (NGOs).

These are also identified as Volage (Voluntary agencies) and AGs (Action groups). The term voluntary association is variously defined. According to Lord Beveridge, A voluntary organization, properly speaking, is an organization that, whether its workers are paid or unpaid, is initiated and governed by its members without external control.

In the words of David L Sills, a Voluntary organization is a group of persons organized based on voluntary membership without state control for the furtherance of some shared interests of its members.

Norman Johnson, in his examination of the various definitions of voluntary social services, points out their four primary characteristics:

i. Method of formation, which is voluntary on the part of a group of people,

ii. Method of government, with the self-governing organization to decide on its constitution, its servicing, its policy, and its clients;

iii. Method of financing, with at least some of its revenues drawn from voluntary sources; and

iv. Motives with the pursuit of profit excluded.

In the Indian context, it is of particular significance for their financial accountability; it is stipulated that only those voluntary associations would be considered for incorporated grants-in-aid and have existed for at least three years.

A formal organization is reflected in the presence of offices filled through established procedures, scheduled meetings, qualifying criteria for membership, and some formalized division and specialization of labor. However, the organizations do not exhibit all these characteristics to the same degree.

Voluntary organizations have to sacrifice their autonomy substantially as there are quite a few restrictions (though regulatory provisions) that they have to accept if they expect public grants. In India, religion, besides politics, is the other social sphere from which they must keep themselves away if they wish to seek public money for participation in nation-building activities.

These Voluntary organizations align with Indian secularism, which prohibits the use of public money for the propagation of any religion; finally, in India, they must be committed to national objectives, namely socialism, secularism, democracy, national unity, and integrity.

Prof MR Inamdar observes, "A voluntary organization to be of durable use to the community has to nurse a strong desire and impulse for community development among its members, to be economically viable to possess dedicated and hardworking leadership and command resources of expertise in the functions undertaken."

Main Characteristics of Voluntary Organization

The definitions of a voluntary organization given above bring out its following main characteristics:

- It is registered under the Societies Registration Act, 1880, the Indian Trusts Act, 1882; the Cooperative Societies Act, 1904, or the Joint Stock Companies Act, 1959, depending upon the nature and scope of its activities, giving it a legal status;
- It has definite aims and objectives and programs for their fulfillment and achievement;
- It has an administrative structure and a duly constituted management and executive committee;
- It is an organization initiated and governed by its members on democratic principles without any external control and
- It raises funds for its activities partly from the exchequer in the form of grants-in-aid and partly in the form of the contributions or subscriptions from the members of the local community and/ or the beneficiaries of the programs.

Factors Motivating Voluntary Action

The factors that motivate people to take voluntary action or the sources of voluntarism may be identified as religion, government, business, philanthropy, and mutual aid. The missionary zeal of religious organizations, the commitments of a government organization to the public interest, the profit-making urge in business, the altruism of the 'social superiors,' and the motive of self-help among fellowmen are reflected in voluntarism. At the operational level, the components mentioned above may not differ much from one another, but each is moved by an impulse with service as the common motivation.

Bouradillon and William Beveridge viewed mutual aid and philanthropy as two primary sources from which voluntary social service organizations would have developed. They spring from individual and social conscience, respectively. The other factors motivating voluntary action could be cited as personal interest, seeking benefits such as experience, recognition, knowledge, prestige, commitment to specific values, etc.

Further, impulses of a great variety move men for their grouping or forming voluntary associations to serve themselves, their fellowmen, or an unfortunate lot of the society. These are idealistic, educative, psychological, and social, operating separately or in varying combinations.

Idealistically voluntary associations preserve democracy and the individuals' personalities and contribute to the general health of society. They are a potent agent of political socialization in a democracy, educate their members about social norms and values, and help combat loneliness. Psychological impulses lead people to join voluntary associations for security, self-expression and satisfying their interests with the decaying of social institutions like family, church, and community.

Sociologists have studied the psychology of membership with the motivating interests in view, namely, community, class, ethnicity, religion, sex, age, etc. They have found that (i) the association gives the individual a feeling of community with his fellowmen, (ii) membership has class bias where socioeconomic interest has motivated the joining of association (iii) membership of a given group is homogenous mainly in terms of class, ethnicity and religion (iv) membership is directly related to socioeconomic status, as measured by the level of income, occupation house ownership, level of living and education.

Greater interest is evinced in joining the voluntary association in urban areas than in rural; men dominate the direction boards of most agencies; women join organizations depending upon their family status and the stage they occupy in the family cycle, and participation in voluntary association declines as people grow old and so on.

Thus, the psychology of joining a voluntary association is a complex phenomenon. It may vary from one individual to another and one group of individuals to another, depending on their culture, social milieu, and political environment.

Social System

The term "system" suggests an orderly arrangement, an interdependence of parts. Every component in the arrangement has a specific location and function. Interaction binds the parts together. To comprehend the operation of a system, such as the human body, one must analyze and identify the subsystems (e.g., circulatory, nervous, digestive, excretory systems, etc.) and comprehend how these various subsystems interact in specific ways to fulfill the organic function of the body.

Similarly, society can be viewed as a system of interconnected, mutually dependent parts that work together to maintain a recognizable whole and achieve some purposes or goals. A social system is a collection of social interactions based on shared norms and values. Individuals make it up, and each has a role and function to play within it.

Meaning of Social System

Talcott Parsons popularized the term "system" in modern sociology. A social system is an orderly arrangement of parts that are interconnected. Every component in the arrangement has a specific location and function. Interaction binds the parts together. Thus, a system denotes the patterned relationship among constituent parts of a structure based on functional relationships, which activates and binds these parts into reality.

Society is a system of conventions, authority, and mutuality founded on the "We" feeling and likeness. Societal differences are not excluded. However, these are subordinated to likeness. It is founded on interdependence and cooperation. It is bound by mutual awareness. It is fundamentally a pattern for instilling social behavior.

It comprises individuals' mutual interaction and interrelationships and the structure formed by their interactions. It is not time-limited. It is distinct from a group of people and the community. "The term society refers not to a group of people, but to the complex pattern of interaction norms that emerge among and between them," writes Lapierre.

When applied to society, the social system can be defined as a collection of social interactions based on shared norms and values.

Individuals make it up, and each has a role and function to play within it. Throughout the process, one influences the other; groups form and gain influence, and numerous subgroups emerge.

But they are all related. They work together to form a whole. Individuals and groups cannot function in isolation. Norms, values, culture, and shared behavior bind them together. The social system is formed by the pattern that emerges.

According to Parsons, a social system is a collection of social actors who interact in a more or less stable manner "according to shared cultural norms and meanings." Individuals are the fundamental units of interaction. However, the interacting units within the system may be groups or organizations of individuals.

According to Charles P Loomis, the social system is composed of the patterned interaction of visual actors whose relationships with each other are mutually oriented through the definition of the pattern of structured and shared symbols and expectations.

Because they are made up of interacting individuals, all social organizations are a 'social system.' Each interacting individual in the social system has a function or role based on their status in the system. Parents, sons, and daughters, for example, are expected to perform certain socially recognized functions or roles in the family.

Similarly, social organizations operate within the constraints of a normative pattern. Thus, a social system requires a social structure composed of various parts that are interconnected to perform its functions.

A social system is an all-encompassing arrangement. It orbits the various subsystems, such as the economic, political, religious, and others, as well as their interrelationships. The environment, such as geography, constrains social systems. This distinguishes one system from another.

Elements of Social System

The elements of the social system are described as under:

1. **Faiths and Knowledge:** Faiths and knowledge promote behavioral consistency. They serve as controlling agencies for various types of human societies. Faiths or beliefs are the results of prevalent customs and beliefs. They enjoy the individual's power and are guided in a specific direction.

2. **Sentiment:** Man does not live solely on logic. Sentiments – filial, social, notional, etc. – have significantly provided society with continuity. It is inextricably linked to the people's culture.

3. **End Goal or Object:** Man is born social and reliant on others. He must meet his requirements and fulfill his responsibilities. Between needs and satisfactions, end and goal, man and society exist. These determine the nature of the social system. They provided a path of progress as well as receding horizons.

4. **Ideals and Norms:** Society establishes certain norms and ideals to maintain the social system and determine the functions of different units. These norms establish the rules and regulations by which individuals or groups can achieve their cultural goals and objectives.

   In other words, ideals and norms are accountable for a society's ideal structure or system. Human behavior does not deviate from them and acts according to societal norms. This system results in order and stability. Folkways, customs, traditions, fashions, morality, religion, and so on are examples of norms and ideals.

5. **Status-Role:** Every individual in society serves a purpose. He believes in the status-role relationship. It can be inherited through birth, sex, caste, or age. It is possible to obtain it based on the service provided.

6. **Role:** Similar to status, society has assigned different roles to different people. Sometimes we discover that there is a role associated with every status. The role is the outward manifestation of the status. Every individual considers their status when performing specific tasks or performing certain activities. This situation results in the social system's social integration, organization, and unity. Statuses and roles of individuals are inextricably linked. They cannot be separated from one another.

7. **Power:** Conflict is a natural part of the social system and aims to maintain order. It follows that some should be given the authority to punish the guilty and reward those who set a good example. The authority exercising power varies by the group; while the father's authority may be supreme in the family, the ruler's authority is supreme in the state.

8. **Sanction:** It denotes confirmation by the superior in the authority of the subordinate's actions or the imposition of a penalty for

the violation of the command. Acts performed or not performed according to norms may result in reward and punishment.

Characteristics of Social System

The social system has specific characteristics. These characteristics are as follows:

1. **The system is linked to a plurality of individual actors:** This means that a system or social system cannot be born as a result of the activity of a single individual. It is the result of various people's activities. The interaction of several individuals is required for the system or social system to function.

2. **Aim and Object:** Individual actors' human interactions or activities should not be aimless or without an object. These activities must be carried out following specific goals and objectives. Human interaction gives rise to the manifestation of various social relations.

3. **Order and Pattern among Constituent Units:** The mere gathering of various constituent units from the social system does not necessarily result in forming a social system. It must follow a pattern, arrangement, and order. The emphasized unity among various constituent units forms a 'social system.'

4. **Functional Relationship is the Foundation of Unity:** We have already seen how different constituent units can work together to form a system. Functional relationships underpin this unity. A social system is formed as a result of the functional relationships that exist between different constituent units.

5. **Physical or Environmental Aspects of Social Systems:** Every social system is linked to a specific geographical area or place, time, society, and so on. In other words, the social system is not the same at different times, in different places, and under different circumstances. This feature of the social system emphasizes its dynamic or changeable nature.

6. **Interconnected with Cultural System:** The social system is also interconnected with the cultural system. It means that the cultural system promotes unity among various members of society based on their cultures, traditions, religions, and so on.

7. **Explicit and Implicit Aims and Objects:** The social system is linked to explicit and implicit goals. In other words, the social

system is the convergence of various individual actors motivated by their goals, objectives, and needs.

8. **Adjustment Characteristics:** The social system has adjustment characteristics. It is a dynamic phenomenon that is influenced by changes in social structure. We have also seen how society's goals, objects, and needs influence the social system. This adjustment means that the social system will only be relevant if it adapts to changing objects and needs. It has been observed that change occurs in the social system due to human needs, the environment, and historical conditions and phenomena.

9. **Order, Pattern, and Balance:** The social system exhibits patterns, order, and balance. The social system is not an integrated whole but a collection of various units. This is coming together does not happen by chance or haphazardly. There is both order and balance. It is so because different units of society do not function as independent entities but as part of a socio-cultural pattern. Different units in the pattern serve different functions and play different roles. It denotes the existence of a pattern and order in the social system.

Social System Functions

A social system is a functional configuration. It would not exist if it did not exist. Its functional nature guarantees social stability and continuity. It is widely acknowledged that the social system faces four major functional issues. They are as follows:

- Adaptation,
- Goal attainment,
- Integration,
- Latent pattern—maintenance.

Adaptation

The ability of the social system to adapt to changing environments is critical. Without a doubt, a social system results from a geographical environment and a long-drawn historical process, which gives it permanence and rigidity by necessity. However, this should not render it wooden and inelastic. It must be a malleable and functional phenomenon.

The economy requires division of labor for better production of goods and effective services and role differentiation for job opportunities. Durkheim emphasizes the role of division of labor and role differentiation in society because they allow for a higher average level of skill than would otherwise be possible.

The social system has frequently been challenged due to a lack of adaptability. It has sparked a revolution, resulting in a system overhaul. The British system demonstrated remarkable adaptability when the continent was under revolution in the nineteenth century. It responded well to the increasing pressures of change. Over time, our system has proven to be highly adaptable.

Goal Attainment

Goal attainment and adaptability are inextricably linked. Both contribute to the preservation of social order. Every social system has one or more goals that must be met through a collaborative effort. National security is perhaps the best example of a societal goal. If objectives are to be met, adaptation to the social and non-social environments is required. However, human and nonhuman resources must be effectively mobilized by the nature of the tasks.

For example, there must be a process to ensure that enough people, but not too many, fill each of the roles at any given time and determine who will fill each. These processes work together to solve the problem of social system membership allocation. We've already discussed the "need" for property standards. Inheritance rules, such as primogeniture, partially solve this problem.

Allocating members and valuable resources is critical for adaptation and goal achievement. The distinction between adaptation and goal achievement is a relative one.

The economy of a society is the subsystem that produces goods and services for a wide range of purposes; the "polity," which includes, above all, the government in complex societies, mobilizes goods and services to achieve specific goals of the entire society viewed as a single social system.

Integration

The social system is essentially a system of integration. In everyday life, it is not society but the group or subgroup in which one feels more involved and interested. Society, in general, does not enter into one's calculations. However, as Durkheim pointed out, we know that the individual is a product of society. Emotions, sentiments, and historical forces are so powerful that it is impossible to break free.

The interaction of these forces is most visible when society faces a domestic crisis or an external challenge. A call to action in the name of society, culture, heritage, patriotism, national solidarity, or social welfare elicits an immediate response. Cooperation in the effort is frequently evidence of integration. It is the foundation of integration.

The spirit of integration is best expressed during regular times by not disregarding the regulative norms. They must be followed, or else the dominance of might over right, of self over society, and the spirit of mutuality based on common welfare will be lost. The command and obedience relationship, as it currently exists, is based on logic and order. If it is not maintained, the social order will crumble.

In almost every social system, including societies, some participants, including entire subgroups, violate relational or regulative norms. Violations of these norms threaten the social system as they meet social needs.

As a result, social control is required. "Social control" refers to the requirement for standardized responses to violations to protect the system's integrity. When there is a disagreement over the interpretation of relational or regulatory norms or the factual aspects of conflicts of interest, there is a need for mutually agreed-upon social arrangements to resolve the disagreement. Otherwise, the social system would be prone to progressive breakdowns.

Latent Pattern—Maintenance

The primary function of a social system is pattern maintenance and tension management. Social order and continuity are impossible to maintain and sustain without reasonable effort in this direction. Every social system has a built-in mechanism for this purpose.

Every individual and subgroup learns the patterns of internalizing norms and values. The socialization process works by imbuing the actors with appropriate attitudes and respect for norms and institutions. It is not enough to simply impart the pattern; it is also necessary to make the actor follow it. In terms of operational social control, this is always a continuous effort.

There may still be times when the components of the social system are distracted and disrupted. Tensions may arise due to internal or external factors, and society may become embroiled in a critical situation. Just as a distressed family uses all its resources to overcome it, society must do the same.

This 'overcoming' process is called tension management. As a family, society is responsible for keeping its members functional, relieving them of anxiety, and encouraging those who would be detrimental to the entire system. The failure of the pattern maintenance and tension management mechanisms has contributed significantly to the decline of societies.

Social Structure

INTRODUCTION

Proper understanding of society depends on the concept of social structure.

In sociology, social structure is the distinct, stable arrangement of institutions through which human beings interact and live together. "Social structure" is frequently used interchangeably with "social change," which refers to the processes that alter society's social structure and organization.

Meaning of Social Structure

Many efforts have been made to define 'Social Structure,' but still, there is no unanimity of opinion on its definition.

Herbert Spencer was the first writer to shed light on the social structure. He referred to society as an organism, but his understanding of society was ambiguous. Emile Durkheim also tried in vain to define it.

According to various perspectives on social structure:
- Social structure is an abstract and intangible phenomenon.
- Individuals are the units of association, and institutions are the units of social structure.

- These institutions and associations are interconnected in a specific arrangement, resulting in the pattern of social structure.
- It refers to the stable external aspect of society instead of the functional or internal aspect of society.
- A social structure is a "living" structure that is created and maintained over time.

Social Structure Elements

In a social structure, humans organize themselves into associations to pursue some object or objects. The goal can only be achieved if the social structure is founded on certain principles **(Fig. 20.1)**.

These principles set in motion the elements of social structure, which are as follows:

- **Normative System:** The normative system presents ideals and values to society. People place emotional value on these norms. According to these standards, institutions and associations are linked. Individuals carry out their responsibilities by societal norms.

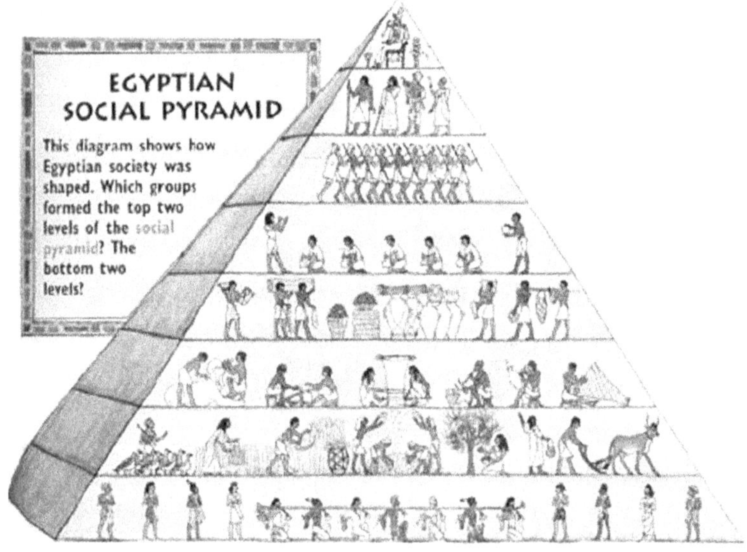

Fig. 20.1: Egyptian social structure in the ancient era.

- **Position System:** The positioning system refers to an individual's status and role. Individuals' desires, aspirations, and expectations are diverse, numerous, and limitless. As a result, these can only be met if members of society are assigned different roles based on their capacities and capabilities. The proper operation of the social structure is dependent on the proper assignment of roles and statuses.

- **Sanction System:** Every society has a sanction system to enforce norms properly. Conformity to social standards is required to integrate and coordinate the various parts of the social structure. Nonconformists are punished by the society based on the nature of their nonconformity.

  It does not, however, imply that there are no nonconformists in a well-organized society. Nonconformity is also an essential aspect of humanity.

  Otherwise, there would be no progress. Nonconformists are less common than conformists. The efficiency of its penalty mechanism determines the stability of a social structure.

- **A System of Anticipated Response:** The anticipated response system calls individuals to participate in the social system, and their preparation sets the social structure in motion. The successful operation of the social structure is dependent on the individual's realization of his duties and his efforts to fulfill these duties.

- **Action Plan:** It is the goal or target that the social organization aspires to achieve. It is the focal point of the entire structure. In action, the core cause of the web of social ties and the mobility of the social structure.

  It should be noted that social structure is an ill-defined concept. It cannot be seen. Its components are dynamic and constantly changing. They are widely dispersed in space, making it challenging to observe them all at once. Any scientific understanding of social structure must take a structural-functional approach.

Types of Social Structure

Talcott Parsons identified four different forms of social structures. His classification is grounded on four social values: universalistic, particularistic, achieved and ascribed.

Universalistic social values are found almost in every society and apply to everybody. For example, every society values expert artisans as, in that case, production is both cheaper and superior, and thus, efficient artisans are selected in every society.

Particularistic social values are the features of particular societies, and these differ from culture to culture. If, for example, the selection is based on caste, religion, state, etc., particularistic social values are considered more important in such societies.

When the statuses are achieved based on efforts, such societies attach importance to achieved social values. When the statuses are hereditary, then society considers ascribed social statuses.

Social Institutions

We may also pay attention to social institutions because they are critical to maintaining the ordered arrangement of social structure. Institutions are modes of collective behavior.

They specify how things should be done. They connect the members of the group. Some people confuse the terms "institutions" and "institutional agencies."

They define "institution" as normative behavioral patterns and "institutional agencies" as the social framework through which these patterns are expressed. Most writers, however, do not distinguish between these normative complexes and the structures that enable them to function because they are so inextricably linked. Societal institutions include the family, school, church, state, and many other institutions.

Types of Institutions

Institutions are classified into five types. These are as follows: (i) the family, (ii) economics, (iii) religion, (iv) education, and (v) the state. Each of the five primary institutions has numerous secondary institutions. Marriage, divorce, monogamy, polygamy, and so on are secondary institutions derived from the family.

Secondary economic institutions include real estate, trading, credit, and banking. Secondary religious institutions include the church, temple, mosque, totem, taboo, and so on. Secondary education institutions include schools, colleges, and universities, among others. Interest groups, party systems, democracy, and other secondary institutions of the state are examples.

Institutions can emerge over time, much like folkways and mores, or as laws are passed; for example, monogamy and polyandry arose in response to people's perceived needs. The number of banks grew in tandem with the demand for borrowing and lending money. Schools and colleges are the results of deliberate decisions and actions. Extending the state's authority over the other four primary institutions is critical for institutional development.

The state now wields more power through laws and rules. Sometimes folkways and customs are incorporated into laws, such as monogamy: other times, new rules are enacted, such as the Hindu Code Bill. The state now regulates and controls the family in a variety of ways. The state has taken over many traditional family functions. The state governs marriage, divorce, adoption, and inheritance. The state's authority has also been extended to economics, education, and religion.

An institution is eternal. Although new institutional norms may replace old norms, the institution remains. For example, the modern family has replaced patriarchal family norms, but the family as an institution persists. When feudalism died, the government did not end. The governmental and economic functions were still carried out by changing norms. Only the institutional norms are new; all primary institutions are thousands of years old.

Functions of Institutions

The functions of institutions are of two types:
i. Manifest and
ii Latent.

Manifest functions are those intended and central functions for which the institution exists primarily. Unintended functions are latent functions. They are by-products rather than primary functions.

Thus, the manifest functions of education are literacy development, occupational training, and the instillation of fundamental social values. However, its latent functions would keep youth out of the labor force, erode parental control, and foster friendships. Religion's obvious functions are God worship and religious ideology instruction. Its latent functions would be to instill attachment to one's religious community, disrupt family life, and instill religious hatred.

Economic institutions' manifest function is to produce and distribute goods, while their latent functions may be to promote urbanization, the growth of labor unions, and the redirection of education. The latent functions may either support or harm the institution's norms.

Inter-relations of Institutions

The stability of a social structure is due to the proper adjustment of relationships among the various institutions. No institution operates in a vacuum. Religion, education, family, government, and business are all intertwined. Thus, education shapes attitudes that influence whether religious dogmas are accepted or rejected.

Religion can elevate education. It allows one to know God's truths or denounce them because they threaten one's faith. Business conditions can have an impact on family life.

Unemployment may have an impact on how many people believe they are capable. Unemployed people may put off marriage until they find suitable work.

Marriage postponement may have an impact on birth rates. The state influences the functions of institutions. It may take over some functions and establish institutional norms for them. Business people, educators, clergy, and officials from other institutions try to influence state actions because any state action can obstruct or help them achieve their institutional goals.

As a result, social institutions are inextricably linked. The interdependence of the various institutions can be compared to a wheel. The family serves as the hub, with education, religion, government, and economics serving as spokes. The community in which the various institutions operate would be the rim.

All institutions face the challenge of constantly adapting to a changing society. Changes in the social environment may affect all institutions. Inflation can significantly impact marriage, death, crime, and education. Economic institution breakdown may have far-reaching consequences for political institutions.

Any change in an institution may cause a shift in other intuitions. Functions may also be transferred from one institution to another. Child care, previously a family function, has now been delegated to the state.

When one organization fails to meet a human need, another frequently steps in to fill the void. There can be no institution if it does not influence or is influenced by others.

Role of Social Welfare Organizations in Maintaining Health

Many voluntary and involuntary organizations assist people in the community to achieve health. The fundamental nature of all humans is to help one another survive in society. Healthcare can be provided by a doctor, physiotherapist, nurse, social worker, psychologist, or others.

These health services are provided in rural slums and urban areas through primary health centers, communities, sub-centers, and hospitals. Their primary objectives are as follows:
- providing affordable healthcare services to all.
- Community-based perinatal care for mothers.
- Reducing infant, antenatal, and postnatal mortality and morbidity rates in high-risk areas.
- Ensuring sanitation.
- Providing safe drinking water, particularly in slums and rural areas.
- Providing electricity and other essential services in rural and urban areas.

These activities help people maintain their health and live in social harmony.

Sociology of Pain

LEARNING OBJECTIVES

☞ Define pain.
☞ How do psychosocial factors affect pain?
☞ How to recognize psychosocial factors impacting pain?
☞ How to address psychosocial factors impacting pain?

■ INTRODUCTION

Pain is the most common reason for patients to see a doctor. Pain is the third leading cause of absence from work. Because each person experiences pain differently, it is a complex experience that is challenging to define or explain.

The International Association for the Study of Pain (IASP) defines pain as "An unpleasant sensory and emotional experience associated with, or resembling that associated with, actual or potential tissue damage".

This definition implies that pain is subjective and multidimensional, involving the sensation of pain and the emotional experience associated with pain. It is not necessary to be associated with noticeable tissue damage or to have an obvious underlying cause.

■ UNDERSTANDING PAIN

Biomedical perspectives have historically dominated theories of pain and focus on its neurophysiological features, both in diagnosis and therapy. The IASP's current definition of pain indicates that this elevation of sensation above emotion in medico-psychological approaches to pain is insufficient because pain is now understood to be both a sensory and an emotional experience.

In the past, scientific medicine saw the feeling of pain as a complex broadcasting system of signals rather than as being influenced by the sociocultural context of the individual.

The Biopsychosocial Model of Pain is the only theory that offers the most thorough justification for why people experience pain and the uniqueness of each patient's experience.

The biopsychosocial approach describes pain and disability as a multidimensional, dynamic interaction among physiological, psychological, and social factors that reciprocally influence one another, resulting in chronic and complex pain syndromes.

Before the biopsychosocial model of pain was developed, many theories and models were offered to explain the experience of pain. Our anatomy and physiology never create pain on their own. Because pain only manifests at the crossroads of bodies, minds, and cultures, recent research has highlighted the need to consider the social environment.

The cultural shaping and patterning of beliefs and responses to pain is part of the social underpinning of pain. It has been discovered through adaptations in pain perception, coping skills, and emotional states that interpersonal connections, support, and diverse social environment factors can have beneficial or negative effects on a person's reaction to chronic pain.

The alternative Gate Control theory model, developed and improved by Melzack and Wall, hypothesizes that psychological and cognitive factors, which are strongly influenced by sociocultural learning and experiences, impact the physiological processes involved in human pain perception and response.

Social pain is from interpersonal loss or rejection, such as being rejected by a social group, being bullied, or losing a loved one. People who have chronic pain physically withdraw from their social networks. Flares of pain can make it difficult to organize and engage in activities and even prevent participation. Social withdrawal might also result from a fear of pain.

Individuals who suffer from chronic pain could experience anxiety or depression. Additionally, they risk abusing drugs and developing other mental illnesses. Sadness, frustration, rage, or a sense of being misunderstood or demoralized are more common emotional reactions to pain. The idea that culture can affect various pain-related aspects is supported by evidence, including but not limited to pain communication styles, empathy for the suffering of others, pain tolerance and intensity, attitudes about and coping mechanisms for pain, and pain catastrophizing.

Chronic pain impairs the quality of life, work and functioning. Chronic pain markedly decreases individuals' health status and quality of life (QoL) and can detrimentally affect patients' families.

CULTURE AND PAIN PERCEPTION

In addition to being embodied and mediated by culture, pain is simultaneously physical, emotional, biological, and phenomenological. The social environment can greatly impact how pain is perceived and expressed.

Culture affects how we perceive and interpret pain and how we react to it. In this way, culture impacts and influences how we perceive pain.

A person's social evaluation is significantly influenced by their emotional displays, including physical and cognitive aspects. When an emotional display deviates from what is considered "socially proper," others may express displeasure. In order to meet social expectations, which are influenced by factors including gender, social class, ethnicity, age, and work, entails altering the quality of perceived emotion.

Helman makes the following arguments:
1. Not all social or cultural groups react to pain in the same way;
2. Cultural factors can greatly affect how people perceive and react to pain, both in themselves and others;
3. Cultural factors can greatly influence how and whether people communicate their pain to medical professionals and other people.

For instance, certain cultural or social groups may value stoicism in the face of pain. Hence, keeping pain private, or expressing it publicly, may be either desirable or undesirable when viewed within the context of a particular social group's belief and value systems. Additionally, cultural values and beliefs could help to "normalize" painful experiences that might seem troubling to others.

GENDER AND PAIN PERCEPTION

The only gender-related issue affecting pain perception that appears to have received any systematic research is the focus on sex differences in "thresholds" and "tolerance levels".

Most likely, there are gender differences in the sensitivity to experimentally generated pain. For instance, a recent experiment that subjected a "normal" sample of undergraduate men and women to noxious heat stimulation found a biological basis for the lower thresholds of the women. The authors said this discovery had the most "logical" explanation, but they also offered another possibility: Men may respond more slowly than women.

Bendelow discovered that both men and women believed that women have a "natural" ability to cope with pain, which is lacking in men. This ability is explained by their biological and reproductive functioning using in-depth interviews and visual imagery to develop a phenomenological approach to understanding pain beliefs.

PAST EXPERIENCES AND PAIN PERCEPTION

The individual's unique past experiences also considerably influence pain perception and response. Some families focus greatly on minor injuries, whereas others tend to minimize or ignore serious ones. There are also differences in the degree and manner to which children are encouraged or discouraged from openly responding to pain. These early experiences influence our sensitivity to potentially painful stimuli and our pain behavior throughout life; as with other areas of social life, we are guided in our interpretations and influenced in our behavior by the interpretations and behavior of others.

STATE OF MIND AND PAIN PERCEPTION

Anxious people are more sensitive to pain than calm people. Anxious patients complain more of pain than others, and pain intensity decreases if anxiety is reduced by giving subjects control over the situation. It is observed that morphine reduces pain only if anxiety is high.

The anticipation of pain and uncertainty regarding its cause tends to raise anxiety, increasing its perceived intensity. Thus, a vicious circle may operate. Pain will be greater for patients who tend to become anxious because pain causes anxiety and, in turn, heightens the pain.

HOW DO PSYCHOSOCIAL FACTORS AFFECT PAIN?

Psychosocial factors affecting pain include marital status, social support, bereavement, home and work environment, social status, and social integration. For example, someone under great stress due to their family life or work stress might have a lower threshold for pain. Conversely, **if a friend is by a patient's side,** they may have a higher threshold for pain.

HOW TO RECOGNIZE PSYCHOSOCIAL FACTORS IMPACTING PAIN?

The interpretation of pain is subjective, and several specific thought processes influence it. Let's review four ways psychosocial factors can affect pain.

a. **Awareness:** Pain is the body's way of alerting us to danger. If we encounter something sharp, we feel pain and move away from it before we experience a more serious injury. If we are paying attention and expecting pain, the feeling of pain may increase. One strategy to help lower pain intensity is to distract the patient with conversation, company, or entertainment. It would not take the pain away, but getting the patient to focus on something else may lower its impact.

b. **Interpretation:** How a patient thinks about pain may also increase their pain. If they expect the worst, their threshold for pain will often lower. Also, if they expected their illness or injury to be healed in a certain timeframe, the disappointment can increase the experience of pain when it continues. It can be helpful to talk through expectations with the patient to ensure they have a realistic understanding of the situation to combat these negative thought processes. If the patient tends to catastrophize, acknowledge their fears, then discuss how they can and will cope even in a worst-case scenario.

c. **Emotional Response to Pain:** Fear, anxiety, depression, and other psychological factors may lower a patient's pain threshold. We must treat these emotional symptoms to reduce how the psychosocial factors affect pain. Cognitive behavioral therapy allows patients to feel heard and provides practical coping techniques to address negative thought patterns. Meditation, physical activity, and time spent outdoors can help increase positive emotions, decreasing the feeling of pain.

d. **Coping Skills:** How a patient approaches pain treatment can affect pain threshold levels. If a patient is prescribed strong pain relievers for relatively mild pain, they lose the opportunity to develop other coping mechanisms. Working with patients on coping mechanisms early in the disease process can help reduce the experience of pain in later stages. That said, when a patient is in the end-stage of a terminal diagnosis and addiction is no longer a concern, the patient's immediate comfort should be the primary goal of treating their pain.

HOW TO ADDRESS PSYCHOSOCIAL FACTORS IMPACTING PAIN?

Improving a patient's psychosocial environment can go a long way in addressing their emotional, spiritual, *and* physical pain. Look for ways to increase the patient's social support. Please encourage them to stay in contact with friends and family regularly. If they live alone, visiting an adult daycare can reduce isolation. Patients receiving hospice care can have volunteers assigned to provide additional companionship.

Physiotherapists and Social workers are key to addressing psychosocial factors by helping the patient with stress management techniques and problem-solving. Family meetings with the physiotherapist/social worker can also help address factors in the family and home that may increase the patient's stress. Addressing a patient's pain is a team effort, and properly assessing the impact of psychosocial factors on pain will provide better overall results.

DISCUSSION

Social and cultural factors always mediate pain's physical reality. Although a person may pay attention to some pain stimuli, these reactions are mediated by the interpretive work of oneself and others, which draws on lay health knowledge and beliefs, giving these stimuli "subjective" interpretations. Additionally, they might differ based on class, gender, and ethnicity issues.

These elements, as mentioned above, influence how pain is perceived and felt and how the body, mind, and emotions respond to it. They have also been demonstrated to impact pain treatments' management and results and other healthcare types. We know that physical experience is inseparable from its cognitive and emotional significance since the mind and body are intertwined in pain. Because of this mind-body relationship, pain can describe physical agony, emotional turmoil, and spiritual suffering.

■ CONCLUSION

Pain, a fundamental part of the human condition, has to be "reclaimed" from the solely biomedical realm and examined at the crossroads of biology and culture.

A more holistic understanding of pain is relevant to medical practice on several levels. It may aid in reducing the stigmatization of the "psychogenic" pain patient at the level of coping with chronic pain for which there is no physical pathology.

Question Bank

LONG ESSAYS

1. Examine the relevance of sociology to health sciences.
2. What does a social group mean? How are the social groups classified?
3. Explain the influence of family on human health.
4. Explain the factors of social change.
5. Define sociology and explain its scope.
6. What is industrialization? What are the problems of industrialization?
7. Explain the role of family in health and disease.
8. Define sociology and explain its scope with special reference to healthcare professionals.
9. What is society? Describe social system explaining its characteristics.
10. Define sociology and bring out the importance of its study in the field of health.
11. Examine the role of family in socialization.
12. Explain the role and importance of a medical social worker.
13. Explain the 'case study method' as a method of sociological investigation.
14. Society as a web of social relationships—explain.
15. Define family and explain the role of family in health and illness.
16. Explain the difference between primary and secondary groups.
17. Describe the factors causing social changes. Briefly point out the negative effect of fast changes in a traditional society like India.
18. Explain the causes for population explosion in India. How does modern Indian Government deal with this problem?

■ SHORT ESSAYS

1. Explain the relationship between sociology and social psychology.
2. Explain the meaning and nature of socialization.
3. Describe the health hazards of tribal people.
4. What is social change? How is it related to stress?
5. Explain the problem of overpopulation in India.
6. Interview is a tool par excellence—substantiate.
7. Discuss the role of primary groups in the hospital and rehabilitation setup.
8. What are the health hazards of ruralities?
9. Explain the relationship of culture and health disorders.
10. Discuss the role of family in health and rehabilitation.
11. What are the merits and demerits of capitalism?
12. Bring out the classification of social groups.
13. What are the social functions of education?
14. Explain any one theory of social change.
15. Mention the differences between custom and law.
16. What is population explosion?
17. Attempt a classification of social groups.
18. How is sociology related to health?
19. Write the demerits of joint family.
20. Explain the health hazards of ruralities.
21. Explain the relationship between culture and health.
22. What do you mean by social security?
23. Alcohol is injurious to health—discuss.
24. Discuss family and nutrition.
25. Bring out the social role of customs.
26. Concept of culture in maintaining health—explain.
27. The process of socialization—discuss.
28. What is population explosion?
29. Features of rural community—explain.
30. Sociology and healthcare professionals.
31. Explain the agencies of socialization.
32. Explain the causes for the disintegration of joint family system.
33. Explain the health effects of industrialization.
34. Explain the health consequences of alcoholism.
35. Interview schedule and questionnaire main differences.

36. Influence of family on health and sickness.
37. Cultural factors in health disorder.
38. Causes for poverty.
39. Social legislation for the disabled in India.
40. Socioeconomic factors of illness.
41. Social survey method.
42. Urban health problems.
43. Tribal community.
44. Medical social works.
45. Stages of aging.

SHORT ANSWERS

1. Define sociology.
2. Mention any four features of joint family.
3. Mention any four factors of social change.
4. Mention any four problems of career women.
5. Write a note on case study method.
6. What is anticipatory socialization?
7. Mention any four psychosomatic disorders.
8. What is meant by juvenile delinquency?
9. Mention any four functions of a medical social worker.
10. What is a social change?
11. What is a primary group?
12. Mention any four characteristics of joint family.
13. What is family planning?
14. Mention any four agencies of social change.
15. Mention four consequences of industrialization.
16. List out four features of association.
17. Define culture.
18. Who is a medical social worker?
19. Consequences of prostitution.
20. Write three problems of overpopulation.
21. Who is beggar?
22. Problems of women in employment.
23. Social security.
24. Mention the types of family.
25. Write three differences between sociology and anthropology.
26. Mention the types of unemployment.

27. Mention the types of socialization.
28. Social psychology.
29. Interview method.
30. Primary group.
31. Concept of health.
32. Types of beggars.
33. Meaning of social work.
34. Social psychology.
35. Meaning of socialization.
36. Define health.
37. Alcoholism.
38. Social security in India.

Bibliography

1. Akram M. Sociology of Health: Rawat Publications; 2014.
2. Alder B, Abraham C, Teijlingen E van, et al. Psychology and Sociology Applied to Medicine: An Illustrated Colour Text: Elsevier Health Sciences; 2009.
3. Armstrong DL. An Outline of Sociology as Applied to Medicine: Elsevier Science; 2015.
4. Barry AM, Yuill C. Understanding the Sociology of Health: An Introduction: SAGE Publications; 2016.
5. Bhushan V, Sachdeva DR. Fundamentals of Sociology: Pearson Education India; 2012.
6. Bid D, Thangamani RA. Sociology for Physiotherapists and Nurses. New Delhi: Jaypee Brothers Medical Publishers; 2015.
7. Clarke A. The Sociology of Healthcare: Taylor & Francis; 2013.
8. Cockerham WC. The Sociology of Medicine: E. Elgar; 1995.
9. Denny E, Earle S, Hewison A. Sociology for Nurses: Polity Press; 2016.
10. French S. Physiotherapy a Psychosocial Approach: Elsevier Science; 2013
11. Giarelli G, Vignera R. Sociology and Sociology of Health: a Round Trip: Franco Angeli; 2012.
12. Khanna P. Sociology for Physiotherapists: AITBS Publishers India.
13. Lohumi S. Sociology for Nurses: Elsevier Health Sciences; 2019.
14. Morrall P. Sociology and Health: An Introduction: Taylor & Francis; 2009.
15. Nagla M. Sociology of Health and Medicine: Rawat Publications; 2018.
16. Neeraja KP. Textbook of Sociology for Physiotherapy Students. New Delhi: Jaypee Brothers Medical Publishers; 2005.
17. Nettleton S. The Sociology of Health and Illness: Wiley; 2021.

18. Pandit N. Sociology and Health for Physiotherapists: BI Publications Pvt. Limited; 2009.
19. Russell L. Sociology for Health Professionals: Sage Publications; 2013.
20. Sujatha V. Sociology of Health and Medicine: New Perspectives: Oxford University Press; 2014.
21. Wainwright D. A Sociology of Health: Sage Publications; 2008.
22. Weiss GL. Sociology of Health, Healing, and Illness: Taylor & Francis; 2015.
23. White K. An Introduction to the Sociology of Health and Illness. Sage Publications; 2002.

Index

Page numbers followed by *f* refer to figure and *t* refer to table.

EU GSPR Authorised Reprsentative
Logos Europe, 9 rue Nicolas Poussin
1700, La Rochelle, France
Phone: +33 (0) 6 67 93 73 78
E-mail: contact@logoseurope.eu

www.ingramcontent.com/pod-product-compliance
Ingram Content Group UK Ltd.
Pitfield, Milton Keynes, MK11 3LW, UK
UKHW020037170726

72141PUK00035B/144